Infection and Immunity

Fourth Edition

John H.L. Playfair

Emeritus Professor of Immunology,
University College London Medical School

Gregory J. Bancroft

Reader in Immunology,
Department of Infectious and Tropical Diseases,
London School of Hygiene and Tropical Medicine

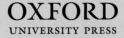
OXFORD
UNIVERSITY PRESS

OXFORD
UNIVERSITY PRESS

Great Clarendon Street, Oxford, OX2 6DP,
United Kingdom

Oxford University Press is a department of the University of Oxford.
It furthers the University's objective of excellence in research, scholarship,
and education by publishing worldwide. Oxford is a registered trade mark of
Oxford University Press in the UK and in certain other countries

© John Playfair and Gregory Bancroft 2013

The moral rights of the authors have been asserted

First Edition copyright 1995
Second Edition copyright 2004
Third Edition copyright 2008

Impression: 1

British Library Cataloguing in Publication Data

Data available

ISBN 978-0-19-960950-5

Printed and bound in China
by C&C Offset Printing Co. Ltd

PREFACE TO THE FOURTH EDITION

Since the third edition of this book (2007) much has been preserved and much has been added. The book is still aimed at students whose undergraduate courses require some knowledge of both microbiology and immunology, and indeed students at any level who, without wishing to study either of these subjects in depth or to buy two heavy textbooks, are interested in a better and more fact-based understanding of the complex world of infectious disease.

The general layout is as before: a section on the infectious organisms, another on the immune system, and a third on the interactions between them. In Parts 1 and 3, we have given their own chapters to insects and other ectoparasites, so crucial in disease transmission. Part 2, besides the obvious updates required by the passage of five years of busy immunological research, now features considerably more emphasis on innate immunity, whose workings are increasingly being uncovered in terms of both beneficial and harmful effects. Throughout Parts 2 and 3 we have introduced occasional Case Studies, to give a more realistic feel to some of the most important disease descriptions. The epidemiology chapter has particularly been expanded to include mankind's two top 'killers': infantile diarrhoea and respiratory disease. For a detailed account of the clinical course of individual infections, the larger textbooks listed under Further Reading should be consulted. A new appendix is devoted to some common laboratory techniques. The tutorial (essay) questions have not dated and are preserved unaltered, but we have added some multiple choice questions of the kind frequently used in exams (see www. oxfordtextbooks.co.uk/orc/playfair4e/).

We hope that students and teachers who have found earlier editions useful will continue to do so, and we thank them and all our colleagues who have contributed by their input, both complimentary and critical.

We encourage any reader with a comment or a complaint to send it in.

London
April 2012

JHL Playfair
GJ Bancroft

New to this Edition

- Two new chapters on insects and other ectoparasites.
- Increased coverage on innate immunity, cell signalling, cancer, and pregnancy.
- Expanded coverage of epidemiology and vaccination: more on HIV, TB, malaria, infantile diarrohea, and respiratory disease.
- New case studies to bring context to the descriptions of disease.
- New appendix on immunological techniques.

PREFACE TO THE FIRST EDITION

Infectious disease is something that affects and surely interests everyone, but for a clear picture of what actually happens during an infection, it is usually necessary to consult one or more large textbooks, since the subject falls across the conventional disciplines of microbiology, immunology, pathology, pharmacology, epidemiology, and medicine.

In this book I have tried to summarize the essentials in a way that can be understood by any student or potential student of science or medicine, including (I hope) the sixth-former and the interested layman. The content of the book corresponds roughly to the second-year BSc course 'Immunity to Infection' run at University College, London, and presupposes no previous knowledge of either microbiology or immunology. The style has been kept as close as possible to actual lectures and tutorials, including an element of self-testing and a guide to the books that can, if desired, be used for delving deeper into the subject.

Both style and content have largely been shaped by the students who have taken the course and made their comments, and I have to thank them for such virtues as it may have. Any errors are, of course, my own, and I would be grateful to be told about them. I also want to thank my colleagues at UCL for many useful suggestions, and my editors at Oxford University Press for their faith in the venture.

London
November 1994

JHL Playfair

ACKNOWLEDGEMENTS

We are grateful to the following colleagues for useful comments and contributions: Quentin Bickle, Dorothy Crawford, Simon Croft, Andy Hall, Helena Helmby, Catherine Hawrylowicz, Paul Kaye, Ulrich Schaible, Silke Schelenz, Debbie Smith, Richard Titball, Brendan Wren. We particularly thank John Raynes for critical reading of Part Two.

The role of the infinitely small is infinitely large.

Louis Pasteur

CONTENTS

PART TWO **The immune system**

PART THREE **The host–pathogen balance**

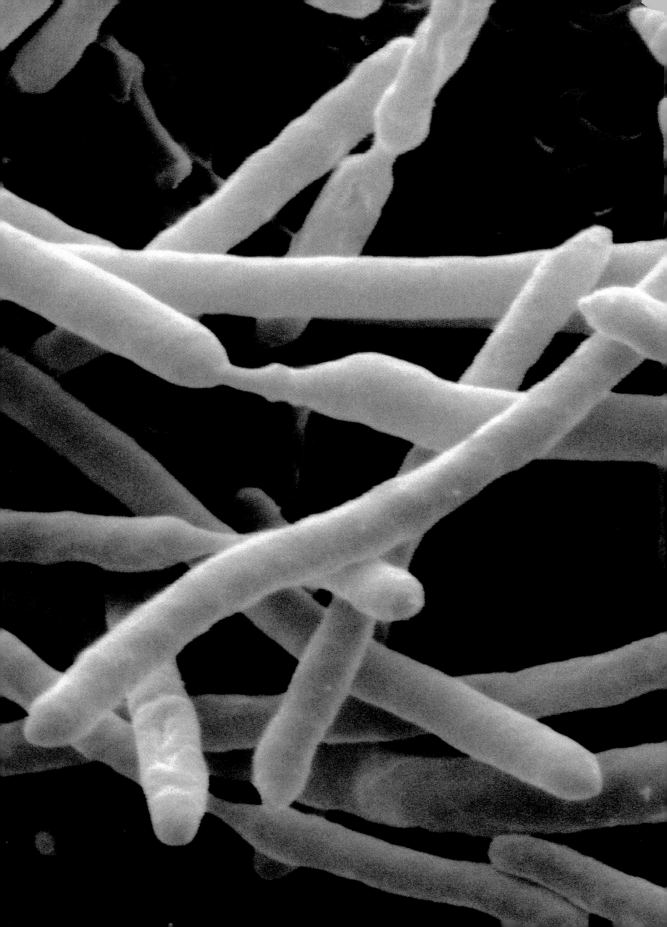

Part 1

The infectious organisms

Chapter 1

Introduction: parasites, pathogens, and immunity

For thousands of years it was known that many of our most serious diseases could be caught from another individual, but only with the invention of the microscope in the seventeenth century and the work of Pasteur and Koch 200 years later was it realized that these *infectious* diseases were caused by the transfer from person to person of infectious *organisms*, invisible parasites living in the body of a much larger host. However, it was also soon realized that the presence of such parasites by no means always caused disease (in this book those that do will generally be referred to as *pathogens*). So before embarking on the study of infectious organisms (microbiology) and the means by which the host can try to control them (immunology) it is worth briefly considering parasitism itself. Why are there parasites? What do they want? Is it better to be a parasite or not? Why do some parasites cause disease while others are harmless?

Our planet is a crowded place, and animals cannot help coming into contact with members of their own and other species. From the very beginning of animal evolution, such contacts have posed important questions, mostly of the yes-or-no type such as 'is it food?' or, in the case of colonial organisms such as corals and sponges, 'to fuse or not to fuse?' (Fig. 1.1). As will be seen later, decisions of this kind, turning on the key distinction between *self* and *not-self*, are still central to immunology, even in the most advanced animals.

With larger animals, the options for interaction are quite numerous. Another species may be treated as prey and taken in as dead meat, or if small enough it may succeed in getting in alive and surviving as a resident. Here the relationship may be convenient to the host (*mutualism*), of neutral value (*commensalism*), or definitely inconvenient (*parasitism*) (Fig. 1.2). The study of infectious disease concerns, for the most part, the last situation. Note that the traditional use of the term 'parasite' to refer only to tropical protozoa and worms is fairly illogical and unhelpful; a virus is no less a parasite (indeed more so) than a roundworm, and, as mentioned above, in this book the term '*pathogen*' will be used for all those microorganisms that get into larger animals and do harm of

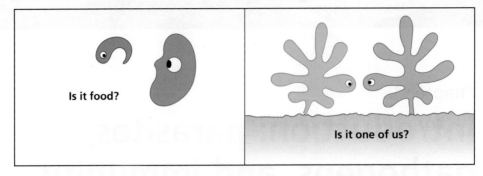

Fig. 1.1 Protozoa considering items of food, or colonies of coral in a position to undergo fusion, make recognition decisions quite similar to those that are the responsibility of the immune system in higher animals.

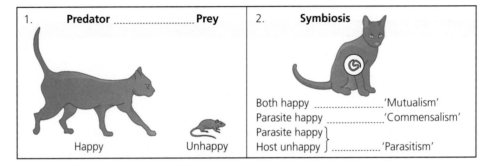

Fig. 1.2 Various two-partner relationships. The study of infectious disease is chiefly about the relationship between host and parasite (pathogen).

some kind. It is interesting that Pasteur's definition of a virus was 'a small obligate parasite requiring energy and information from a host organism'.

■ Pathogens

You do not need to be an expert microbiologist to understand infection, but you do need to know certain facts about the five classes of pathogen that cause infectious disease: the *viruses*, *bacteria*, *fungi*, *protozoa*, and *helminths* (worms), together with those strange bits of infectious protein, the *prions*. A sixth class, the insects inhabiting or invading the skin (ectoparasites) will be considered too, since although they generally remain outside the body, they can engage the attention of the immune system. Some insects and other animals will also feature in later sections as *vectors* or alternative hosts for some pathogens.

In fact, the terms 'microorganism' and 'microbe' are slightly ambiguous, implying something you need a microscope to see, which does not apply to most of the parasitic worms. It is interesting to compare the sizes of the major parasites of interest to humans, which range over nine orders of magnitude (Fig. 1.3). Note

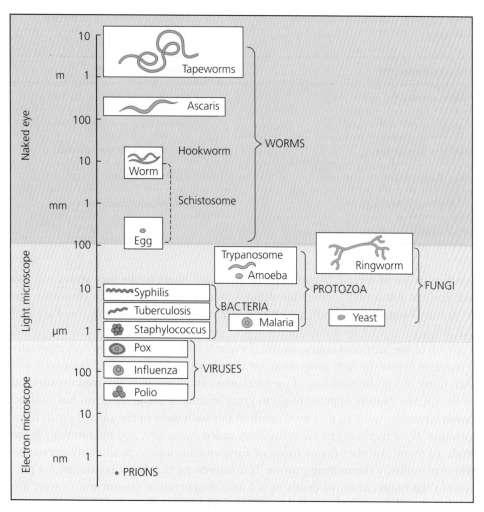

Fig. 1.3 Parasites of humans range in size over more than nine orders of magnitude, from viruses only visible in the electron microscope to worms easily visible to the naked eye. One important distinction is between those too big to be taken in by phagocytes (worms and the largest fungi) and those small enough to be disposed of in this way (all the rest). Another is between those incapable of independent existence (e.g. viruses) and the rest.

that the largest ones are much closer in size to humans than they are to the smallest ones, so it is not surprising that they too have their parasites, right down to the bacteria, which can be infected with special viruses known as bacteriophages.

Some of the advantages of being a parasite are obvious. As a parasite you are protected from the hostile conditions of the outside world (heat, cold, injury, etc.); you are provided with many of your nutritional needs and synthetic pathways; you can travel over relatively great distances without exertion (many tropical parasites use insects for this purpose); you can therefore devote much of your efforts to reproduction. On the downside, you are obliged to go where your host goes; your diet has to be chosen from what your host eats; you may have to use ingenuity to enter the host, to migrate through its tissues to your chosen location, and to exit

Table 1.1 Both infection and immunity are influenced by particular features of the pathogen concerned

Affecting infection	Affecting immunity
Means of entry and spread	Habitat (intracellular or extracellular)
Rate of multiplication (if any)	Susceptibility to immune mechanisms
Ability to damage tissue	Ability to escape immune mechanisms
Ease of transmission to other hosts	Ability to damage the immune system
Existence of animal reservoir	Suitability for vaccination
Drug therapy (if any)	

again in order to spread; if your host dies you are likely to die too; above all, you are likely to encounter formidable defence mechanisms designed to eliminate you or at least keep you in check, which is where immunology comes in (see Part 2 of this book).

Death of the host is of course a critical event for the host organism too, especially if it occurs before the next generation has been born and safely raised, because it will then result in a permanent loss of parental genes and ultimately threaten the survival of the species. Nature appears to go to great lengths to avoid this, and has evolved powerful mechanisms to minimize death at this early age. In the case of death from infection, these mechanisms are collectively called *immunity*, and immunology is the study of them. Another major cause of early deaths, injury, is similarly prevented where possible by the *healing* process. It is interesting that the mechanisms for preventing the main causes of death in old age, degenerative disease and cancer, are much less well developed, which is perfectly logical when it is considered that, with the possible exception of humans, elderly members of most animal species are usually a burden, in terms of consumption compared with productivity.

The five classes of organism mentioned above display a huge range of variation, between and within classes. Some of the characteristics of an organism that can influence the pattern of infection it causes and the effectiveness or otherwise of immunity are listed in Table 1.1. Those that facilitate infection are often lumped together as *virulence factors*, and we shall return to these in Chapter 9.

■ Infectious disease

As mentioned above, death of the host constitutes a grave risk for the parasite, but what about *disease*? One could argue that the ideal parasite would not cause its host to die or develop disease, and certainly there are examples of this idyllic coexistence, including the millions of bacteria that reside harmlessly, and even beneficially, in our intestinal tract. But the parasites we are most interested in are precisely those that *do* cause disease, the pathogens, which unfortunately are very numerous and widespread and a major cause of death worldwide. Their impact on a population can be evaluated in several ways: average life expectancy, disability adjusted life years (DALY), and economic cost (care and medicines, loss of workforce). By all these criteria, it is tropical countries that bear the major burden (see Table 1.2). Why have these diseases not achieved the 'ideal' state? This is a very deep question to which there is no easy answer. It used to be assumed that all parasite–host combinations would, given time, evolve towards the ideal state, or at least to a state where they did not kill the host. According to this theory, parasites that frequently did kill their hosts were simply not yet properly 'adapted'. Again, examples can be found, such as the fact that the often fatal human malaria parasite, *Plasmodium falciparum*, appears to have got into humans (probably from birds) more recently than the other three milder species of malaria, which reached us via other primates. So *P. falciparum* would be expected to evolve towards lesser virulence given time. A similar argument is based on 'zoonotic' infections, such as plague, Lassa fever, and the immunodeficiency viruses, that are still mainly restricted to animals and so have not had to adapt to humans. When they do infect humans they are very often fatal; in one of these, human immunodeficiency virus (HIV), we have had the dubious privilege of actually being able to follow the genetic evolution of the virus as it spread from primates to humans. However, experts in this field, modelling millions of years of host–parasite evolution on their computers, no longer accept the old generalization. Each parasite–host combination has to be looked at separately; sometimes disease may be the result of the parasite ensuring its own spread through the tissues or its transmission

Table 1.2 Infectious diseases are a much more important cause of death in low-income than in more prosperous areas. Total deaths per year (in brackets: per cent of all deaths)

Cause of death	World	High and middle	Low income
Circulatory (heart, CNS)	13.4 (23.6)	12.4 (26)	1.0 (11.0)
Cancer	7.6 (13.8)	5.6 (12)	2.0 (22)
Infantile respiratory disease	3.46 (6.1)	2.42 (5.1)	1.05 (11.3)
Infantile diarrhoeal disease	2.46 (4.3)	1.68 (4.4)	0.76 (8.2)
AIDS	1.75 (3.1)	1.03 (2.7)	0.72 (7.8)
TB	1.34 (2.4)	0.93 (2.4)	0.4 (4.3)
Malaria	1.1 (1.2)		0.48 (5.2)
All 5 above infections	9.7 (17.1)	6.1 (14.6)	3.4 (36.8)

Source, WHO 2008. All figures approximate.

AIDS, acquired immune deficiency syndrome.

to another host, and the occasional death is the price paid for this. Nevertheless, it does appear to be a reasonably safe statement that, in the long term, the more successful parasites are those that cause their hosts less distress.

■ Immunity

In this book, immunity will be considered in its broadest sense, including the devices by which hosts try to keep parasites out as well as those they use against the ones that get in. You will see that these devices are very numerous and tailored to different requirements: some act fast, others are more accurate but take time; some have a fairly broad spectrum, whereas others display the most exquisite specificity against individual microbial molecules. You will also see that, not surprisingly, all successful parasites, whether or not they are pathogens, have evolved counterdevices to prevent themselves being eliminated. Often these escape mechanisms are even more remarkable than those deployed by the host immune system. After all, parasites have been evolving for longer than we have, and at a vastly higher rate. However, you will perhaps be surprised to learn that, in many cases, the actual symptoms of an infectious disease are caused by the immune system itself rather than by the parasite, emphasizing the point that immune defence mechanisms are very potent, and are not absolutely guaranteed against doing damage to innocent parties such as host tissues (*immunopathology*).

You will see that this raises other very interesting questions, to which immunologists devote a lot of their time, such as: What are the limits to immunity? What regulates the activity of the immune system? How does it know which devices to use against which infection? How can it distinguish friend from foe, or in immunological parlance *self* from *not-self*? By bearing such questions in mind, you can sometimes see more clearly why one infectious disease takes a particular course, or another proves difficult or even impossible to get rid of. Note that the famous 'postulates' of Robert Koch (1891)*, which laid down the rules for attributing a particular disease to a particular organism, did not take account of the role of the immune system and other host elements (or of multiple infections) in pathology and, though generally valid, are no longer regarded as sacrosanct.

Pursuing this idea of seeing infection from the parasite's viewpoint, it is useful to consider all infectious disease as a sort of 'obstacle course' in which the parasite's objective is to enter and survive in a host and, when appropriate, spread to another. Meanwhile the host's objective is to prevent this process by all available means. Figure 1.4 is a simple 'map' of the resulting conflict, showing the main host strategies

---

*Koch's postulates state that:

1. The organism should be found in all cases of the disease, in the same location as the pathological lesions, and not in healthy individuals.
2. The organism should be grown in pure culture.
3. The culture should reproduce the disease when introduced into another susceptible host.
4. The organism should be isolated from this host and recultured.

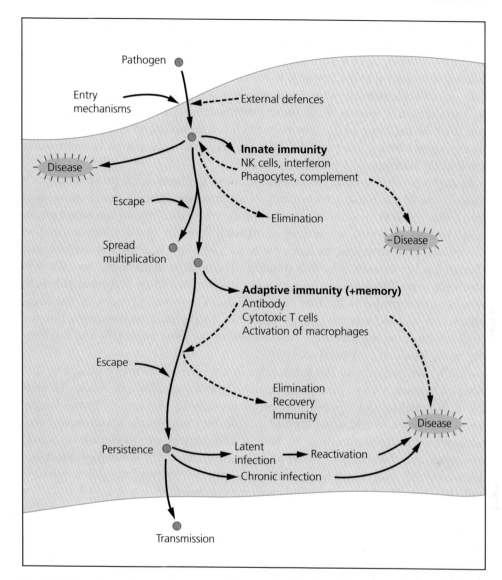

Fig. 1.4 The various stages and outcomes of a generalized infection, showing the main strategies available to the pathogen (left) and the host (right), leading to elimination of the pathogen or damage to the host (extreme right). NK cell, natural killer cell.

(i.e. defences) and the potential strategies for avoiding them as practised by pathogens. Most of this book consists of a description of these competing mechanisms, emphasizing that not all are involved equally, or involved at all, in every single disease, which is why different infectious diseases appear so different, just as different battles do, but also bringing out the underlying similarity. As you proceed through the book you may find it useful to refer back to this figure to check on how far along the obstacle race you have gone.

An increasingly important group of individuals consists of those whose immune system is faulty for some reason, not only because they may be more susceptible to certain infections than the rest of us, but also because a lot has been learned from them, and from animals that have been deliberately made *immunodeficient*, about the workings of the normal system. It is true in immunology as in any other branch of biology that the best way to find out the real importance of some organ, cell, or molecule is to see what happens when it is missing, or when you remove it. The alternative approach—to assume that because two events happen together, one must be the cause of the other—is much less reliable, and immunology is full of examples where some powerful immune response turns out to be quite unrelated to the outcome of a particular infection.

In Part 3 we shall look at some applications of immunological principles, which include one of the finest achievements of all medicine, namely, *vaccination*. It is ironic that this was introduced into Europe over 200 years ago by a country physician (Jenner) at a time when neither microbiology nor immunology existed as disciplines, and was given its scientific basis 100 years later by a microbiologist (Pasteur) when immunology was thought of as a part of microbiology. We will also take a passing look at *chemotherapy*, the brainchild of a chemist (Ehrlich) who is often regarded as the first immunologist. The moral, perhaps, is that disciplines and specialties come and go according to the pace of discovery, but the study of infection and immunity remains one of the most important and fascinating in the whole of biological science.

Finally, we integrate all this knowledge in a review of the major infectious diseases of humans, viewed microbiologically, immunologically, and medically, ending with a look ahead at what new problems may be awaiting us in the future. These are numerous and worrying and include, for example, the emergence of new pathogens, whether naturally or by human intervention, the development of drug resistance, and the effects of travel and climate change. The control of infectious disease is, and always will be, a continuing process requiring the fullest possible understanding of all its aspects and constant vigilance.

SUMMARY

- Infectious disease is caused by parasites (pathogens) capable of damaging their host.
- These include some, but not all, members of the viruses, bacteria, fungi, protozoa, worms, and prions.
- Infections are held in check, where possible, by the immune system, operating at several levels, depending on the evasion strategies adopted by the pathogen.

Chapter 2
Viruses

Viruses were discovered just before 1900 and used to be known as 'filtrable viruses' to emphasize their small size, all but the largest being visible only in the electron microscope. It is debatable whether they should really be considered as living organisms, since they consist merely of nucleic acid wrapped in a coat of protein and depend entirely on a host cell for their metabolism and multiplication (just as 'computer viruses' need the computer's hardware before they can wreak their havoc; for once the analogy is a rather good one). But living or not, viruses are the most widespread of all pathogens, capable of infecting every species of animal from mammals down to insects, protozoa, and even bacteria, as well as plants (the well-known tobacco mosaic virus was the first virus to be transmitted experimentally, in 1876, although its nature was not understood at the time). It has been estimated that there are more species of virus than of all other creatures put together. By no means all are harmful; indeed their ability to act as 'mobile genes' is thought to have influenced the genetic make-up and evolution of higher organisms. In fact their resemblance to the genes of higher animals that can 'jump' from one chromosome to another may be a clue to their origin: many experts now believe that they are descended from bacterial *plasmids*, which are little packets of genes lying outside the bacterial chromosomes and capable of being transferred to another bacterium (see Chapters 3 and 29 for a discussion of the role of plasmids in antibiotic resistance). Another less-favoured theory is that viruses are degenerate bacteria that have given up the free-living lifestyle. Recently viruses have come to play an important role in the development of *gene therapy* because of the ease with which they can enter cells, taking in with them a selected gene to replace one missing in the recipient.

In this chapter we shall consider the basic biology of viruses; details of the individual diseases they cause will be found in Part 3, Chapter 31 (the same pattern is followed in Chapters 3–8).

■ Viral structure, replication, and function

Although they vary greatly in size and complexity, viruses have certain features in common. Figure 2.1 shows the organization of a typical virus particle. Because the genome consists only of DNA or RNA, but not both, the way in which viruses replicate themselves varies from virus to virus, depending on the nature of its genome, the object in every case being to make viral proteins plus more copies of the viral genome. DNA viruses are the simplest, since the host cell's RNA polymerase can make mRNA which can then be translated on host ribosomes to make viral proteins. RNA viruses have to provide their own RNA polymerase to make mRNA, and in the case of so-called negative-sense RNA viruses an additional transcriptional step is required to make positive-sense RNA. Yet another approach, used by (RNA) retroviruses, which carry the enzyme *reverse transcriptase*, is to make their own DNA which is then inserted into the host genome (Fig. 2.2). The replication of viral nucleic acid, the synthesis of viral proteins, and their assembly into new viral particles may take place in the host cell's nucleus (e.g. influenza, measles) or, less often, in the cytoplasm (e.g. rabies, herpes), depending on the virus.

A remarkable feature of most viruses is the symmetrical structure of their protein coat, built up of one or more subunits packed in a way that recalls a chemical crystal more than a form of life. Figure 2.3 illustrates two kinds of symmetry favoured by viruses. Viruses unfortunately do not lend themselves to the branched system of classification used for most animals, and are usually classified on the basis of their *nucleic acid* and whether or not they possess a lipid *envelope* outside their protein coat (Table 2.1). This envelope is acquired by the virus from the host cell in the process of making its exit—a process known as *budding*—which enables the virus to survive outside the cell sufficiently long enough to spread elsewhere via the bloodstream. Whether a particular virus spreads in this way or directly from one cell to its immediate neighbour has a considerable bearing on both the pattern of infection and the development of immunity. Thus an enveloped virus can leave its host cell without destroying it, whereas the non-enveloped sort will rupture the cell (cytolysis); the latter are known as *cytopathic* viruses because of

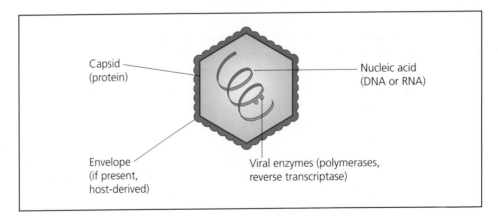

Fig. 2.1 Basic structure of a typical virus (diagrammatic).

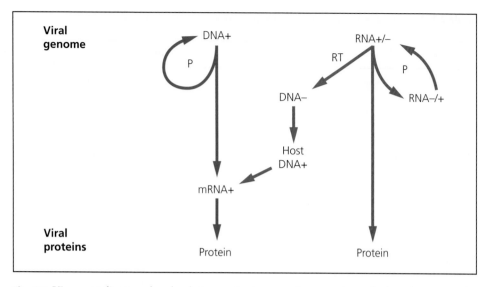

Fig. 2.2 Viruses replicate and make their proteins by several routes, depending on the nature of their genome. + and − refer to the sense of the DNA or RNA; P is polymerase, which may be host- or virus-derived; RT is reverse transcriptase, an enzyme found in retroviruses.

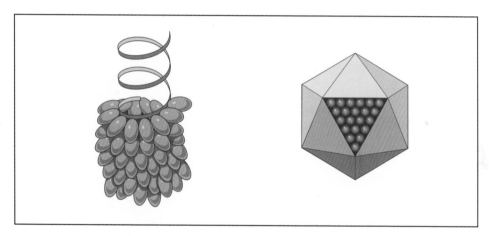

Fig. 2.3 The two most common types of viral symmetry. Left: helical (e.g. mumps, measles). The RNA is shown at the top and the surrounding capsid units (capsomeres) below. Right: icosahedral (e.g. polio). Ten of the 20 faces of the capsid are shown and 21 of the 252 capsomeres.

their ability to damage cells and tissues; that is, cause *pathology*. Figure 2.4 illustrates these two means of spread.

Receptors

Having left one cell, a virus must enter another in order to multiply. Viruses are not simply taken into cells as water is, but must first attach to a *receptor* on the cell surface. Each virus has its specific receptor, usually a vital component of the cell surface: if it were not, the cell could simply shed the receptor or stop making

Table 2.1 A simple classification of the principal viruses infecting humans

	DNA	RNA
Enveloped	Herpesviruses	Orthomyxoviruses
	1, 2	Influenza
	3 (VZV), 4 (CMV)	Paramyxoviruses
	5 (EBV), 6, 7, 8	Measles, mumps,
		Respiratory syncytial virus
	Pox viruses	Rhabdoviruses
	Smallpox	Rabies
	Hepadna viruses	Retroviruses
	Hepatitis B	HIV, HTLV-1
		Togaviruses
		Rubella
		Chikungunya
		Flaviviruses
		Yellow fever, dengue
		Hepatitis C
		West Nile virus
		Coronaviruses (colds)
		SARS
		Arenaviruses
		Lassa fever virus
		Bunyaviruses
		Hanta virus
		Filoviruses
		Marburg virus
		Ebola virus
Non-enveloped	Adenoviruses (colds, etc.)	Picornaviruses
		Rhinoviruses
	Parvoviruses	Enteroviruses
	Papovaviruses (warts, etc.)	Polio, Coxsackie, hepatitis A, Echo
		Reoviruses
		Rotavirus
		Caliciviruses
		Norovirus

CMV, cytomegalovirus; EBV, Epstein–Barr virus; HIV, human immunodeficiency virus; HTLV, human T-lymphotropic virus; VZV, varicella zoster virus.

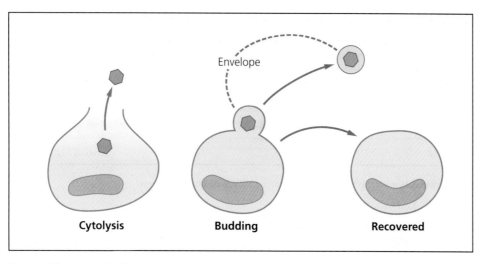

Fig. 2.4 The two methods of viral escape from the infected cell have very different effects on the cell.

Table 2.2 For some viruses, the cell-surface receptor required for attachment and subsequent entry is known, but for many others it remains to be discovered

Virus	Receptor
EBV	B-cell complement receptor CR2
HIV	T cell, macrophage CD4, CCR5, CXCR4
Rhinovirus	Adhesion molecule ICAM-1
Rabies	Acetylcholine receptor
Vaccinia	Epidermal growth factor receptor
Influenza	Neuraminic acid (also on red blood cells)
Reovirus	β-Adrenergic hormone receptor
Poliovirus	Adhesion molecule CD155
Echo, Coxsackie	Complement inhibitor CD55/DAF
Measles	Complement inhibitor CD46

ICAM, intercellular adhesion molecule.

it, and thus resist infection. Some examples of known virus–receptor pairs are shown in Table 2.2. It is the distribution of these receptor molecules on host cells that largely determines the cell-preference (or *tropism*) of individual viruses. For example, the human immunodeficiency virus (HIV) infects mainly T lymphocytes and macrophages because only they carry a surface molecule known as CD4

Table 2.3 Viral infection can lead to several different outcomes for the infected cell

Lysis (cytopathic)	Persistence (carrier state)	Latency (reactivation)	Transformation	
			Benign	Malignant
Adenovirus	Hepatitis B	Herpesviruses	Warts	Hepatitis B
Influenza	EBV	(HSV, VZV, CMV)		(liver cancer)
Poliovirus				(Burkitt's lymphoma)

CMV, cytomegalovirus; HSV, herpes simplex virus; VZV, varicella zoster virus.

(where CD stands for cluster of differentiation; see Appendix 3), whereas Epstein–Barr virus (EBV) infects B lymphocytes carrying the complement receptor CR2.

Effects of infection

Infection of a cell by a virus can have one of several effects. Many viruses cause no harm or disease whatever. But as mentioned above, the cell may be lysed as the viral particles burst out and spread elsewhere: a *lytic* infection. Eventually, if host immunity operates effectively, the virus-infected cell may be killed by the host, leading to interruption of the virus cycle and cure of the infection. Not all viruses are got rid of so easily. They may persist in the cell without damaging it, giving rise to the *carrier* state, in which an apparently cured patient can still be infectious to others. Or they may survive in a non-infectious form that can become reactivated to cause a second infection; this is called *latency*. Table 2.3 lists some well-known examples of these different outcomes.

Viruses and cancer

Finally, the viral DNA (or DNA copied from viral RNA) may become integrated into host DNA, with effects on the control of cell growth that can in some cases lead to *transformation*, in other words a tumour. However, integration does not always lead to transformation, nor is it essential for tumour formation. The association of viruses with tumours in animals was first suspected 90 years ago but only in the 1960s was a virus (EBV) shown convincingly to be associated with a human tumour (Burkitt's lymphoma). Table 2.4 illustrates some key dates in the gradual unfolding of the virus–cancer link. Currently it is estimated that about 15% of human cancers are virus-related. The mechanism by which viruses push cells into the uncontrolled growth characteristic of tumours appears to involve *oncogenes*, of either viral or host origin. In some cases these genes code for growth factor or hormone receptors on the cell surface; in other cases the virus inhibits the cell's tumour-suppressor genes or the normal process of cell suicide (apoptosis), and sometimes other factors come in. One of the most complex pathways is that by which heavy EBV infection, malaria infection, and the translocation of the cellular oncogene *c*-myc to a site active in B lymphocytes all come together to

Table 2.4 Landmarks in the understanding of tumour viruses

1908	Bang, Ellerman	Chicken leukaemia transmitted by filtrable particle
1911	Rous	Chicken sarcoma transmitted by filtrable particle
1930	Shope	Rabbit skin tumours transmitted by filtrable particle
1936	Bittner	Mouse breast cancer transmitted by milk factor
1962	Burkitt	Human lymphoma due to infection?
1964	Epstein, Barr	Virus extracted from Burkitt's lymphoma
1977	Blumberg	Liver carcinoma due to hepatitis B virus
1980	Gallo	HTLV-1 causes T-cell leukaemia
1984	Zur Hausen	HPV viruses cause cervical cancer
1987	Zur Hausen	Hepatitis C viruses cause liver carcinoma
1994	Chang, Moore	HHV-8 causes Kaposi's sarcoma; some HPV types cause cervical and skin cancer

HHV, human herpesvirus; HPV, human papilloma virus; HTLV, human T-lymphotropic virus.

induce the B-cell tumour known as Burkitt's lymphoma. This happens mainly in Africa while, surprisingly, in China EBV is associated with a completely different tumour, nasopharyngeal carcinoma.

■ Viral spread

As well as replicating themselves in the host, most viruses need to spread to another host, since the original host may either die or eliminate the infection (how this happens will be described in later chapters). The main routes of spread are listed in Table 2.5. Meanwhile, in order to survive long enough to spread to another host, viruses may often need to escape the attentions of the immune system. How they do this is described in detail in Chapters 13 and 22 where you will see that some of their strategies are very sophisticated, such as repeatedly changing their surface molecules or switching off immune responses. A special category of viruses is those that cause disease only when the immune system is deficient in some way; these are called opportunists, and *opportunistic infection* is one of the main problems in patients with, for example, AIDS. How individual viruses and the immune system interact to set the pattern of disease is described in Chapter 31.

■ Control of viruses

The pattern of viral disease has been altered radically by the introduction of *vaccines*. Many of the really successful vaccines are against viruses, and one

Table 2.5 The principal routes of viral spread

Route	Examples
Skin contact	HPV (warts)
Respiratory	Cold viruses, influenza, measles, mumps, rubella
Faecal–oral	Polio, echo, Coxsackie, hepatitis A, rotavirus
Milk	HIV, HTLV-1, CMV
Transplacental	Rubella, CMV, HIV
Sexual	Herpes 1 and 2, HIV, HPV, hepatitis B
Insect vector	Yellow fever, dengue, Chikungunya
Animal bite	Rabies

CMV, cytomegalovirus; HPV, human papilloma virus; HTLV, human T-lymphotropic virus.

Table 2.6 Some zoonotic viruses

Virus	Animal reservoir
Influenza	Birds, pigs, horses
Rabies	Bats, dogs, foxes
Lassa and Hanta viruses	Rodents
Ebola and Marburg viruses	Monkeys
HIV-1 and -2	Chimpanzees, monkeys
Newcastle disease	Poultry
West Nile virus	Birds

disease—smallpox—has been completely eliminated (1980). It is hoped that several other viruses, such as polio and measles, will follow. This is just as well because the development of antiviral drugs still has far to go. Further details are given in Chapters 28 and 29. Nevertheless, there are unfortunately a number of viruses that at present do not seem promising candidates for vaccines. In addition, apparently 'new' viruses crop up from time to time, usually by spreading from an animal in which they are well adapted to humans in which they are not; these *zoonoses* include some of the most frightening and acutely fatal of all virus diseases (Table 2.6 and Chapter 37).

SUMMARY

- Viruses have a genome of RNA or DNA which can replicate, but rely on a host cell for their metabolism. Thus they are obligate intracellular parasites.

- Viruses enter cells by attaching to receptors, which are usually cell-surface molecules needed for normal cell function.

- Once in the host cell, they replicate and usually leave the cell, to infect others. This exit may be by budding or by lysis.

- Some viruses may lie dormant, to be reactivated later, or they may transform the host cell into a benign or malignant tumour.

- There are some drugs against viruses, but the best control has been by vaccines.

Chapter 3
Bacteria

With the bacteria, we enter the world of cellular organisms, capable of fully independent existence and within range of the ordinary light microscope. Bacteria were almost certainly the first truly living things on our planet, representing a high degree of organization within a single cell. Some are parasitic, but the majority live free in soil, water, etc., while some can live free or as parasites as it suits them. However, bacteria differ fundamentally from all other cellular organisms, whether unicellular like the fungi and protozoa or multicellular like worms (and humans), in that they are *procaryotic* rather than *eucaryotic*. The distinction between these two forms of cellular organization is important to the understanding of how they respond to the immune system, and also, as Chapter 29 will show, to therapeutic drugs. The principal features of the two types of cell are illustrated in Fig. 3.1.

■ Classification; the cell wall

One part of the bacterium with a special significance for both disease and immunity is the *cell wall*, and bacterial classification starts with the distinction between three types of cell wall that vary greatly in their structure (Fig. 3.2). Conveniently for microbiologists, a simple iodine/crystal violet-based technique, the Gram stain, identifies two fundamentally different types: *Gram-positive* (stained), with a thick sugar amino-acid polymer (peptidoglycan) outside a single cell membrane, and *Gram-negative* (unstained) with a thinner peptidoglycan layer between two cell membranes. A third group, the mycobacteria, have waxy outer layers that resist

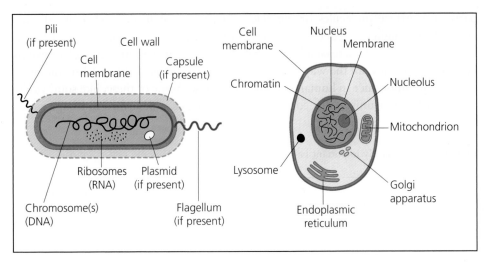

Fig. 3.1 Procaryotic and eucaryotic cells compared. Left: a typical (procaryotic) bacterium. Right: a typical eucaryotic cell.

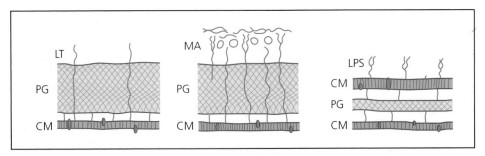

Fig. 3.2 Three types of bacterial cell wall, showing the single or double cell membrane (CM). Left: Gram-positive (e.g. *Staphylococcus*); the exposed peptidoglycan (PG) is accessible to host lysosomal enzymes; LT, lipoteichoic acid. Centre: mycobacterium (e.g. *Mycobacterium tuberculosis*); the surface coat of the lipid mycolic acid (MA) confers resistance to acid, alcohol, and many immune killing mechanisms. Right: Gram-negative (e.g. *Salmonella*); the lipopolysaccharide (LPS) inserted in the outer cell membrane is an important virulence factor.

the Gram stain and can be visualized using a fuchsin-based stain (Ziehl–Neelsen or ZN). Their tough wall has earned them the name acid-fast bacilli (AFB).

The cell wall has a considerable influence on bacterial survival; thus peptidoglycan is resistant to digestion by bile but sensitive to the enzyme *lysozyme* (and also to penicillin; see Chapter 29), whereas the waxy mycolic acids of mycobacteria enhance long-term survival in dry conditions. Other external features of some bacteria are the capsule (see below) and long processes that facilitate motility (flagella) or attachment to host cells (pili).

Beyond this level, bacteria are classified according to shape into the roughly spherical *cocci* and the long thin *rods*, plus an assorted group of 'atypical' bacteria. Further subdivisions are made on the basis of growth requirements, possession of particular surface molecules or *antigens* (a term you will meet when we discuss antibody in Chapter 17), and the sequences of their proteins and nucleic acids; ribosomal RNA is used increasingly as a reliable index of evolutionary relationships between organisms, all the way from bacteria to mammals. Table 3.1 lists the main bacteria of importance in human and animal disease. Some of these, like some of the viruses, are opportunists. The corresponding diseases are described in Chapter 32.

Table 3.1 The medically important bacteria

	Gram-positive	Gram-negative
Cocci (spherical)	Staphylococci	*Neisseria*
	Streptococci	*Meningococcus*
		Gonococcus
Bacilli (rod-shaped)	*Bacillus anthracis*	Enteric
	Clostridium tetani	*Salmonella*
	Clostridium perfringens	*Shigella*
	Clostridium botulinum	*Escherichia*
	Corynebacterium diphtheriae	*Yersinia*
	Listeria	*Pseudomonas*
	Mycobacterium tuberculosis	*Vibrio cholerae*
	Mycobacterium leprae	*Campylobacter*
		Helicobacter
		Brucella
		Haemophilus
		Bordetella
		Legionella
		Bacteroides
Filamentous	Actinomycetes	
Spiral		*Spirochaetes*
		Treponema
		Leptospira
		Borrelia
Obligate intracellular		*Chlamydiae*
		Rickettsiae
Lacking cell walls	*Mycoplasma*	

Those in the group below the line are often referred to as 'atypical' (see text). Note that the Gram-positive cocci and the Gram-negative rods are responsible for the majority of severe bacterial disease. The asterisked organisms are not normally identified by the Gram stain, but share characteristics of the Gram-positive or Gram-negative groups as shown.

Unlike eucaryotic cells, bacteria have no clear-cut nuclei, their DNA being in the form of a single, usually circular, chromosome without introns. A system of repressor, inducer, and co-repressor molecules ensures economical regulation of the genes coding for bacterial enzymes appropriate to the available substrates (see below). Further DNA may be present in the form of small circular *plasmids*, which carry genes for adaptive functions such as toxin production and antibiotic resistance (see below). Sometimes a plasmid is large enough to be considered as a second chromosome (e.g. in *Vibrio cholerae*); indeed, it is thought that eucaryotic chromosomes may have evolved from plasmids that became segregated into nuclei.

■ Bacterial metabolism

Parasitic bacteria, unlike plants and some free-living bacteria, lack chlorophyll and cannot obtain energy from photosynthesis. Instead, they use various inorganic molecules and glucose, from which they derive energy by glycolysis (fermentation); some can go further and use oxygen (respiration). The *mitochondria* of higher animals are believed to have originated from bacteria that were taken up and used by early eucaryotes to enable them to respire (in a similar way, the *plant* cell probably evolved from the uptake of photosynthetic bacteria). This distinction between aerobic and anaerobic bacteria shows up in certain infections. For example, the aerobic tubercle bacillus grows well in the (well-oxygenated) lungs, whereas the anaerobic clostridia that cause tetanus and gas gangrene flourish in the oxygen-starved environment of deep wounds.

■ Atypical bacteria

Not all bacteria fit neatly into the foregoing classification. *Spirochaetes* are unusual in being helically coiled, highly motile, and resistant to Gram-staining. *Actinomycetes* are filamentous, and were formerly considered to be fungi. Poised between viruses and typical bacteria are the *Rickettsiae* and *Chlamydiae*. Like bacteria they have both DNA and RNA, but like viruses they are obligate intracellular parasites because they lack some of the biosynthetic pathways for independent existence. *Mycoplasmas*, on the other hand, can survive extracellularly, despite their lack of a cell wall. Table 3.2 lists those important as human pathogens; see Chapter 32 for further details.

■ Bacterial genetics and reproduction

Bacterial replication normally occurs by simple binary fission and may be extremely fast (every 20 min for some staphylococci) or very slow (around 2 weeks for the leprosy bacillus); for comparison, a time of 24 h would be considered rapid for mammalian cells.

Table 3.2 The major pathogenic atypical bacteria

Group	Examples	Human disease
Actinomycetes	*Actinomyces israelii*	Actinomycosis
Spirochaetes	*Treponema pallidum*	Syphilis
	Leptospira interrogans	Weil's disease
	Borrelia recurrentis	Relapsing fever
	B. burgdorferi	Lyme disease
Rickettsiae	*Rickettsia typhi*	Typhus
	Coxiella burnetii	Q fever
Chlamydiae	*Chlamydia trachomatis*	Trachoma
	C. psittaci	Psittacosis
Mycoplasma	*Mycoplasma pneumoniae*	Atypical pneumonia

Gene expression

Bacterial DNA is transcribed into RNA which is translated into protein by pathways similar to those used by higher organisms. Special features of gene expression include (1) the occurrence of several genes together in *operons* that ensure the efficient production of complex elements such as pili or toxins, and (2) rapid regulation of gene expression to meet new conditions by *regulons*, which coordinate the expression of several genes or operons.

Variation

Far from being the fixed entities of the older textbooks, bacteria are constantly evolving, even within species. Genes may be lost, gained, or altered. *Gene loss*, or 'genome decay', occurs when genes are no longer required, for instance when a free-living bacterium becomes an intracellular parasite: rickettsia are an extreme example of this. Avoidance of immune attack may be another stimulus for gene loss, e.g. flagellar proteins in *Shigella*. It is thought that mitochondria represent ancient bacteria that have lost almost all their genes. *Gene gain* can occur by duplication or by horizontal gene transfer from bacteria of the same or a different species. Genes can be transferred by bacteriophages (bacterial viruses), by the exchange of extra-chromosomal plasmids, or by clusters of chromosomal genes known as pathogenicity islands, which often carry several different genes for virulence factors (see Fig 3.3 and Chapter 9).

Another method for bringing about rapid changes in genes is *phase variation*, by which mispairing of repeat sequences causes the synthesis of important proteins to be switched on or off.

	Transformation	Transduction	Conjugation
Form of DNA transferred	Naked (small pieces)	In bacteriophage	In plasmid
Transfer			
Integration			
Example	'Competent' strains only e.g. *Streptococcus pneumoniae*	Many toxin genes	Antibiotic-resistance genes

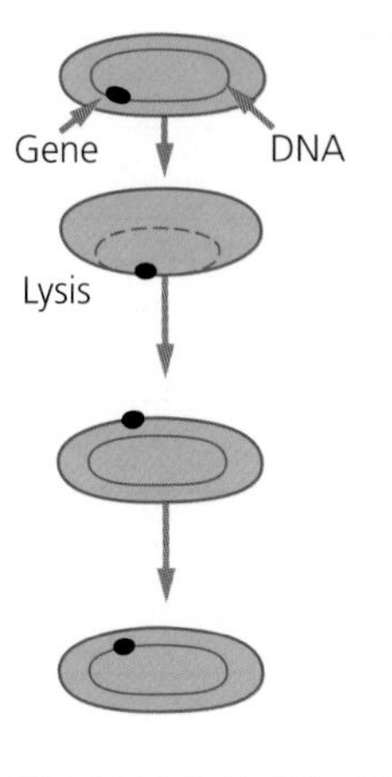

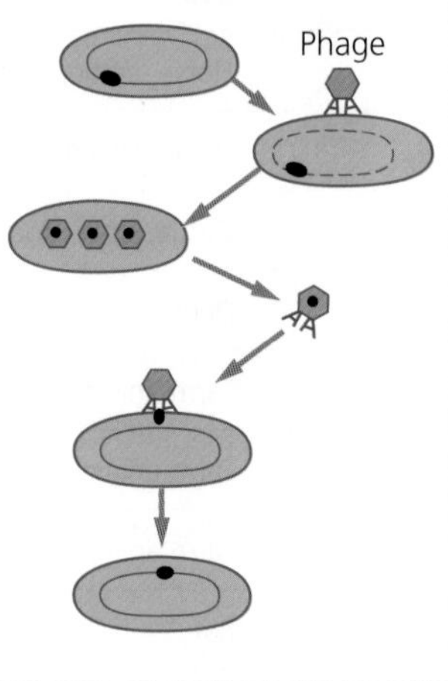

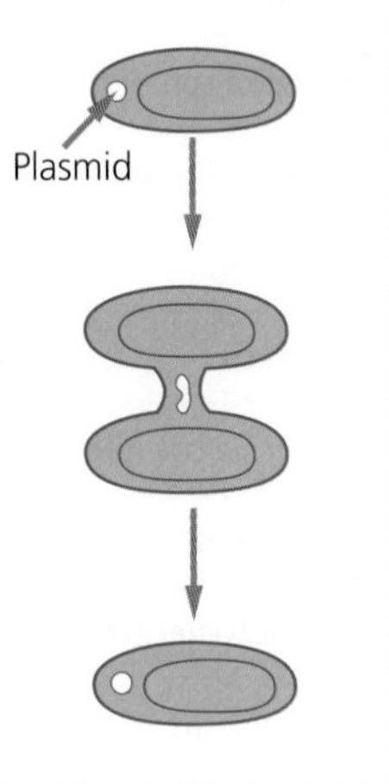

Fig. 3.3 Bacteria can acquire new genes in several ways.

These strategies, combined with rapid replication, frequently allow bacteria to keep 'one jump ahead' of their environment; one topical example of this is the continuous emergence of staphylococci resistant to many or even all antibiotics: the dreaded 'hospital staphs' or methicillin-resistant *Staphylococcus aureus* (MRSA; see Chapter 29). Some bacteria can halt their growth altogether under adverse conditions and form *spores*, which can lie dormant for years until the conditions for growth reappear. This is how, for example, tetanus bacilli are able to survive in the soil, and cause rapid infections if they get into a wound.

■ Disease and immunity

Bacteria do not always cause disease, in fact the intestine of a healthy adult contains about 10^{14} bacteria (more as you move down the bowel) with perhaps another 10^{12} on the skin. The value of this 'normal flora' has been the subject of much argument, but it does appear that interfering with it can be dangerous; for

Table 3.3 Some zoonotic bacterial infections

Bacterium	Animal reservoir	Disease
Mycobacterium bovis	Cattle	Tuberculosis
M. avium	Birds	Pneumonia
Leptospira spp.	Horse, cattle, dog	Weil's disease
Clostridium tetani	Horse, sheep, cattle	Tetanus
Brucella spp.	Cattle, goat, dog	Brucellosis
Borrelia spp.	Deer	Lyme disease
Escherichia coli (EHEC)	Farm animals (meat, milk)	Food poisoning
Salmonella spp.	Farm animals (eggs)	Food poisoning
Campylobacter spp.	Farm animals	Food poisoning
Yersinia pestis	Rat	Plague
Bacillus anthracis	Farm animals	Anthrax

example, by allowing other more harmful organisms to establish themselves. However, some bacteria do unfortunately cause very severe disease, as will be described in Chapters 9 and 32. Gastrointestinal disease, much of it bacterial, is a major infective cause of death worldwide, with tuberculosis not far behind (see Table 1.2).

Like all parasites, bacteria have evolved numerous mechanisms for avoiding elimination by the immune system. Strategies of particular relevance to bacteria include the production of a *capsule*—a slimy polysaccharide coat that covers the cell wall—various ways of inhibiting phagocytic cells, and other ingenious devices to be described later (Chapters 10, 13, and 22). As a result, bacteria are responsible for several chronic infections; for example, tuberculosis, leprosy, and brucellosis. Another common feature of bacteria is the production of *toxins*, which can cause some of the most acute and serious diseases, including tetanus, cholera, and gas gangrene. Toxins will be discussed in detail in Chapter 9, and the immunology of particular bacterial diseases in Chapter 32.

As with viruses, many bacteria can be acquired from animals, in which they may be better adapted and so less pathogenic (see Table 3.3).

■ Control of bacteria

With respect to therapy, the situation with bacteria is almost the opposite of that with viruses. The control of bacterial disease by *antibiotics* (Chapter 29) has been

Table 3.4 Some useful functions of bacteria

Soil	Nitrogen fixation, biodegradation
Cattle rumen	Digestion
Human intestine ('normal flora')	Compete for space with pathogens, (some) vitamin synthesis
Dairy industry	Fermentation (e.g. cheese, yoghurt)
Energy industry	Methane ('natural gas'), recycling of waste
Pharmaceutical industry	Production of enzymes and antibiotics
Biotechnology	Plasmids as vectors

one of the twentieth century's success stories, although we are not nearly as optimistic as we were (see hospital staphs, above). On the other hand, there are not many really good bacterial *vaccines* (Chapter 28 explains why this is so) and certainly very few bacterial diseases that look like candidates for elimination. Since the eucaryotic pathogens, described in the next three chapters, are generally more common in tropical countries, it seems likely that in the years to come bacteria will be the major cause of infectious disease in the developed world.

■ Useful bacteria

We should not forget the remarkable number of ways in which bacteria, far from being pathogenic, are useful and even essential to humans and animals. Table 3.4 lists a few of these useful functions.

SUMMARY

- Bacteria are single free-living prokaryotic cells, a few of which can parasitize humans and cause disease.

- The bacterial genome consists of a single loop of DNA, analogous to a chromosome. The cell is contained within a membrane and a more rigid cell wall. Some 'atypical' bacteria lack a cell wall or certain metabolic pathways, obliging them to be parasitic. Others can be free-living or parasitic.

- Bacterial genes can vary by mutation and transfer between bacteria by several routes: transport by phage, transport of plasmids, conjugation. This enables them to adapt rapidly to external threats.

- Bacteria can cause disease by secreting toxins or by inducing harmful immune responses.

- Some bacteria are useful to their hosts or to plants, or have been exploited for our benefit, for example in making antibiotics, yoghurt, and cheese.

- The most successful control of bacteria so far has been by drugs (antibiotics). There are also a few good bacterial vaccines.

Chapter 4
Fungi

When one thinks of mushrooms and toadstools, the idea of a fungus parasitic on humans seems rather improbable, but most fungi are not this large, existing as single cells (yeasts) or slender filaments (moulds), while some exist as a mixture of both (dimorphic). Out of a total of some 70 000 species, about 300 are parasites of animals, and of these a few (shown in Table 4.1) are of major importance as human pathogens.

Table 4.1 The principal medically important fungi

	Yeasts	Dimorphic	Filamentous
Superficial infection	Candida	Malassezia	Microsporum Trichophyton
Subcutaneous		Sporothrix	Madurella
Systemic dissemination	*Cryptococcus *Candida †Pneumocystis	Histoplasma Blastomyces Coccidioides Paracoccidioides	*Aspergillus *Zygomyces *Fusarium

*Opportunists; that is, pathogenic only in immunodeficient individuals.
†A single-celled opportunist, but taxonomic status uncertain.

■ Structure and morphology

Unlike bacteria, fungi are eucaryotes, with a basic cell design very similar to our own except for their complex cell wall stiffened by the addition of polysaccharides such as chitin, glucans, and mannans. Another difference is that in most cases the plasma membrane contains ergosterol in place of cholesterol (Fig. 4.1).

Yeasts and moulds differ mainly in their means of reproduction: a process of *budding* in yeasts and *apical extension* in moulds (Fig. 4.2). Dimorphic fungi behave as moulds at environmental temperatures but switch to the yeast form at body temperature. Most fungi are acquired from soil or decaying plants via inhalation of spores or from animals (e.g. *Microsporum* from cats and dogs; *Cryptococcus* from bird droppings) or other humans (e.g. *Trichophyton*).

In size, the single-celled fungi lie between bacteria and mammalian cells, and are therefore small enough to be taken in by host phagocytes (for a description of these important host defence cells, see Chapter 12) in which they sometimes manage to survive. This has the result that some fungal diseases, or *mycoses* (e.g. histoplasmosis), closely resemble diseases caused by bacteria with a similar lifestyle (e.g. the tubercle bacillus), although the organisms themselves are totally different in structure and physiology. When you consider that some protozoa behave similarly, you will appreciate that the precise taxonomic status of the microbe is not all that matters in pathogenesis; its habitat in the body, the immunity it evokes, and how it escapes this are quite as important in dictating the outcome. Indeed, one microorganism, *Pneumocystis carinii*, a major cause of disease in immunodeficient patients (that is, an opportunist), has recently had to be reclassified on the basis of its ribosomal RNA as a fungus, having hitherto been accepted as a protozoan!

The eucaryotic parasites pose particular problems to the host because their cells resemble those of the host much more closely than do bacteria (or indeed viruses). When we come to consider the way in which the immune system recognizes the presence of an invading microbe, you will appreciate why fungi, protozoa, and

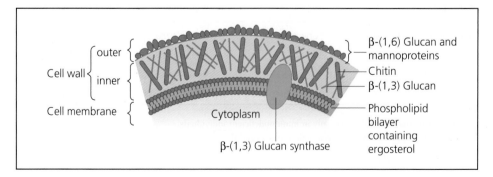

Fig. 4.1 The typical structure of the fungal cell wall. Note the importance of the stiffening components of the cell wall.

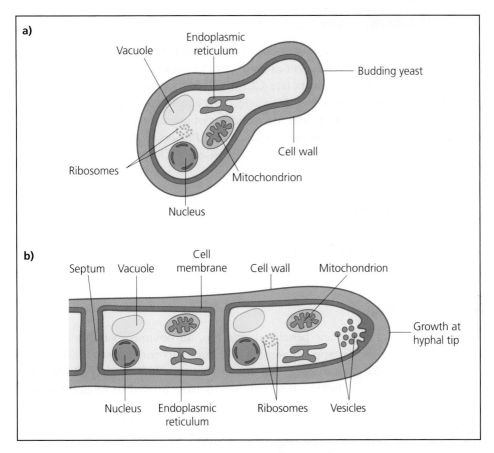

Fig. 4.2 Reproduction in fungi. (a) A budding yeast cell; (b) the growing tip of a filamentous mould.

worms are usually hard to get rid of and, by the same token, hard to eliminate by chemotherapy.

■ Cutaneous and superficial mycoses

Known collectively as dermatophytes, these fungi grow on skin, nails, and hair. *Trichophyton* and *Microsporum* spp. cause tinea (capitis, corporis: ringworm; pedis: athlete's foot). *Malasezzia* causes pityriasis. The yeast *Candida albicans* is a normal commensal of the gut and moist skin sites, but can overgrow in the mouth and vagina, causing thrush, particularly following long-term antibiotic treatment which disturbs the normal bacterial flora.

■ Subcutaneous mycoses

Sporothrix, common in gardeners, causes the ulcerating nodules of sporotrichosis. *Madurella* causes the swollen and destructive lesions of Madura foot.

■ Systemic mycoses

Mostly acquired by inhalation of spores, *Histoplasma*, *Blastomyces*, *Coccidioides*, and *Paracoccidioides* are a frequent cause of pneumonia in parts of Central America. In immunocompromised patients (see Chapters 15, 25, and 26 for a discussion of the causes of immunodeficiency) these infections can become widely disseminated and may be fatal. The same is true for a number of normally less pathogenic fungi, notably *Aspergillus*, *Cryptococcus*, *Candida*, and *Pneumocystis*. What this teaches us about the role of the immune system is discussed in Chapter 33.

■ Control of fungi

Fungal infections are not easily controlled. There are some quite effective antifungal drugs (see Table 29.5) but, at present, no vaccines for human use.

■ Useful fungi

Yeasts, of course, have their beneficial side too, an obvious example being the ability of *Saccharomyces* spp. in aerobic conditions to convert sugars into CO_2 (which helps bread dough to rise) and, in anaerobic conditions, alcohol (the basis of the wine and beer industry). Recently, yeasts have proved to be good cells in which to insert foreign genes so as to manufacture large amounts of a pure protein; the current hepatitis B vaccine is made in this way. And of course one should not forget that penicillin was originally obtained from the mould *Penicillium notatum*. Some species of fungi live symbiotically with algae and bacteria as *lichens*, which have been used as food, wool dyes, and in folk medicine. Recently lichen extracts have been shown to degrade prions (see Chapter 8).

SUMMARY

- Fungi are eucaryotes, differing from typical animal cells in having a cell wall stiffened with chitin.
- Fungal infection is a common cause of skin disease, and of pneumonia from inhalation of spores.
- Fungi are particularly invasive in immunocompromised patients, in whom they can give rise to severe opportunistic infection.
- Control of fungi by drugs is limited by toxicity.
- Fungi have useful industrial roles in the fermentation of alcohol, the rising of bread, the production of antibiotics, and in biotechnology.

Chapter 5
Protozoa

The protozoa (the name means 'first animals') are single-celled eucaryotes of amazing diversity and sophistication. The vast majority live free, employing a range of special structures for moving, adhering, killing other organisms, etc., but a few are parasites of humans or domestic animals and some of these are major pathogens. Their medical importance is heightened by the fact that they are very successful as parasites, hard for the immune system to dislodge, and hard to design effective drugs against. Most of the really severe protozoal diseases are restricted to the tropics because they depend on an insect or other *vector* and often an *animal reservoir* which is only found there.

Like bacteria and fungi, protozoa can be extracellular or intracellular parasites, as is shown in Table 5.1 together with an indication of how they are generally classified. Their impact on the affected areas can be judged from Table 5.2. One of them, the malaria parasite, has a life cycle of remarkable complexity (see below), but this is unusual, and most protozoa have relatively simple life cycles.

As might be predicted from their success as parasites, protozoa have very well-developed mechanisms for eluding the immune system of their hosts, often by varying their antigens and/or suppressing immunity; how these affect the course of disease will be described in the last Part of this book (Chapter 34). Some, such as *Toxoplasma*, are opportunists, normally harmless but pathogenic in those who are immunodeficient. It seems likely that, with the increasing numbers of immunodeficient individuals (see Chapters 25 and 26), the difficulty in making effective protozoal vaccines (see Chapter 28), the development of drug resistance (see Chapter 29), and the prospect of climate changes through global warming, protozoa will become increasingly important as human pathogens.

Table 5.1 The protozoa of medical significance

| | Habitat | |
Means of spread	Extracellular	Intracellular
Insect-borne*	African trypanosome (blood)	*Plasmodium* (liver, red blood cell)
		Leishmania (macrophage)
		South American trypanosome
		(macrophage, muscle, nerve)
Water-borne or other routes	Amoeba (gut)	†*Toxoplasma* (macrophage)
	Giardia (gut)	
	†*Cryptosporidium* (gut)	
	Isospora (gut)	
	Trichomonas (urogenital)	

*The protozoa carried by insect vectors are mainly confined to the tropics by the distribution of the vectors.
†*Toxoplasma* and *Cryptosporidium* are important opportunists.

Table 5.2 Approximate annual incidence and mortality for the major protozoal diseases

Disease	Incidence	Mortality
Giardiasis	500 000 000	–
Malaria	300 000 000	1 100 000
Trichomoniasis	180 000 000	–
Toxoplasmosis	100 000 000	250 000 (in AIDS)
Amoebiasis	500 000	50 000
Leishmaniasis	2 000 000	50 000
Trypanosomiasis		
African	500 000	400 000?
South American	300 000	50 000

■ Malaria

The malaria parasite, *Plasmodium*, has a life cycle whose origin almost defies imagination, with successive stages in the mosquito gut and salivary glands, via a mosquito bite to human blood, the liver, the blood again, with a repeating ('*asexual*') cycle through the red blood cell, and thence via another bite back to the mosquito (Fig. 5.1). An unusual feature is the development in the host red blood

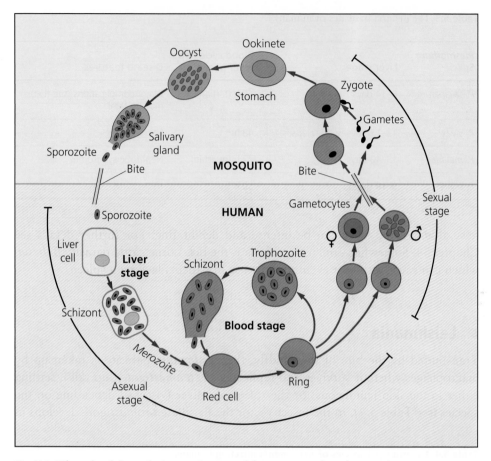

Fig. 5.1 Life cycle of the malaria parasite, one of the most complex of any pathogen.

cell of male and female gametes, which fuse to complete the *sexual* stage in the mosquito. The advantage to the parasite is rapid reassortment of genes, with the slight disadvantage that the host is not infectious at all times. From the host's point of view, this complex cycle means that a confusing sequence of different *antigens* is presented to the immune system, further complicated by the fact that many of them are highly polymorphic. The many species of *Plasmodium* that infect animals and birds are not infective for humans; thus there is no animal reservoir for human malaria.

Four species of *Plasmodium* infect humans, each with slightly different characteristics (Table 5.3). In terms of mortality, *Plasmodium falciparum* (malignant tertian) is by far the most important, being responsible for at least a million deaths per year. These result chiefly from *anaemia* and *cerebral malaria*, the latter being associated with the phenomenon of *sequestration*, in which parasitized red blood cells become attached to the vascular endothelium in the brain and other organs. Other complications include glomerulonephritis, hypoglycaemia, and pulmonary oedema. *Plasmodium vivax* does not show sequestration and complications are

Table 5.3 The malaria parasites of humans

Plasmodium Species	Liver stage	Blood cycle and fever peaks	Disease features
P. falciparum	6–14 days	48 h (tertian)	Major complications (see text); may be fatal
P. vivax	12–17 days (with relapses)	48 h	Seldom fatal
P. malariae	13–40 days	72 h (quartan)	Nephrotic syndrome
P. ovale	9–18 days	50 h	

few, although the fever can be intense and debilitating. For further details see Chapter 34. Somewhat similar to malaria is the tick-borne cattle parasite *Babesia*, which can cause severe or even fatal disease in patients lacking a spleen.

■ Leishmania

Transmitted by the bite of the sandfly, the *Leishmania* parasite is taken up by macrophages where it survives and replicates as an *amastigote* ('no tail'), settling either in the skin (cutaneous) or the spleen and liver (visceral) depending on the species (see Table 5.4). In the insect vector the flagellate *promastigote* develops in

Table 5.4 The principal species of *Leishmania* infecting humans

Species	Areas affected	Disease pattern
L. donovani	Old World (Africa, India, Middle East)	Visceral
L. infantum	Old World (Africa, India, Middle East)	Visceral
L. major	Old World (Africa, India, Middle East)	Cutaneous
L. tropica	Old World (Africa, India, Middle East)	Cutaneous
L. aethiopica	Old World (Africa, India, Middle East)	Cutaneous
L. mexicana	New World (Central and South America)	Cutaneous
L. braziliensis	New World (Central and South America)	Cutaneous
L. peruviana	New World (Central and South America)	Cutaneous
L. venezuelensis	New World (Central and South America)	Cutaneous
L. chagasi	New World (Central and South America)	Visceral

Stage		Leishmania	T. brucei	T. cruzi
Insect form (promastigote)	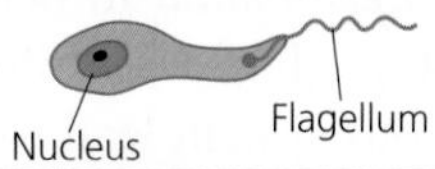 Nucleus — Flagellum	Sandfly	Tsetse fly	Reduviid bug
Blood form (trypomastigote)	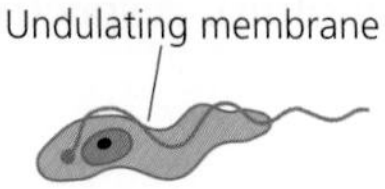 Undulating membrane	—	Free in blood	Free in blood (brief)
Intracellular/tissue form (amastigote)	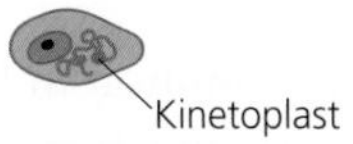 Kinetoplast	Host macrophage	Choroid plexus	Heart, CNS

Fig. 5.2 *Leishmania* and two types of *Trypanosoma* compared. CNS, central nervous system.

the gut for reinfection of the human host (Fig. 5.2). The cutaneous disease runs a chronic course with eventual healing, but visceral leishmaniasis can be fatal, with massive splenomegaly and liver failure. Dogs and rodents are the main reservoir of infection.

■ Trypanosomes

Trypanosomes belong to the same order as *Leishmania* and resemble them in appearance (Fig. 5.2). The species of *Trypanosoma* infecting humans differ in their geographical distribution, vector, and life cycle (Table 5.5).

African trypanosomes

Trypanosoma brucei is unusual in living and multiplying free in the blood of its mammalian hosts, which include humans and many species of cattle. This lifestyle necessitates sophisticated immune-evasion strategies, as described in Chapter 22. Involvement of the central nervous system (CNS) leads to the characteristic coma of *sleeping sickness* (see Chapter 34).

Table 5.5 The human trypanosomes

Trypanosoma species	Areas affected	Vector	Disease pattern
T. brucei gambiense	West Africa	Tsetse fly	Parasite free in blood: sleeping sickness
T. brucei rhodesiense	East Africa	Tsetse fly	Parasite free in blood: sleeping sickness
T. cruzi	South America	Reduviid bug	Macrophages, heart; Chagas' disease

South American trypanosome

Trypanosoma cruzi somewhat resembles *Leishmania* in being predominantly an intracellular parasite, after a brief blood stage (Fig. 5.2). Infection of cardiac muscle and the ganglia of the autonomic nervous system lead to chronic heart failure and dilated organs (megaoesophagus, megacolon), respectively.

■ Toxoplasma

Toxoplasma gondii, an intracellular parasite, common in both farm and domestic animals (particularly cats), causes symptomless infection of up to 50% of human populations, who acquire it through contaminated water, food, or faeces. The parasite can survive in the form of cysts, which can be reactivated if the host becomes immunodeficient (see Chapters 26 and 34). An active infection can be transmitted from mother to fetus via the placenta, leading to fetal damage, particularly to the brain and eye, or death. It has been claimed that toxoplasmosis can act as a trigger for schizophrenia through effects on brain neurotransmitters.

■ Amoebae

Entamoeba histolytica is the cause of the well-known amoebic dysentery and occasionally of abscesses in brain, liver, and lung. The cyst form is acquired via contaminated water and develops into trophozoites in the intestine (Fig. 5.3).

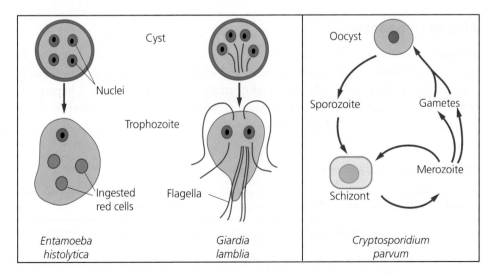

Fig. 5.3 Water-borne intestinal parasites of humans. Note the resemblance of the *Cryptosporidium* life cycle to that of malaria, except that no insect vector is involved.

■ Giardia, Cryptosporidium, Trichomonas

Giardia lamblia has a similar life cycle to that of *Entamoeba*, but its effects are normally limited to the intestine. Giardiasis is one of the commonest causes of diarrhoea in the developed world. Many farm and wild animals can act as reservoirs.

Cryptosporidium parvum has a more complex life cycle, which includes a sexual stage (Fig. 5.3). Like *Toxoplasma*, it is an important opportunist in immunodeficient patients, particularly those with AIDS (as is the rather similar *Isospora belli*), but also causes outbreaks of diarrhoea in otherwise healthy individuals following breakdown of water-purification procedures.

Trichomonas vaginalis is a sexually transmitted parasite of the vagina and urethra and a common cause of vaginitis and occasionally urethritis.

■ Control of protozoa

A variety of drugs are available to kill protozoa, many of them quite toxic to the host and prone to the development of resistance (see Table 29.6). There are no effective vaccines for human use (but see Chapter 27).

SUMMARY

- Protozoa are single-celled eucaryotes. Only a few are parasites of humans.

- Those transmitted by insects, including malaria, are major causes of disease and mortality in tropical areas. Malaria kills over a million people a year, mainly in Africa.

- Those transmitted by water or from animals can occur anywhere.

- Immunity following protozoal infection is minimal or absent, and there are no vaccines in standard use. Treatment is by drugs.

Chapter 6
Helminths (worms)

Worms represent the limit as far as parasite size is concerned, some of the largest ones being almost as long as their hosts (though fortunately not as bulky!). The vast majority are free living, and only three classes of worm include pathogens of humans; these are listed in Table 6.1.

Table 6.1 The major helminths of medical significance

Means of spread	Roundworms (nematodes)	Tapeworms (cestodes)	Flukes (trematodes)
Intermediate host	Filariae		Schistosoma (snail)
	Onchocerca (fly)		Paragonimus (crab)
	Wuchereria (mosquito)		Clonorchis (fish)
	Brugia (mosquito)		
	Loa loa (fly)		
Food, water, or other	Ascaris	Taenia	
	Hookworm	Echinococcus	
	Toxocara	('hydatid')	
	Trichinella		
	*Strongyloides		

*Mainly important as an opportunist.

■ General structure and function

Worms are unlike other parasites in several respects. To begin with, they are of course *multicellular* animals, with well-developed organs, digestive and nervous systems, and usually very tough outer coats, which makes them virtually impossible for the immune system to dislodge. However, they do induce vigorous immune responses, with an unusual emphasis on eosinophils and IgE antibody (see Chapters 17 and 35). Another difference is that with a few exceptions they do not replicate within their human host, but either free or in another host (insect, snail, etc.). From the human point of view, this means that a single worm, once acquired, remains a single worm, rather than multiplying into thousands or millions like viruses, bacteria, or protozoa. Thus the final weight of infection is directly proportional to the original number of infecting organisms (although they may increase substantially in size). This in turn has important effects on the design of preventive measures.

Although their sheer size makes worms difficult to get rid of, they also have some very sophisticated mechanisms for eluding the immune system. A striking example is the blood fluke *Schistosoma*, which manages to camouflage itself by picking up a surface coating of molecules from the blood of the host (see Chapter 22). Because they represent a huge amount of foreign material yet survive for long periods (years in some cases), parasitic worms represent some of the largest sustained challenges to the immune system. Unfortunately, a large sustained challenge frequently leads to overstimulation of the system, with harmful effects to the host. This is called *immunopathology*, and will be discussed in Chapters 23 and 35. Here, three examples of it may be quoted: the lymphoedema of the limbs caused by prolonged responses to the filarial worm *Wuchereria bancrofti*, leading to the terrible deformities of elephantiasis, the river blindness caused by another filarial worm *Onchocerca volvulus*, which unfortunately likes to visit the eye, and the potentially fatal liver cirrhosis caused by the eggs of *Schistosoma mansoni*. Not only in numbers, but also in terms of prolonged human suffering, worms must rank as the most unwelcome parasites of all (Table 6.2).

■ Schistosomes and other trematodes (flukes)

Three species of the blood fluke *Schistosoma* are important human pathogens, with a worldwide distribution (Table 6.3) and complex life cycles involving an aquatic snail as an intermediate host (Fig. 6.1).

Schistosomiasis (also known as bilharzia) probably originated in the Nile valley, and has been identified in Egyptian mummies. Other flukes causing less serious disease include the gut flukes *Metagonimus* and *Heterophyes*, and humans may be infected by the sheep liver fluke *Fasciola* and the intestinal fluke *Fasciolopsis*.

The lung fluke *Paragonimus westermanii* has a life cycle similar to that of the schistosomes but more complex, involving two aquatic vectors: snail and crustacean

Table 6.2 Approximate worldwide prevalence of the major helminth infections

Nematodes	
Filarial	150 000 000
Intestinal	4 200 000 000
Tapeworms	175 000 000
Flukes	
Blood	200 000 000
Lung	20 000 000
Intestinal	200 000
Liver	20 000 000

Table 6.3 Major characteristics of the human blood flukes

Schistosoma species	Geographical distribution	Disease features
S. mansoni	Africa, Middle East, South America	Dermatitis ('swimmer's itch')
		Abdominal pain, diarrhoea
		Eggs in liver → portal fibrosis → portal hypertension → haematemesis
		Eggs also in lung and CNS
S. japonicum	China, Japan, Philippines	Eggs also in lung and CNS
S. haematobium	Africa, Mediterranean	Eggs in bladder → haematuria, bladder cancer

(crab). The adult worms settle mainly in the lungs, forming cysts and occasionally causing bronchopneumonia.

■ Nematodes (roundworms)

Filarial nematodes

These thread-like worms have a simple life cycle, involving a sexual stage giving birth to microfilarial larvae in the mammalian host, and an insect vector in which the larval stages develop (Fig. 6.2). The four major filarial pathogens of humans differ mainly in the vector and in the sites at which larvae, adult worms, and microfilaria become deposited (Table 6.4).

Other filarial nematodes causing human infection are *Mansonella streptocerca*, *Mansonella perstans*, and *Mansonella ozzardi*, but these are of little medical importance.

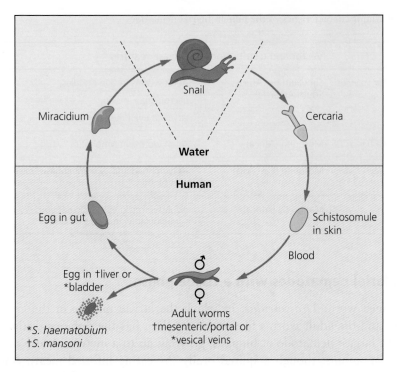

Fig. 6.1 The schistosome life cycle.

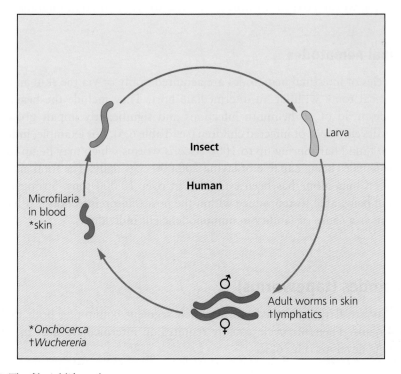

Fig. 6.2 The filarial life cycle.

Table 6.4 Major characteristics of the human filarial nematodes

Species	Vector and distribution	Disease features
Onchocerca volvulus	Simulium fly (Africa, South America)	Adult worms in skin nodules, microfilariae in skin, larvae in eye ('river blindness')
Wuchereria bancrofti	Mosquito (Africa)	Adult worms in lymphatics
Brugia malayi	Mosquito (East Asia)	→ lymphoedema → elephantiasis, microfilariae in blood
Loa loa	Mango fly (Africa)	Adult worms in eye, subcutaneous, microfilariae in blood → CNS

Non-filarial nematodes with a tissue phase

The Guinea worm *Dracunculus*, in which the larvae mature in the crustacean *Cyclops* and the adult worms live under the skin, has the dubious distinction of being the largest nematode of humans, growing up to a metre or more in length. *Trichinella spiralis*, though acquired orally (by eating infected meat), causes its main pathology when the larvae encyst in striated and (rarely) cardiac muscle. A somewhat similar process, affecting several tissues (liver, brain, eye), occurs with the dog worm *Toxocara canis*, giving rise to 'visceral larva migrans'.

Intestinal nematodes

Most species of intestinal nematodes are acquired orally or via the skin and spread by the faecal route without an intermediate host. They include the heaviest and most widespread of all helminth infections and significantly impair growth and cognitive development of infected children (see Table 6.5). For example, individuals have been found harbouring up to 1000 *Ascaris* worms which may be up to 30 cm long, the females being capable of laying 200 000 eggs daily. The total annual egg output for China alone has been estimated at over 10 000 tons. Strongyloides is unusual in being able to reproduce within the host ('autoreinfection'). It has come to the fore as a cause of fatality in immunodeficient individuals.

■ Cestodes (tapeworms)

The adults are flat, segmented worms, each segment containing both male and female organs. Their life cycle usually requires an intermediate host in which a cystic stage develops (Fig. 6.3).

Table 6.5 Major characteristics of the human intestinal nematodes

Species	Site infected	Principal pathology
Ascaris lumbricoides	Small intestine, with migration to liver, heart, lungs, and back to gut	Intestinal obstruction, allergic pneumonitis
Trichuris trichiura	Colon, caecum	Diarrhoea, rectal prolapse
Enterobius vermicularis	Caecum, rectum	Anal pruritus
Ancylostoma duodenalis (hookworm)	Small intestine, attached to mucosa	Anaemia, itch
Necator americanus	Small intestine, attached to mucosa	Anaemia, itch
Strongyloides stercoralis	Small intestine, attached to mucosa, with migration to lungs	Malabsorption, may disseminate in immunodeficient individuals

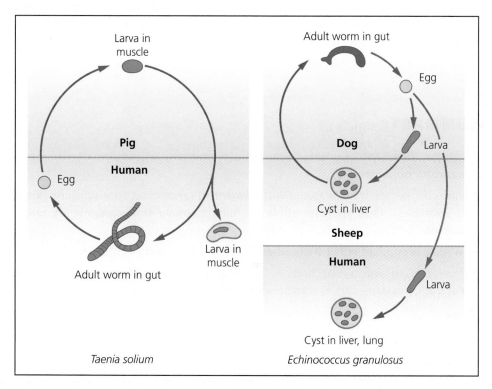

Fig. 6.3 Cestode life cycles. Left: tapeworms; right: hydatid worm.

Adult tapeworms in the gut, although they may reach up to 10 m in length, usually cause only mild digestive symptoms. However, in two cases the cystic larval stages can be pathogenic when they infect vital organs.

1. *Taenia solium* (the pork tapeworm): the adult tapeworm lives in humans and the normal intermediate host is the pig, which becomes infected by swallowing eggs from human faeces. However, humans may also act as an intermediate host. After swallowing eggs, these release larvae in the duodenum which are carried via the blood to muscle, CNS, and eye where they form cysts with pain, fever, and neurological symptoms.

2. *Echinococcus granulosus*: the adult worms are found in dogs and the larval cysts in the liver and other organs of sheep and humans. These *hydatid* cysts may contain 'daughter' cysts and several litres of fluid, and in addition to pressure effects they can induce immunopathology if they rupture (see Chapters 23 and 35). *Echinococcus multilocularis* produces rapid-growing invasive cysts; the normal animal hosts are foxes and rodents.

■ Control of helminths

As with protozoa, helminths can be to some extent controlled by drug treatment (see Table 29.7) but there are no effective human vaccines, so that public health measures are of the greatest importance.

SUMMARY

- Worms (helminths) are large multicellular animals, only a few of which are parasites of humans.
- Parasitic worms are nematodes (roundworms), tapeworms (cestodes), or flukes (trematodes). They are responsible for huge amounts of disease, mainly in the tropics.
- Worms are spread either by food and water or by insect or other vectors.
- Immunity to worm infections is minimal or absent. There are no human vaccines, but drug-cure is sometimes possible.

Chapter 7
Ectoparasites

Ecto- ('outside') parasites are arthropods that live on or in the skin, often feeding on blood. They can cause intense itching and inflammation, and can be very hard to get rid of (see Chapter 36), but medically their main importance is as vectors for many major diseases (Table 7.1).

Mites

Mites are not insects but *arachnids* (like spiders), which parasitize a wide range of animals and plants. The most important medically are *Sarcoptes scabei*, the cause of scabies, and *Dermatophagoides pteronyssinus* (the house-dust mite) a common cause of dermatitis and asthma. The scabies mite burrows into the skin, where the female lays eggs which hatch and spread locally.

Ticks

Ticks are also arachnids. They live on the skin surface and feed on blood. They have a complex life cycle, part of which occurs in animals such as deer, sheep, domestic pets, and rodents. Ticks are vectors for a number of serious diseases.

Lice

Lice are wingless insects, parasitic on a variety of animals. Three species of human lice live and feed on particular regions of the skin: *Pediculosis capitis* (head lice), *P. corporis* (body lice), and *Phthirus pubis* (pubic lice).

Table 7.1 Arthropods as disease vectors

Vector	Pathogen	Disease
Tick	*Borrelia burgdorferi*	Lyme disease
	Borrelia recurrentis	Relapsing fever
	Rickettsia typhi	Typhus
	Dermacentor (rickettsia)	Rocky Mountain spotted fever
	Flaviviruses	Encephalitis
	Various arboviruses	Haemorrhagic fevers
Flea	*Rickettsia typhi*	Typhus
	Yersinia pestis	Plague
Mosquito	Flaviviruses	Yellow fever
		Dengue fever
	Chikungunya virus	Chikungunya disease
	Plasmodium spp.	Malaria
	Wuchereria, Brugia	Elephantiasis
Sandfy	Leishmania spp.	Leishmaniasis
Tsetse fly	*Trypanosoma gambiense*	Sleeping sickness
	Trypanosoma rhodesiense	Sleeping sickness
Simulium fly	*Onchocerca volvulus*	Onchocerciasis
Reduviid bug	*Trypanosoma cruzi*	Chagas' disease

■ Fleas

Fleas are insects, wingless but notorious for their phenomenal jumping ability. They feed on blood, and their bites can cause itching and severe inflammation. *Pulex irritans* is a vector for typhus and plague in humans, and a large variety of bacterial and rickettsial diseases in animals are also flea-borne.

■ Other insect vectors

Where human populations are scattered over wide areas, flying insects are an ideal means of spread. Without mosquitoes, malaria (see Fig 5.1) would disappear, but the high hopes of mosquito eradication with insecticides following the Second World War proved to be short-lived because of (1) the development of resistance and (2) damaging effects on the environment. The enormous role of mosquitoes in tropical ill-health can be judged from Table 7.1. On a smaller scale, tsetse flies, sandflies, and blackflies (*simulium* spp) also contribute.

Chapter 8
Prions

Several separate observations during more than 70 years led to the identification of a novel form of pathogen: the prion. The name, coined by Stanley Prusiner in 1982, represents the existence of a *protein* that is *in*fectious, and the current concept is that prions are proteins of about 50 kDa in molecular mass, present in normal brain tissue and in an altered form in a variety of neurodegenerative diseases characterized by spongy vacuolation and amyloid plaques in grey matter (see Chapter 31). Since many of these diseases were hitherto attributed to 'slow viruses' and since it was extremely hard to eliminate the possibility of a minute amount of nucleic acid associated with the protein (the virion theory), a few authorities are still unconvinced, but the evidence for prions as pathogens is now fairly overwhelming. Table 8.1 shows some of the key steps in the development of the prion theory.

The really novel biological aspect of this remarkable sequence of events is the idea that protein *conformation*, for example, the proportion of α-helix to β-pleated sheet, with an excess of the latter, rather than just amino-acid sequence, can determine function, including the initiation of fatal degenerative diseases. It focuses attention on the role of *chaperones*: the molecules that regulate the folding of proteins into their secondary and tertiary structure. Perhaps this will be the clue that leads eventually to the development of drug-based therapies.

A striking feature of the pathology of prion diseases is the apparent lack of immune responses to the damaged brain tissue. This is not because prion proteins (PrPs) are not immunogenic—indeed, an antiserum to the 27–30 kDa fragment of PrP^{Sc} (the form of PrP in prion disease) was used to detect it in suspected prion diseases—but probably because, in the absence of inflammation and breaching of the blood–brain barrier, brain antigens do not make contact with lymphocytes. However, the use of a vaccine that induced immune responses in the vicinity of altered prions would clearly be a risky matter. Avoidance of the known routes of spread and vigorous sterilization of possibly contaminated equipment with strong NaOH, appear to be the best approach to reducing the numbers of cases. An interesting breakthrough may be the discovery that lichen-derived enzymes can apparently degrade prion proteins.

Table 8.1 A brief history of prion biology

1920–1	Creutzfeldt and Jakob described a form of dementia (CJD) characterized by spongiform encephalopathy
1930	CJD shown to be familial (i.e. genetic) as well as infectious
1947	Scrapie (a similar disease of sheep) transmitted by an agent resistant to heat and formalin (which inactivate viruses)
1954	Scrapie attributed to a 'slow virus'
1959	Kuru (a similar disease restricted to brain-eaters in New Guinea) attributed to a slow virus
1960	Scrapie agent shown to be resistant to ionizing radiation
1966	Kuru transmitted to primates from diseased human brain
1968	CJD transmitted to primates from diseased human brain
1970	Scrapie agent shown to be resistant to ultraviolet light (which destroys DNA)
1978	CJD agent shown to be resistant to ultraviolet light
1982	Scrapie agent shown to be susceptible to proteolytic treatments; named 'prion' or prion protein (PrP)
1984–6	Two forms of PrP described: PrP^c (in normal cell membranes) and PrP^{Sc} (in prion disease), differing in conformation. PrP^{Sc} is richer in β-pleated sheets and poorer in α-helices, is deposited as fibrils, and converts neighbouring PrP^c to PrP^{Sc}: a true infectious process; antibody raised in mice to a 30 kDa fragment of PrP
1985–6	Amyloid fibres in prion disease shown to be composed of PrP
1986	BSE described in British cattle (spread from sheep scrapie by bone/meat feeding?)
1988	UK ban on contaminated cattle feed
1989	Familial prion disease shown to be due to a mutation in the PrP gene; UK ban on 'specified offal' in beef for human consumption
1993	Deletion of PrP gene in mice prevents induction of prion disease; peak of BSE epidemic in UK
1993–7	CJD transmitted by human growth hormone, pituitary gonadotrophin, in dura mater grafts
1995	A new form, new-variant CJD (vCJD), described in young humans, spread from cattle BSE by eating beef; European Union bans British beef
1994–7	Prion-like proteins found in yeast and other fungi
1998	Last recorded death from kuru
2004	Disease induced by synthetic prion protein
2006	Cattle genetically engineered to resist BSE

Table 8.1 (*Continued*)

2009	PrP^c prions contribute to Alzheimer's disease?
2010	Detection of PrP^{sc} in blood samples
2010	Prions able to evolve and adapt?
2011	Prions transferred by aerosol
2011	Lichen enzyme degrades prions

BSE, bovine spongiform encephalopathy; CJD, Creutzfeldt-Jakob disease.

SUMMARY

- Prions have only recently become accepted as agents of disease: the transmissible spongiform encephalopathies.
- Prions are believed to consist of protein, without nucleic acid. Infectious prions 'reproduce' by inducing conformational changes in surrounding normal prion proteins.
- Spread is normally animal–animal, but animal–human spread has occurred.
- No treatment has yet been devised.

Chapter 9

Disease: virulence and susceptibility

The term 'infectious disease' implies the existence of not merely a parasite but a *pathogen* that makes people ill; that is, they develop symptoms, which may even be fatal. This is a sign that somewhere tissue has been damaged, either grossly in terms of structure or more subtly by a disturbance of function. This is the realm of *pathology*. The question why a parasite should induce pathology was discussed in Chapter 1; here we describe how it can occur.

■ Virulence factors

The answer is not as obvious as it might seem, and in Chapters 14 and 23 you will learn the surprising fact that in many infections it is actually the immune system that causes much of the pathology. However, in this chapter we will discuss those elements in the pathogen that predispose to disease, which are collectively known as *virulence factors*. Some of these have been mentioned in Chapter 3 in relation to bacteria, but as Table 9.1 shows, there are many others. Virulence factors fall into two main categories: (1) pathogen mechanisms directly or indirectly causing host damage; (2) pathogen mechanisms aimed at escaping host protective mechanisms, including immunity.

■ Genomics and virulence

Recent molecular biological advances have facilitated the precise identification of large numbers of microbial virulence factors and other important molecules,

Table 9.1 Some important virulence factors

Mechanism	Result	Example
Cytopathic organism	Destruction of host cells	Lytic viruses: polio, influenza; malaria
Release of exotoxins	Various (see Table 9.6)	Staphylococci, tetanus, cholera
Endotoxin in cell wall	Macrophage stimulation, cytokine release, shock	*Salmonella*, Meningococcus
Infect lymphocytes and dendritic cells	Inactivate immunity	HIV, measles
Capsule	Block phagocytosis	*Staphylococcus, Streptococcus, Haemophilus*, Meningococcus
Adhesion factors	Prevent removal	*E. coli, Mycoplasma, Neisseria* (pili)
Ciliary toxin	Inhibit cilia in bronchi	*Bordetella pertussis*
Antigenic variation	Escape from immunity	Influenza, HIV, *Borrelia, Trypanosoma*
Plasmid exchange	Resist chemotherapy	*Staph. aureus*
Protease	Destroys IgA	*Neisseria*
Protein A	Blocks IgG	*Staphylococcus*
Urease	Protects against acid	*Helicobacter*
Elastase	Inhibits complement	*Pseudomonas*
IL-10-like molecule	Inhibits other cytokines	EBV
Reduce MHC	Avoid cytotoxic T cells	CMV
Inhibit killing mechanisms	Intracellular survival	TB, *Listeria, Brucella*
Induce granuloma	Elude immune system	TB
Induce cyst formation	Elude immune system	*Echinococcus*

IL, interleukin; TB, tuberculosis.

predominantly those consisting of proteins (Table 9.1). Using microarrays of DNA or synthetic oligonucleotides on glass or silicone, exposed to labelled DNA probes, up to 300 000 genes can be scanned for simultaneously. Host gene expression can be studied in a similar way by measuring cDNA from a sample in question, and more recently by RNA-Seq – the process of high throughput sequencing of cDNA to define the transcriptome of an organism; see Table 9.2 for a list of some novel terminology in this area. Since 1995 over 1000 bacterial and over 3000 viral genomes have been completely sequenced, the principal aim being to identify potential candidates for vaccine or drug development, concentrating on molecules

Table 9.2 The language of molecular microbiology

Term	Meaning
Genome	The full set of genetic material (DNA) in an organism
Core genome	Genes present in all members of a species
Genomics	Analysis of the genome
Plasmid	Extrachromosomal DNA in bacteria
Bacteriophage	Bacterial virus able to transmit DNA to other bacteria
Horizontal gene transfer	Transfer of DNA to a cell other than offspring
Transposon	A cluster of genes transmissible horizontally
Pathogenicity island	A transposon carrying one or more virulence genes
Transcriptome	The set of mRNA transcripts in a particular situation
Transcriptomics	Analysis of the above
Proteome	The set of proteins expressed in a particular situation
Proteomics	Analysis of the above
Metabolome	Molecules, protein or otherwise, made in a particular situation
Immunomics	Analysis of molecules interacting with the immune system

likely to be exposed to the immune system (e.g. surface proteins) or released (e.g. toxins) while avoiding those with similarities between pathogen and host that might give rise to adverse reactions if targeted by vaccines or antibiotics. Some examples of genome sizes are shown in Table 9.4.

Importantly we now have genome sequences of many different strains or geographical isolates of each organism. In the process, much has been learned about the generation of diversity in pathogens, enabling more accurate predictions to be made about their possible future evolution (look back to Chapter 3 for some basic facts about the mechanisms of bacterial variation). Table 9.3 lists some examples of pathogens where 'genomic' concepts have been applied to infectious disease, and the case studies below illustrate three situations where this approach has proved of practical value.

Establishing the whole genome sequence for a pathogen was very expensive and time-consuming, although both aspects have been dramatically reduced by recent advances in sequencing technology. For comparing strains within a species, the technique of DNA microarray is also used. A large number of either 'reporter genes' or of synthetic oligonucleotides are tested for hybridization with the DNA under study. In this way the variability, the evolutionary history, and the source

Table 9.3 Some applications of genomics to the study of infectious diseases

Analysis	Applications	Examples
Genome (DNA)	Discovery of genes:	
'comparative genomics'	new families,	Lipid metabolism in *Mycobacterium tuberculosis*
	unknown function,	*Escherichia coli*
	'core genome'	*M. tuberculosis, Brucella, Plasmodium*
	Comparison of genes:	
	strains versus species,	*M. tuberculosis*
	pathogen versus host	*Staphylococcus, Streptococcus, M. tuberculosis*
	Evolutionary studies:	
	of pathogen,	*Neisseria, Yersinia*, MRSA
	of host range	*Yersinia, Listeria, M. tuberculosis*
	Virulence factors	Many
	Vaccination	DNA vaccines (many pathogens)
Transcriptome (mRNA)	Response to external factors:	
'expression genomics'	environmental stress,	*Salmonella, Campylobacter*
	site of infection,	*Streptococcus pneumoniae*
	oxygen,	*M. tuberculosis*
	host defences	*Helicobacter pylori*/acid, *M. tuberculosis*/macrophages, trypanosomes/antigen variation
	Drugs and drug resistance	*M. tuberculosis*, etc.
Proteome (proteins)	Protein studies:	
	identifying new drug targets,	*Plasmodium*, etc.
	mechanisms of drug resistance,	Many
	vaccine candidates,	Many
	diagnostic tools,	Many
	immune serum,	Malaria, etc.
	T cells	*Leishmania, M. tuberculosis*, etc.

of new genes (e.g. by mutation or lateral transfer) can be analysed, as has been done, for example, for MRSA, mycobacteria, and *Neisseria*.

Virulence factors that are mainly carbohydrate or lipid cannot, of course, be directly deduced from the genome, but some of their structures are well established, for example bacterial lipopolysaccharide (LPS; see Fig. 14.1), a molecule

Table 9.4 Some important species whose genomes have been sequenced

Organism	Disease	Genome size (MB)
Homo sapiens		≈2900
Mus musculus (mouse)		≈2500
Danio rerio (zebrafish)		≈1700
Schistosoma mansoni	Schistosomiasis	≈270
Caenorhabditis elegans		97
Aspergillus fumigatus	Aspergillosis	≈30–35
Plasmodium falciparum	Cerebral malaria	23
Entamoeba histolytica	Amoebic dysentery	≈20
Trypanosoma brucei	African sleeping sickness	≈35
Mycobacterium tuberculosis	Tuberculosis	4.4
Mycobacterium leprae	Leprosy	3.1
Vibrio cholerae	Cholera	4.0
Neisseria meningitidis	Meningitis	2.18
Streptococcus pyogenes	Toxic shock/rheumatic fever, necrotizing fasciitis	1.85
Helicobacter pylori	Peptic ulcer, gastric cancer	1.66
Borrelia burgdorferi	Lyme disease	1.44
Treponema pallidum	Syphilis	1.14
Mycoplasma genitalium	Urethritis	0.58
Hepadnaviridae	e.g. Hepatitis B	0.003
Poxviridae	e.g. Smallpox	≈0.2
Filoviridae	e.g. Ebola	0.012 (RNA)
Retroviridae	e.g. HIV	0.003–0.009 (RNA)

with a number of variants that has so far eluded attempts to attack it through drugs or a vaccine.

Other applications of genomics

Apart from the identification of virulence factors, genome sequencing is becoming widely used for epidemiological studies on isolates, being both more precise and more rapid than older methods. Massively high throughout DNA sequencing—so called deep sequencing'—is also being used to probe the huge complexity of the commensal organisms that live within us (particularly in the gut) defining our 'microbiome', and our 'metagenome'.

■ Genetics of host susceptibility

Genetic differences on the host side also contribute to the occurrence and severity of disease, although these are frequently multigenic and more difficult to investigate than when they can be accounted for by a single gene, as is sometimes the case. Many of these genes affect entire innate or adaptive immune mechanisms (e.g. complement, antibody) and these will be discussed in the chapters on primary immunodeficiency (Chapters 15 and 25). But some show their effects on only one or a few infections (Table 9.5). A hint of this will be given if the disease, or some element of it, segregates in a Mendelian fashion, as was observed in mice with susceptibility/resistance to a range of intracellular infections (bacille Calmette–Guérin – BCG, *Leishmania*, *Salmonella typhimurium*), which was narrowed down

---

CASE STUDY 9.1 Genomics applied to infectious disease

Clostridium difficile, an evolving pathogen

Only in the last 30 years has *C. difficile* become recognized as a major human pathogen, particularly after antibiotic therapy. Detailed genome sequencing of six virulent and less virulent strains suggested that antibiotic resistance had emerged several times rather than clonally from a single lineage, probably mainly under the selection pressure of increased antibiotic use. Horizontal gene transfer and recombination appeared to be the main mechanisms employed by the bacteria.

A tuberculosis outbreak

A large outbreak of tuberculosis in a developed country was studied by the usual methods of contact tracing and social network analysis, which suggested a clonal origin, as expected. However, genome analysis showed that it was in fact due to the simultaneous flare-up of two separate lineages of *M. tuberculosis* which had diverged five years earlier, pointing towards an additional environmental factor for this particular outbreak. An increase in addictive drug use was considered the most likely trigger.

Liver gene expression in Hepatitis C infection

About 80% of infected individuals fail to clear Hepatitis C Virus (HCV) completely (as compared to about 10% with Hepatitis B). Of these, at least 10% will develop liver cirrhosis requiring transplantation. In the absence of a vaccine, interferon (IFN) α is widely used in therapy. However, experiments in chimpanzees using RNA extracted from the liver showed that while all animals expressed IFN α or IFN α-dependent genes during the acute infection, only animals that expressed IFN γ as well completely cleared the virus, and genes responsible for T cell responses were also up-regulated. In HCV-infected humans, increased TNFβ gene expression and reduced IL-12 correlated with progressive fibrosis, while in patients with hepatocellular cancer, increased oncogene expression was detected. Studies like these should help in diagnosis, prognosis, and treatment of this virus.

Table 9.5 Some human disease susceptibility/resistance genes

Gene	Disease association
HbS (sickle cell)	*Plasmodium falciparum* malaria
Duffy blood group negativity	*Plasmodium vivax* malaria
CCR5, *CCR2* (chemokine receptors)	HIV/AIDS resistance; West Nile virus susceptibility
Interferon γ receptor; IL-12	Disseminated BCG, *Salmonella*, atypical mycobacteria
MBL-2, *FcγRII*	Acute bacterial infection
HLA class I	HIV (B27 protective, B8 rapid progress)
HLA class II	TB, leprosy, hepatitis B, malaria
CSF, IL-4, IL-5, IL-9, IL-13 region	Egg output in schistosomiasis
Vitamin D receptor, *SLc11a1*	TB
Fucosyl transferase 2	Norovirus

CSF, colony-stimulating factor; IL, interleukin; TB, tuberculosis.

to a gene now known as Slc11a1 (formerly NRAMP-1), a cation-protein transporter. In the case of humans, very large studies are often needed (at least 1000 cases) but important effects, particularly of major histocompatibility complex (MHC) alleles, have been established for several diseases (Table 9.5). This contribution by the host as well as the pathogen to disease severity reopens, to a certain extent, the old argument of 'seed' versus 'soil' (see Box 9.1). An encouraging recent discovery is the extraordinary similarity between the human and mouse genomes, which should allow the effects of human genes, alone or in combination, to be modelled in the laboratory with greater confidence. No human example has yet been discovered as dramatic as the selection of Australian rabbits resistant to myxomatosis virus, originally introduced to control their numbers. However, a reduction in virus virulence also played a part in this, and a similar process is presumably responsible for the gradual lessening in virulence of the 'childhood' viruses in human populations since the Middle Ages.

■ Disease directly due to the pathogen

As can be seen from Table 9.1, in two situations disease is caused directly by the pathogen:

1. pathogens that destroy cells (*cytopathic*), predominantly viruses;
2. pathogens that release *toxins*, predominantly bacteria.

Cytopathic infections

In Chapter 2 (see especially Fig. 2.4) we described how some viruses spread by killing the host cell. Sometimes the damage is mainly in the cytoplasm, with inhibition of essential nucleic acid or protein synthesis, sometimes mainly in the cell membrane, resulting in lysis. Sometimes the cell is merely 'rounded up', separated from its neighbours and washed away, leaving a very sore mucous membrane; this is what happens to the nose and throat with the common cold viruses. Pathologists recognize the signs of cell damage as *cloudy swelling*, the presence of *inclusion bodies*, or the formation of multicellular *giant cells* and *syncytia*. It was also mentioned in Chapter 2 that some viruses can *transform* cells into a tumour, which should clearly be included as a form of pathology, though on a much slower time scale.

Cytopathic effects are not restricted to viruses: they are also seen in infection with other intracellular organisms such as *Chlamydia*, *Rickettsia*, *Mycoplasma* and, over a longer period of time, mycobacteria, although in the last case the cell involved (the macrophage) is readily replaceable and this is not the main cause of the pathology, most of which is immunological. The malaria parasite is unusual in growing inside and at first destroying liver cells and subsequently red blood cells; the damage to the liver is insignificant but the destruction of red blood cells can lead to severe anaemia. Hookworms feeding on blood from the intestinal epithelium can also cause a remarkable degree of anaemia.

Most extracellular parasites are too small to cause trouble by their simple presence, but some of the worms are large enough to obstruct vital organs. Examples are the roundworms *Ascaris* (intestine, bile duct) and *Wuchereria* (lymphatics), while the 'hydatid' cysts formed by the tapeworm *Echinococcus* can cause mechanical problems in the liver and lung.

Toxins

Several of the most acute and dangerous bacterial diseases are caused not by the bacteria themselves but by the toxins they secrete. Secreted toxins are known as *exotoxins*, as distinct from the *endotoxins* that are an integral part of the cell wall (see LPS, Fig. 3.2); the way endotoxins cause pathology will be discussed later (see Chapter 14).

Bacterial exotoxins are interesting for a number of reasons. They include some of the most toxic molecules in existence; for example, 1 mg of botulinum toxin (beloved of detective story writers) is calculated to be enough to kill a million guinea-pigs. Vaccines against the exotoxin of tetanus and diphtheria are among the most successful vaccines available, and must have saved hundreds of millions of lives from these rapidly fatal diseases. Toxins are often coded for by extrachromosomal DNA, sometimes in the form of plasmids, sometimes of bacterial viruses (phages). Because of their well-studied mode of action, several toxins have become valuable laboratory reagents, one—botulinum (Botox)—having even found its way into the beauty industry. Finally, there is the question, why should bacteria secrete molecules, some of which are almost guaranteed to kill their host?

Box 9.1 'Seed' versus 'soil' theories; a brief historical survey

Contagion

Smallpox and syphilis were just two diseases where the close proximity required for spread to occur suggested the presence of infectious material of some kind. The Tartars understood this when in 1347 they catapulted plague corpses into the besieged town of Caffa. But in the minds of most, the infectious agent was an ill-defined 'miasma'. The clear tendency of, for example, tuberculosis to 'run in families' was considered evidence that the disease was inherited.

Microorganisms

During the seventeenth and eighteenth centuries the old theory of 'spontaneous generation' was disproved by careful experiments with meat and maggots. In the following century, mainly thanks to Louis Pasteur, it was disproved for yeasts too, using his famous swan-necked flasks open to the air. Bacteria were soon added to the list of organisms that could not arise from nowhere, but only from other similar organisms.

Bacteria cause disease

Henle in Berlin and Pasteur in Paris proposed that bacteria were a cause of disease, and further that particular bacteria caused particular diseases. This was first conclusively proved by Robert Koch, working with anthrax bacilli in a corner of his consulting room at Wollstein: a far cry from today's high-containment facilities! He went on to add cholera and tuberculosis to the list of diseases associated with identifiable bacteria, and laid down the famous 'four postulates' of the germ theory.

Seed or soil?

Not everybody was convinced, however. Rudolf Virchow, the founder of modern pathology, while accepting that bacteria were found in increased numbers in many diseases, considered them to be effect rather than cause, maintaining that the 'soil' (the body) had more influence than the 'seed' (the microbe) on the pattern of disease. Disease was a breakdown of intrinsic cellular health. Max von Petternkofer, in Munich, despised the 'germ theory' to the extent of drinking a culture of cholera and surviving. Nevertheless, as further disease-linked pathogens were discovered, germ theory as proposed by Koch came to be accepted as dogma throughout most of the twentieth century.

Susceptibility

In its original form the germ theory did not explain the obvious fact that even during epidemics, with virtually universal exposure, not everyone gets infected. Moreover if they do, not all display the same symptoms. Then it was discovered that the severity, and even the occurrence, of certain diseases was influenced by host genes, the first clear-cut example, in 1954, being the effect of the sickle-cell gene in protecting against severe *P. falciparum* malaria. Subsequently the protective effect of mutations in the CCR5 cytokine receptor in HIV infection, and the growing links between individual human leucocyte antigen (HLA) alleles and disease susceptibility/resistance, have opened up the field of host genetic studies, facilitated by rapid improvements in the analysis of human genes. It seems safe to say that in many cases, while the 'seed' is necessary, it is not always sufficient.

To take the last point first, some exotoxins undoubtedly help the bacteria to spread through the tissues or to get out of the body (Table 9.6). For bacteria that are not normally parasitic (e.g. tetanus) one could argue that death of the host is irrelevant. The impression remains that some toxin-secreting bacteria are 'overdoing it' a bit, and it will be interesting to see how those bacteria fare whose toxins

Table 9.6 Some exotoxins are of potential benefit to the organisms that secrete them

Organism	Toxin	Benefit to organism
Streptococcus	Streptokinase	Spread through tissues
	Hyaluronidase	Spread through tissues
	Streptolysin	Destroys phagocytes
Staphylococcus	Leucocidin	Destroys phagocytes
	Enterotoxin	Diarrhoea → spread
Bordetella pertussis	Toxin	Blocks bronchial cilia
Clostridium perfringens	Phospholipase (α toxin)	Spread through tissues
Shigella	Enterotoxins	Diarrhoea → spread
Cholera, *Escherichia coli*	Enterotoxins	Diarrhoea → spread
Entamoeba histolytica	Toxin	Penetrates gut wall

have been genetically engineered away, as is now being done in molecular biology laboratories; for example, with the deletion of the α toxin from *Clostridium perfringens*, which considerably reduces its virulence.

The modes of action of exotoxins are very diverse, but can be classified under five main headings. Table 9.7 illustrates these, bringing out the fact that some toxins consist of more than one subunit, usually one to bind (B) to a cell-surface receptor and one to act (A) inside the cell. Advantage has been taken of this recently, in that by replacing the binding subunit by some other molecule with very precise cell specificity (monoclonal antibodies are generally used), the toxic subunit can be directed to a particular cell such as a cancer cell: the 'magic bullet' therapy. Possibly in the future the same approach might be used to attack recalcitrant pathogens.

Another way for bacterial toxins and enzymes (e.g. from *Salmonella*, *Shigella*, and *Yersinia*) to gain entry to cells is by the formation of tubular structures in the membrane: a Type III ('syringe and needle') secretion mechanism by which as many as 20 different proteins can be injected at once into host cells. Many bacteria carry not only toxins and secretion systems but also other virulence factors together in their genome or on plasmids; these *pathogenicity islands* constitute the main difference between virulent and non-virulent strains.

A few non-bacterial organisms also produce exotoxins. In one case, the protozoan *Entamoeba histolytica*, the toxin may assist the parasite to penetrate the intestinal wall and form its characteristic 'amoebic' abscesses. In another example, the fungus *Aspergillus flavus*, the toxin (aflatoxin) may contaminate food sources such as grain and nuts, and has been incriminated in the development of liver damage and liver cancer. Note that some secreted toxins (e.g. TSST-1 from *Staphylococcus aureus*) act indirectly by over-stimulating the production of cytokines by the host; that is, behaving like endotoxins (see Chapter 14).

Table 9.7 Bacterial exotoxins produce their effects in a variety of ways

Mode of action	Example
Lysis of cell membranes	
(1) by enzyme action	*Clostridium perfringens* (phospholipase C)
(2) by pore formation	*Staph. aureus* (α toxin)
Lysis of connective tissue and fibrin	*Streptococcus pyogenes* (streptokinase, hyaluronidase)
Inhibition of protein synthesis	*Corynebacterium diphtheriae* (diphtheria toxin, B unit binds, A unit blocks ribosome function)
Raise cAMP levels leading to fluid loss	*Vibrio cholerae* (cholera toxin, B unit binds, A units raise cAMP)
	Escherichia coli, *Shigella* similar, anthrax (also kills macrophages)
Blocking of nerve–muscle transmission	
(1) by blocking acetylcholine release	*Clostridium botulinum* ($\rightarrow$ flaccid paralysis)
(2) by overstimulation	*Clostridium tetani* ($\rightarrow$ spastic paralysis)

cAMP, cyclic adenosine monophosphate.

■ Diarrhoea and vomiting

These common complications of intestinal infection with toxin-producing organisms are worth separate comment. Symptoms following within hours of a meal (food poisoning) are usually due to toxins already present in the food, whereas if the food is merely contaminated with organisms, symptoms take a few days to appear (Table 9.8). In both cases, the symptoms can be viewed as a logical attempt on the part of the host to get rid of the cause, but they can also be life-threatening, the death from dehydration that can occur within 24 h of the onset of cholera being an extreme example. From the bacterial point of view, of course, this is an

Table 9.8 Vomiting and diarrhoea can be due to a wide variety of infectious organisms. Often the time between exposure and symptoms is a guide to the likely cause

Organism	Common sources	Time of onset
Food poisoning (toxin in food)		
Staphylococcus aureus	Cream, meat	1–6 h
Bacillus cereus	Reheated food	1–20 h
Clostridium perfringens	Reheated meat	8–20 h
Clostridium botulinum	Tinned food	12–36 h

Table 9.8 (*Continued*)

Infectious gastroenteritis (organisms in food)		
Rotaviruses	Faecal–oral	2–5 days
Enteroviruses	Faecal–oral	2–5 days
Shigella	Faecal–oral	1–4 days
Vibrio cholerae	Faecal–oral	1–2 days
Escherichia coli	Faecal–oral	1–4 days
Salmonella	Eggs, meat	1–2 days
Campylobacter	Eggs, meat	1–2 days
Yersinia	Animals	Gradual
Giardia lamblia	Faecal–oral	1–2 weeks
Entamoeba	Faecal–oral	Gradual
Cryptosporidia	Animals	Gradual

excellent method of spread. Note, however, that not all diarrhoea is caused by bacteria; it may be due to viruses, protozoa, drugs, poisons, non-infectious disease of the bowel, and even nervousness.

SUMMARY

- Virulence describes the tendency of a pathogen to cause disease.
- A wide range of 'virulence factors' have been identified, ranging from the release of toxins to the evasion of host immune defences. A full analysis of both pathogen and host genome (DNA), expressed DNA (transcriptome, RNA), and expressed proteins (proteome) should ultimately enable all virulence factors to be characterized and suitable targets for vaccines and chemotherapy to be identified.
- The host genome also contributes to disease susceptibility and severity.
- Most host susceptibility differences are multigenic, affecting elements of the immune system, but some are single-gene effects. In many cases, the MHC plays a key role.

Tutorial 1

At this point you should have a sufficient understanding of the major pathogens and their direct effects on their host to attempt an essay on each of the topics below. Make a list of the headings you would base your essay on and a suitable order to present them in, and compare your version with the specimen lists given in the section at the back of the book (p. 370).

1. Comment on this (fictional) press release.

   The malaria virus threatens to make a comeback in Northern Europe, a junior Health Minister warned yesterday on his return from Nairobi, advising his audience to have their vaccine boost and avoid uncooked meat when abroad.

2. We would be better off without bacteria. Discuss.

3. Viruses are not really living organisms—or are they?

4. No parasite needs to make its host ill. Discuss.

5. The evolution of higher animals has not significantly affected the world of microorganisms. Discuss.

Further reading and information

Textbooks

Goering, R., Dockrell, H., Zuckerman, M., Roitt, I., Chiodini, P. L., Mims, C. A. *Medical Microbiology*. Saunders, 5th edn., 2012.

Madigan, M. T., Martinko, J. M., Stahl, D. A., Clark, D.P. *Brock Biology of Microorganisms*. Pearson Education, 13th edn., 2011.

Mims, C. A., Nash, A., Stephen, J. *The Pathogenesis of Infectious Disease*. Academic Press, 5th edn., 2001.

Web sites

http://www.hhmi.org/biointeractive/ (Topics in microbial pathogenesis, with video clips.)

http://www.microbeworld.org/ (general American Society for Microbiology sponsored site on current topics in microbiology. See also ASM home page at www.asm.org.)

www.sanger.ac.uk/ (The Wellcome Trust Sanger Institute. Sequencing of microbial genomes.)

www.tigr.org/ (The Institute for Genomic Research (TIGR). Sequencing of microbial genomes.)

Recent reviews and articles

Burgner, D., Jamieson, S. E., Blackwell, J. M. 'Genetic susceptibility to infectious diseases: big is beautiful, but will bigger be even better?' *Lancet Infect Dis.*, 2006, Oct 6 (10): 653–63.

Chapman, S. J., Hill, A. V. 'Human genetic susceptibility to infectious disease'. *Nat Rev Genet*. 2012, Feb 7; 13 (3): 175–88.

Cho, I., Blaser, M. J. 'The human microbiome: at the interface of health and disease'. *Nat Rev Genet*. 2012 Mar 13; 13 (4): 260–70.

Clemente, J. C., Ursell, L. K., Parfrey, L. W., Knight R. 'The impact of the gut microbiota on human health: an integrative view'. *Cell*. 2012 Mar 16; 148 (6): 1258–70.

Florens, L., Washburn, M. P., Raine, J. D., Anthony, R. M., Grainger, M., Haynes, J. D., Moch, J. K., Muster, N.,

Sacci, J. B., Tabb, D. L., Witney, A. A., Wolters, D., Wu, Y., Gardner, M. J., Holder, A. A., Sinden, R. E., Yates, J. R., Carucci, D. J. 'A proteomic view of the Plasmodium falciparum life cycle'. *Nature*, 2002, Oct. 3; 419 (6906): 520–6.

Gagneux, S. 'Host-pathogen coevolution in human tuberculosis'. *Philos Trans R Soc Lond B Biol Sci.* 2012 Mar 19; 367 (1590): 850–9.

Gardner, M. J., Hall, N., Fung, E., White, O., Berriman, M., Hyman, R. W., Carlton, J. M., Pain, A., Nelson, K. E., Bowman, S., Paulsen, I. T., James, K., Eisen, J. A., Rutherford, K., Salzberg, S. L., Craig, A., Kyes, S., Chan, M. S., Nene, V., Shallom, S. J., Suh, B., Peterson, J., Angiuoli, S., Pertea, M., Allen, J., Selengut, J., Haft, D., Mather, M. W., Vaidya, A. B., Martin, D. M., Fairlamb, A. H., Fraunholz, M. J., Roos, D. S., Ralph, S. A., McFadden, G. I., Cummings, L. M., Subramanian, G. M., Mungall, C., Venter, J. C., Carucci, D. J., Hoffman, S. L., Newbold, C., Davis, R. W., Fraser, C. M., Barrell, B. 'Genome sequence of the human malaria parasite Plasmodium falciparum'. *Nature*, 2002, Oct. 3; 419 (6906): 498–511.

He, M., Sebaihia, M., Lawley, T. D., Stabler, R. A., Dawson, L. F., Martin, M. J., Holt, K. E., Seth-Smith, H. M., Quail, M. A., Rance, R., Brook, K., Churcher, C., Harris, D., Bentley, S. D., Burrows, C., Clark, L., Corton, C., Murray, V., Rose, G., Thurston, S., van Tonder, A., Walker, D., Wren, B. W., Dougan, G., Parkhill, J. 'Evolutionary dynamics of Clostridium difficile over short and long time scales'. *Proceedings of the National Academy of Sciences USA*. 2010 Apr 20; 107 (16): 7527–32.

Mueller, K., Ash, C., Pennis, E., Smith, O. 'The gut microbiota'. *Science*, 2012, 336:1245.

Mutreja, A., Kim, D. W., Thomson, N. R., Connor, T. R., Lee, J. H., Kariuki, S., Croucher, N. J., Choi, S. Y., Harris, S. R., Lebens, M., Niyogi, S. K., Kim, E. J., Ramamurthy, T., Chun, J., Wood, J. L., Clemens, J. D., Czerkinsky, C., Nair, G. B., Holmgren, J., Parkhill, J., Dougan, G. 'Evidence for several waves of global transmission in the seventh cholera pandemic'. *Nature*. 2011 Aug 24; 477 (7365): 462–5.

Pannifer, A. D., Wong, T. Y., Schwarzenbacher, R., Renatus, M., Petosa, C., Bienkowska, J., Lacy, D. B., Collier, R. J., Park, S., Leppla, S. H., Hanna, P., Liddington, R. C. 'Crystal structure of the anthrax lethal factor'. *Nature*, 2001, Nov. 8; 414 (6860): 229–33.

Parkhill, J., Wren, B. W. 'Bacterial epidemiology and biology – lessons from genome sequencing'. *Genome Biology*, 2011, Oct 24; 12 (10): 230.

Rowell, J. L., Dowling, N. F., Yu, W., Yesupriya, A., Zhang, L., Gwinn, M. 'Trends in population-based studies of human genetics in infectious diseases'. *PLoS One*. 2012;7 (2): e25431.

Sebaihia, M., Wren, B. W., Mullany, P., Fairweather, N. F., Minton, N., Stabler, R., Thomson, N. R., Roberts, A. P., Cerdeno-Tarraga, A. M., Wang, H., Holden, M. T., Wright, A., Churcher, C., Quail, M. A., Baker, S., Bason, N., Brooks, K., Chillingworth, T., Cronin, A., Davis, P., Dowd, L., Fraser, A., Feltwell, T., Hance, Z., Holroyd, S., Jagels, K., Moule, S., Mungall, K., Price, C., Rabbinowitsch, E., Sharp, S., Simmonds, M., Stevens, K., Unwin, L., Whitehead, S., Dupuy, B., Dougan, G., Barrell, B., Parkhill, J. The multidrug-resistant human pathogen Clostridium difficile has a highly mobile, mosaic genome. *Nat Genet.*, 2006, Jul.; 38 (7): 779–86.

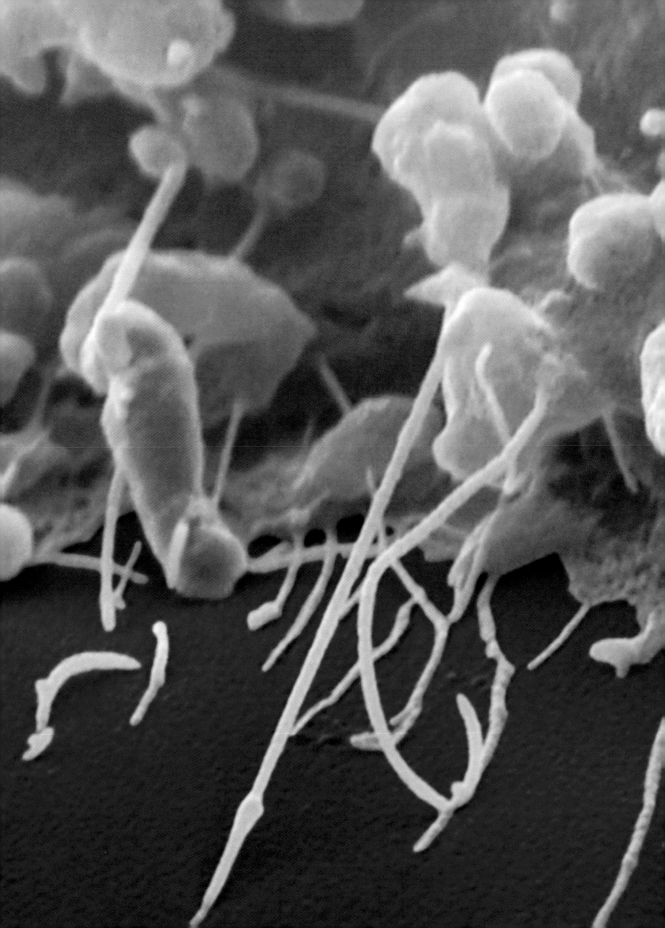

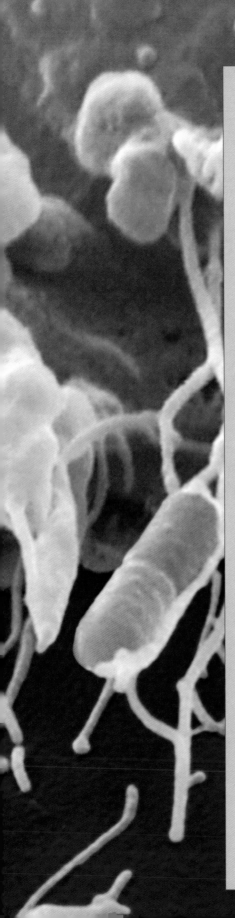

Part 2

The immune system

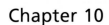

Chapter 10

Defence, immunity, the immune system

That the body has the resources to heal itself from injury must have been obvious to our earliest ancestors, but the concept of built-in defences against infection is a relatively modern one. As recently as 1755, in Samuel Johnson's *Dictionary*, immunity was defined simply as 'discharge from any obligation'. Today, two and a half centuries later, its successor the *Oxford English Dictionary* relegates this definition to second place, the principal meaning now being 'the ability . . . to resist a specific infection, toxin, etc.' Between these two dates lies the development of a whole new understanding of the causes and effects of infectious disease and how to treat it, and of two new disciplines—microbiology and immunology—together with the gradual identification of a body-wide repertoire of organs, cells, and molecules devoted to controlling infection: the immune system. Table 10.1 lists some landmarks along the way and further details can be found in Box 10.1.

■ Three levels of defence

You will see from Table 10.1 that the understanding of infection and how the body deals with it did not proceed in a smooth logical fashion. Discoveries in microbiology, immunology, chemotherapy, and public health, and theories to explain them, emerged only gradually, from different quarters and accompanied

Table 10.1 Key events in the development of modern ideas about infectious disease and immunity

Date	Event
1796	Edward Jenner: the first scientific vaccine (against smallpox)
1847–1869	Ignaz Semmelweiss, Joseph Lister: antisepsis
1855	John Snow: cholera spread by water
1860	Louis Pasteur: fermentation caused by microorganisms (yeast)
1876	Robert Koch: anthrax caused by a bacillus
1881	Louis Pasteur: anthrax vaccine (sheep)
1882	Elie Metchnikoff: phagocytosis
1888	Pierre Roux, Alexandre Yersin: diphtheria caused by toxin
1890	Emil Von Behring, Shibasaburo Kitasato: antitoxin (antibody)
1890	Paul Ehrlich: receptor ('side chain') theory
1910	Paul Ehrlich: chemotherapy (salvarsan for syphilis)
1929–1940	Alexander Fleming, Howard Florey, Ernst Chain: penicillin
1935	Gerhard Domagk: sulfanilamide
1952	Ogden Bruton: immunodeficiency (antibody)
1957	Alick Isaacs, Jean Lindenman: interferon
1959	James Gowans: lymphocytes
1959	Macfarlane Burnet: clonal selection theory of adaptive immunity
1960	Peter Medawar: tolerance
1961	Jacques Miller: thymus and immunity
1965	Angelo Di George: immunodeficiency (lymphocytes)
1972	Jean Borel: cyclosporin (immunosuppressive drug)
1980	World Health Organization: smallpox eradicated
1981	AIDS recognized

by frequent and sometimes violent disputes (Box 10.1). However, we can now agree on a generally accepted description of how infectious organisms cause disease and how the host defends itself. The causes of disease (*pathogenesis*) will be discussed in Chapters 14, 23, and 24; here we are concerned with the host's defence mechanisms.

The problem of defence against a pathogen is fairly analogous to that faced by a country at war or fighting its own internal criminals—namely, how to avoid damage by hostile agents—and in fact the solutions arrived at by nature and by

Box 10.1 Discoveries and controversies in many disciplines have contributed to the understanding of infectious disease

See also Table 10.1 and Box 9.1.

The role of microorganisms

Bacteria had been seen in the seventeenth-century microscopes of Hooke and Leeuwenhoek, but were not convincingly linked to disease until the work of Koch and Pasteur two centuries later, and even then the idea of 'one bacterium one disease' was not at first universally accepted; the great pathologist Rudolf Virchow maintained until his death (1902) that the 'soil' was more important than the 'seed': that is, the body itself rather than the microbe determined the pattern of disease. The identification of the malaria parasite as a *protozoan* (Laveran, 1880), and its transmission by mosquitoes (Ross, 1897), and of the first human *virus* (yellow fever by Reed and Carroll in 1900), unveiled a wider range of pathogens, the latest of which is the still mysterious *prion* (Prusiner, 1982).

The immune system

Another long-running dispute, over the relative importance of *phagocytes* and *antibody* in immunity, was ultimately resolved by the discovery of opsonization (Wright, 1900), in which both collaborated. Further understanding had to wait until the 1950s and 1960s with the structural analysis of antibody by Porter and Edelman, the identification of the *lymphocyte* as the key cell of adaptive immunity by Gowans, and the key role of the thymus, leading to the classification of lymphocytes into two types, T and B. The discovery of *interferon* (1957) revealed the importance of small chemical messenger molecules, the *cytokines*.

The idea that immunity can be enhanced goes back to the pioneer *vaccine* of Jenner, which had to wait a hundred years for a sequel (Pasteur: anthrax, rabies). New vaccines, mostly viral, were added during the twentieth century. However, already it had been shown (Porter, Richet 1902) that too much immunity (*hypersensitivity*) could be a bad thing, especially if it was directed against 'self' (*autoimmunity*: Coombs, 1945).

At the other end of the scale, insufficient immunity (*immunodeficiency*) was identified as the cause of unexplained susceptibility to infection, whether endogenous (Bruton, 1952; DiGeorge, 1965) or due to infection itself (AIDS, 1981). Meanwhile, the need to inhibit immunity in cases such as organ transplantation, for example, led to the discovery of *immunosuppressive drugs*, notably corticosteroids and cyclosporin.

Chemotherapy and antibiotics

Paul Ehrlich's imaginative extrapolation from his early work with dyes to the synthesis of 'pathogen-specific' compounds led the way to the *chemotherapy* industry. Meanwhile, Fleming's chance observation and the work of Florey and Chain on penicillin revealed the power of naturally occurring *antibiotics*. Drugs against other classes of pathogen (viruses, fungi, protozoa, worms) followed, although without such a dramatic success rate as the antibacterials. Unfortunately the evolution of *drug resistance* by pathogens is proving a severe limitation to this form of disease control.

Epidemiology and public health

Well before the role of microorganisms was understood, it was known that many diseases were infectious. Washing a surgeon's hands reduced post-operative mortality. Cholera was spread by water. Improved housing and nutrition led to a drop in tuberculosis before streptomycin or the

> **Box 10.1 (*Continued*)**
>
> BCG vaccine. Even today it is estimated that clean water supplies would save more lives worldwide than vaccines and chemotherapy.
>
> **Theories of immunity**
>
> Among many extraordinary ideas to explain the phenomena of immunity (specificity, memory, the rarity of autoimmunity), two great mental leaps stand out. Ehrlich—again drawing on his chemical background—proposed that cells carried *receptors* (side chains) that enabled them to recognize foreign material; when released, these constituted the antibody response. Seventy years later Macfarlane Burnet, reflecting on the genetic basis of antibiotic resistance in bacteria, proposed that individual lymphocytes are pre-programmed to carry different receptors, being selected by foreign material to expand into clones: the *clonal selection theory*. The rival *instructive theory*, despite the championship of double-Nobel laureate Linus Pauling, never succeeded in explaining the facts.

governments are remarkably similar, so the often-used 'war/police' analogies, though they *are* only analogies, will be called upon quite often in our discussions. Nature's method operates at three levels:

1. to keep pathogens out by setting up effective *external defences*;

2. if they get in, catch and dispose of them rapidly, using an always ready and available army of cells and molecules: the *innate immune system*;

3. if this fails, devote a specialized set of cells to each pathogen, able to identify it, mark it for disposal, and retain memory of its details for the future: the *adaptive immune system*.

■ External defences

These are the easiest defence mechanisms to understand, corresponding roughly to the various strategies by which a medieval city might be defended: thick walls, arrow slits, vats of boiling oil, etc. Nature's rather more subtle equivalents will be described in the next chapter.

■ The immune system

This term covers the complex network of organs, cells, and molecules scattered throughout the body, whose function is to deal with infectious organisms that penetrate the external defences. They fall into two broad categories: *innate* and *adaptive*. To work properly, an immune system requires three sets of components:

1. a *recognition* system to identify the presence of the invader: this is carried out at the molecular level by various recognition molecules;

2. a *disposal* system to kill or otherwise eliminate the threat from the invader: disposal is carried out at both molecular and cellular levels;

3. a *communication* system to coordinate the activities of the various recognition and disposal elements, and to limit damage to the host and return the system to its previous condition (homeostasis).

As already hinted, this is very much the way a country defends itself against enemy agents: (1) trained observers identify them, (2) weapons knock them out, and (3) radio keeps everyone in touch. And in a very similar way to an army, all these immune components are characterized by a high degree of *mobility*, a feature unique to the immune system. This makes sense, considering that it is impossible to know in advance where the invader will choose to attack.

Recognition molecules

Pursuing the analogy with the armed forces, one can imagine that an invader could be recognized simply because it 'looks unusual', or because it is clearly 'foreign', or because it corresponds to a precise 'known face' in some central filing system. At the same time, care must be taken not to mis-recognize and dispose of members of our own side. In immunological jargon, 'our own side' is referred to as *self* (e.g. self molecules, self cells, etc.), and everything else as *non-self*. Recognition is thus essentially a problem of distinguishing self from non-self. Unfortunately no single recognition unit can achieve this, nor is there any infallible way of distinguishing harmful from harmless microorganisms. Recognition molecules that recognize a variety of foreign invaders are sometimes referred to as *non-specific* (although *less*-specific would be a more accurate term), whereas those that can unerringly pick out one individual from thousands of others are called *specific*: both these terms are relative.

In later chapters you will see that the 'less-specific' recognition is characteristic of the *innate* immune system, exemplified by the phagocytic cells, while highly specific recognition is typical of the *adaptive* immune system, based on the lymphocyte. Thus the recognition receptors of the innate system are quite efficient in identifying a pathogen as a virus, bacterium, or fungus, etc., and guiding the appropriate response, while it usually requires the lymphocytes to make the fine distinction between, for example, one virus and another. You will also see that the distinction of self from non-self is a more serious problem for the adaptive system, because of its millions of different recognition molecules, which are individually able to recognize virtually any type or shape of molecule, harmless or otherwise, whereas those of the phagocytes seem to be particularly responsive to microbial molecules that spell danger (see Chapters 12 and 13 for more on this).

Not all the recognition molecules are equally well understood. Those of the adaptive immune system have been studied very thoroughly; they are proteins and a great deal is known about their genes, amino acid sequences, three-dimensional shapes, etc. The recognition molecules of the innate immune system have only been identified recently and the list is probably still incomplete. Much more will

Table 10.2 The principal recognition molecules of the immune system

Molecule and location	Nature	Structures recognized
Receptors on phagocytic cells	Mostly protein	General microbial features, e.g. bacterial sugars; most foreign or denatured molecules, e.g. carbon, effete red cells; microbial DNA, RNA
Receptors on natural killer cells	Protein	Virus-infected cells and some tumour cells
Complement	Numerous proteins	(1) Some bacterial cell walls; (2) antibody bound to antigen
MHC molecules	Protein	Short intracellular peptides (transported to cell surface and presented to T cell)
T-cell receptor (on T cells)	Protein	Short peptides bound to MHC; glycolipids bound to CD1
Antibody (on B cells)	Protein (immunoglobulin)	Three-dimensional shape of proteins, carbohydrates, etc.

Note that some of these molecules act together; for example, antibody and complement, the T-cell receptor and MHC molecules.

be said about these molecules in later chapters. Meanwhile Table 10.2 summarizes their main features. You will see that between them they are able to recognize virtually every component of any conceivable pathogen.

Disposal mechanisms

The need to dispose of foreign material goes back to the earliest forms of cellular life. For example, an amoeba swimming in the sea needs to eat, and eating involves (1) recognition of what is food, and (2) some process for getting it inside the amoeba (endocytosis). As animals increased in complexity, developing internal cavities and a blood circulation, not every cell needed to take in food particles in this way; instead a population of specialized cells has been retained, with properties remarkably like the primitive amoeba. In vertebrates these are the *phagocytes* (or 'eating cells'), perhaps the single most important component of our defence system. As Table 10.2 indicates, phagocytic cells have their own recognition molecules built into their surface, but also take advantage of more recently evolved recognition molecules that circulate in the blood, such as complement and antibody (see Chapters 12 and 17).

Phagocytic cells are particularly effective in disposing of bacterial and fungal infection, less so with protozoa, and of course are far too small to take in worms. They are also relatively ineffective against viruses, which spend so much of their time inside the cells of the host. Two further developments go some way to filling this gap. Some phagocytes, and also some non-phagocytic cells, are able to attach to their target and kill it from the outside; this is often referred to as *extracellular killing*, and, when the attachment is mediated by antibody, as *antibody-dependent cellular cytotoxicity* (ADCC). The latter may operate against worms, but this is still controversial. In the case of virus-infected cells, extracellular killing is carried out by two specialized types of cell: the natural killer (NK) cell and the cytotoxic T lymphocyte, often known as the CTL. How these cells detect the presence of viruses inside a host cell and how they then kill both cell and virus is described in Chapters 18 and 20.

When the object to be disposed of is a molecule rather than a whole microbe, for example a bacterial toxin, it is often sufficient merely to *neutralize* it. This task falls to the adaptive system, since *antibody* is the best-studied neutralizing molecule, although there are others (Table 10.3).

Communication: cell contact and cytokines

Few cells in the immune system act entirely on their own; much of what they do is under the influence of signals from other cells: to divide, to stop dividing, to migrate, to differentiate into effector cells, to secrete antibody, etc. These signals are delivered in two distinct ways: (1) by the interaction of cell-surface molecules brought together by cell–cell contact, and (2) by soluble molecules that can act at a distance, in which case the immune system functions rather like the endocrine system, with its set of hormones to regulate the activities of other cells. In the case of the immune system, these hormone-like molecules are called *cytokines* (Fig. 10.1), a term that covers a growing list of molecules with a bewildering array of overlapping functions.

Table 10.3 The principal disposal mechanisms

Disposal mechanism	Effective against
Phagocytosis, intracellular killing	Bacteria, fungi, some protozoa
Extracellular killing	
(1) NK cells	Intracellular viruses
(2) CTLs	Intracellular viruses and bacteria
(3) Antibody-dependent	
by granulocytes	Worms
by natural killer cells	Intracellular viruses (?); other infections (?)
Neutralization by antibody	Exotoxins, viruses, bacteria
Lysis	
by complement	Some bacteria, viruses, protozoa
by high-density lipoprotein	Some trypanosomes

Note that phagocytosis is not always followed by killing, since some bacteria, fungi, and protozoa have specialized mechanisms for avoiding this (see Chapter 13).

Table 10.4 summarizes what they have in common, and a list of the main cytokines of relevance to infectious disease can be found in Tables 12.4, 19.1, 20.1.

For historical reasons, cytokine nomenclature is not very logical; thus the *interferons* were named because they interfere with virus replication, *tumour necrosis factor* because it causes (some) tumours in mice to shrivel up, the *colony-stimulating factors* because they affect the growth of bone-marrow cells in culture, and *chemokines* because they induce cell movement (chemotaxis) towards them; however, all these molecules have several other important activities as well. Most new cytokines added to the list are nowadays called by the more non-committal name *interleukin* (meaning between white cells) plus a number, and if they were to be discovered now, probably they would all be called interleukins. An up-to-date list of cytokines is given in Appendix 2.

Their effects are so widespread that cytokines will be mentioned in practically every chapter from now on. However, one rather unexpected finding is worth

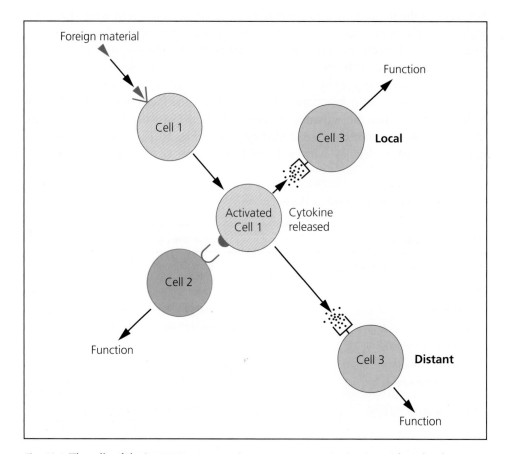

Fig. 10.1 The cells of the immune system are in permanent communication with each other, either by contact or through a network of small molecules called cytokines. In the example shown here, cell 1 has recognized foreign material and become activated, and is sending cytokine signals to cell 3 to dispose of it. This can occur locally (top) or at a distance via the bloodstream (bottom). Meanwhile cells 1 and 2 are communicating via surface-bound molecules.

Table 10.4 Cytokines, the communication molecules of the immune system, have several properties in common

1.	They are proteins or glycoproteins, with molecular weights generally in the 10–30 kDa range.
2.	Each of them can be produced by more than one type of cell, but usually in response to a stimulus.
3.	They do not specifically recognize particular microbial molecules, thus their effects are non-specific with respect to the pathogen.
4.	They bind to cell-surface receptors on the 'target' cell, which send signals to the nucleus and induce various functions.
5.	Each cytokine has effects, often different, on several target cell types; however, two cytokines can sometimes have identical effects.
6.	They often enhance each other's effects (synergy) or oppose each other.
7.	There are soluble inhibitors (often free receptors) to restrict their effects to the immediate microenvironment of the producing cell.

Note that cytokines somewhat resemble hormones, but not in all respects (see points 2, 5, and 7).

mentioning here, which is that there seems to be a link between these molecules and certain parasites. For example, some bacteria, protozoa, and worms appear to respond to cytokines, generally by increased growth. Even stranger is the fact that some viruses contain genes for cytokines or cytokine receptors, which they use to send confusing signals to the immune system. Immunologists are only half-joking when they complain that parasites know more about immunology than they do!

Communication by cell–cell contact is of course something the endocrine system *cannot* carry out, since its cells are fixed in the endocrine organs. Indeed the immune system is the only one whose cells are constantly on the move. You will read much more about cell interactions and mobility when we consider the T and B lymphocytes in Chapters 17–20.

■ Innate and adaptive immunity

As already mentioned the immune system divides conveniently into two parts—the *innate* and the *adaptive* immune systems—which differ in a number of important ways. A comparison (Table 10.5) shows that with innate immunity the emphasis is on disposal, while recognition is comparatively broad in its specificity. On the other hand adaptive immunity, which evolved much more recently, features an extremely high degree of specificity of recognition, different for individual cells, while adding relatively less in the way of new disposal mechanisms, often leaving this task to the innate system. In the following chapters, these two types of immunity will be described in considerable detail, but it should be borne in mind that in vertebrates, which possess both, the two systems are integrated, interacting with

Table 10.5 The division of the immune system into innate and adaptive components is based on several important differences

	Innate immunity	Adaptive immunity
Evolutionary origin	Earliest animals, all invertebrates and vertebrates	Vertebrates only
Principal cells	Phagocytes	Lymphocytes
Principal molecules	Complement, cytokines	Antibody, cytokines
Specificity of recognition	Broad	Very high*
Speed of action	Rapid (minutes, hours)	Slow (days)
Development of memory	No	Yes*

*High specificity and memory are the hallmarks of adaptive immunity.

each other at many levels and employing both cell–cell contact and cytokines to do so. A further complication is that between the two extremes of the innate–adaptive spectrum (e.g. macrophages–T cells) are a number of cells with intermediate properties, inhabiting a sort of grey area in terminology. The best example of this is the natural killer (NK) cell, to be described in Chapter 12, but there are others, including some sub-populations of T lymphocytes that do not carry the 'normal' T-cell receptor molecules as well as some 'innate' B cells.

Evolution and the time element

Two other important differences between innate and adaptive immune processes have to do with the *time* factor. The innate system has evolved extremely slowly, from species to species over hundreds of millions of years (see Box 10.2), but when it goes into action it does so very rapidly. In contrast the adaptive immune system is evolutionarily recent (dating from the earliest vertebrates) while its recognition molecules complete their evolution in a matter of days, within the lifetimes of each individual animal; however its responses, because they involve an element of cell proliferation, tend to be slower off the mark. To take two examples, the activation of complement, and of phagocytosis by macrophages (innate), occur within minutes, while the production of antibody (adaptive), which requires two different kinds of lymphocyte and several cycles of cell division, can take a week or more. Fortunately lymphocyte responses display *memory*, ensuring that a subsequent response to the same pathogen occurs much faster. Thus the adaptive immune response is more flexible and vigorous, so much so that it requires quite sophisticated *regulatory* mechanisms to stop it going on too long or causing damage to its possessor, also a possibility with some innate mechanisms (see Chapters 14 and 21). We shall discuss the workings of adaptive immunity in detail in Chapters 16–20.

Box 10.2 The evolution of immunity can be traced back to the earliest living forms

Microorganisms

Bacteria can be infected by viruses (bacteriophages) and bacterial endonucleases probably evolved to destroy these. The uptake of nutrients by single-celled organisms is mediated by receptors analogous to those used by the phagocytes of higher animals.

Sponges and corals

Multicellular life involves recognition systems to prevent inappropriate colony formation: the distant forerunner of adaptive cellular immunity. Quite sophisticated antibacterial and antiviral mechanisms are also seen in plants.

Later invertebrates

Soluble antimicrobial molecules in the body cavities of arthropods and molluscs play the part of humoral immunity in later animals. Phagocytosis by specialized cells, first observed in the starfish by Metchnikoff, has remained essentially similar ever since. Other advanced invertebrates show graft rejection and precursors of some cytokines.

Early vertebrates

Lymphocytes first appear in the jawless fishes (hagfish, lamprey), together with the first immuno-globulin (antibody) molecule; the real beginning of adaptive immunity.

Sharks and fishes

The appearance of the thymus and of a multi-allelic histocompatibility gene system (the MHC), and further elaboration of the antibody molecule, bring adaptive immunity closer to its most developed mammalian form.

Birds

A specialized organ for maturing B lymphocytes, the Bursa, appears to be unique to birds. In mam-mals this function remains located to the fetal liver and the bone marrow.

Mammals

The main immunological differences between and within modern-day mammalian species lie in the huge diversity of their MHC, immunoglobulin, and T-cell receptor genes. One must bear in mind, however, that any surviving species, however primitive its defence mechanisms may seem, is by defi-nition adequately protected against the pathogens it is likely to encounter.

Since higher animals possess both innate and adaptive immune systems, it was always assumed, very reasonably, that both systems are important for optimal resistance to infection. But the degree to which they are interactive and interde-pendent has only been appreciated recently. Nowadays the relationship can be studied directly by using animals (usually mice) deficient in one or other system, or both. This can be engineered by the technique of *gene knock-out*. Observations can also be made on humans lacking various immune components (immunodeficient).

The effect of such deficiencies varies considerably from infection to infection, but a generalized picture might look something like Fig. 10.2, which shows the growth of an imaginary pathogen in three kinds of host: (a) deficient in most

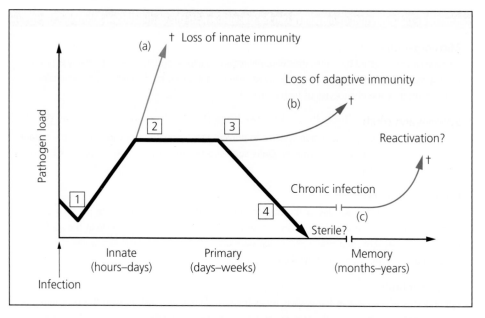

Fig. 10.2 Time course of typical infections in (a) mice lacking phagocytic cells or innate cytokines, (b) mice lacking T and B lymphocytes, (c) normal mice, illustrating that innate immunity is required for early control and adaptive immunity for eventual recovery. † denotes death of host. Note that if sterile immunity is not achieved, residual organisms may persist for years and re-emerge to cause disease.

phagocytic cells, (b) deficient in lymphocytes, and (c) normal. Looking along the time axis, you can see four distinct stages: (1) the first few hours, in which pathogen numbers fall because some are removed by macrophages resident in the tissues while others simply fail to survive the change to a new environment; (2) a period of growth which is checked, though not completely stopped, by mobile phagocytes together with complement, cytokines, and inflammatory responses, in the absence of which it may progress to death; (3) a period of a week or more in which pathogen numbers are brought down by adaptive responses which may in the long term result in (4) complete cure or, in the absence of this, (5) persistence of some pathogens with the possibility of reactivation and relapse. We shall consider human immune deficiencies in more detail in Chapters 15 and 25; these unfortunate individuals have been most useful in defining exactly which parts of which immune system are responsible for controlling which infection.

Complexity: a warning and a reassurance

Having read this chapter, you might come away with the feeling that immunology is not as complicated as you might have been led to believe. On the other hand, pick up a modern immunology textbook (they are usually very heavy!) and you might easily conclude that the subject is impossibly complex: dozens of cell types, subtypes, and sub-subtypes, hundreds of molecules with mysterious names and numbers, whose functions overlap, everything apparently interacting with everything else and every theory controversial.

Please don't despair. In this book we have concentrated on the essentials of immunology as it relates to infectious disease, theories and controversies being kept to a minimum, except where they seem to us sufficiently lively to interest the average student at undergraduate or diploma level. Almost every statement in the book could probably be followed by 'at least this is what most people in the field believe', or 'actually there are a few exceptions to this rule'. If you feel at some point lost or confused, re-read the troublesome chapter(s) and particularly the Summaries. If you are still stuck, you are most welcome to write to the authors.

SUMMARY

- Immunity is defined as resistance to infectious disease.
- It operates at three levels: external defences, innate immunity, and adaptive immunity. The latter two are the responsibility of the immune system.
- Innate and adaptive immunity use different cells and molecules, but interact extensively. They differ mainly in speed of action (innate is fastest), specificity of recognition, and the development of memory (adaptive only).
- Both require mechanisms for recognition, disposal, and communication.
- Recognition operates through molecules free in body fluids or bound to cells.
- Disposal operates mainly through phagocytic and cytotoxic cells, although small molecules such as toxins can be disposed of by molecules such as antibody.
- Communication operates through cell contact and soluble signalling molecules known as cytokines.

Chapter 11

External defences: entry and exit

■ External defences can be physical or chemical

The healthy body is surrounded by an intact layer of skin (outside) and mucous membranes (lining the hollow viscera). These are a very effective barrier against invasion by most pathogens, although some are able to get through. Those which do are referred to as *invasive*; those which remain on body surfaces are *noninvasive* and usually cause no trouble. However, if the continuity of the surface barrier is lost, entry into the tissues of organisms normally resident on the surface can occur; painful examples are the development of staphylococcal skin infections following a wound or burn, and the frequent occurrence of post-operative infections. Alternatively, if the pathogen manages to infect a biting animal, insect etc., entry is obviously facilitated, sometimes (e.g. a mosquito bite) directly into the bloodstream (see Table 11.1).

■ The skin

The skin is more than just a barrier. The secretions of its various glands contain powerful antimicrobial proteins, such as lysozyme, lactoferrin, defensins, and peroxidases. These may be produced by epithelial cells themselves, by specialized

Table 11.1 The skin is generally an efficient barrier to pathogens, but several pathogens do enter by this route, some of which (*) can also enter via the respiratory tract

Intact skin	
Direct attachment	Pox viruses
	Papova (wart) virus
	Dermatophytes (fungi)
From water	*Leptospira*
	Schistosoma
	Hookworm (via faeces)
Insect bite	Yellow fever
	Typhus
	Borrelia (Lyme disease)
	Plague*
	Malaria
	Trypanosomes (African, South American)
	Leishmania
	Roundworms (e.g. *Onchocerca*)
Animal bite	Rabies
Abrasions, wounds, burns	Staphylococci
	Streptococci
	Clostridium tetani (tetanus)
	Clostridium perfringens (gas gangrene)
	Anthrax*

glands, or by phagocytic cells such as neutrophils and macrophages that have migrated to the site. Their action may be directly antimicrobial by enzymatic digestion of the pathogen (e.g. phospholipases) or by forming pores in the membrane (e.g. antibiotic peptides). Many of these substances are present constitutively in normal tissues, but their concentration can be increased greatly following challenge with a pathogen. Each has a broad but not unlimited antimicrobial spectrum, with activity mainly focused on bacteria, fungi, or some viruses. Simultaneous production of several different substances therefore provides coverage against a wide range of pathogens. These components of the defence system are particularly suited for dealing with the small numbers of invading organisms encountered during everyday life. Larger numbers of pathogens that overwhelm this local killing capacity have to be dealt with by other elements of the innate and adaptive immune systems and the skin contains specialized cells that recognize foreign material such as microbes and initiate immune responses against them, as described in later chapters.

Even in health, large numbers of harmless microorganisms inhabit the skin—up to an estimated 200 bacterial species and some fungi. These are referred to as the *normal flora* and owe their survival to the normally low pH (3–5) of the skin surface and their own antimicrobial secretions which they are adapted to resist, and their presence helps to inhibit the growth of more pathogenic organisms.

Unlike the skin, the linings of the respiratory, intestinal, and urogenital tracts are delicate membranes, designed to allow the exchange of substances across them. They are therefore rather more vulnerable to penetration by parasites, and require special mechanisms to prevent this, which have to be considered separately.

■ The respiratory tract

The inhalation of viruses, bacteria, and fungi is unavoidable. It is estimated that a normal person inhales at least 10 000 microbes daily, and a wide range of infections are acquired by this route (Table 11.2). However, it is a remarkable fact that in healthy life the terminal parts of the respiratory tract—the alveoli, where gases are exchanged—are sterile. This is achieved by a combination of mucus secretion in the lower bronchial tree and the upwardly beating action of cilia, which constantly waft this mucus up towards the pharynx, to be coughed out or swallowed; this has been vividly termed the *muco-ciliary escalator*. Its importance is illustrated by the serious lung infections suffered by patients with *cystic fibrosis*, a genetic disorder in which the mucus is too viscid to be cleared properly, resulting in distended and chronically infected airways, a condition known as bronchiectasis. Some microbes can defeat the 'escalator' either by forming firm attachments to the bronchial membranes (viruses and some bacteria) or by inhibiting the action of the cilia (mainly bacteria); see Table 11.3. Needless to say, these are among the most successful parasites of the respiratory system, responsible for many serious chest infections.

The alveolar spaces also contain the hydrophilic surfactant proteins SP-A and SP-D which can recognize the surface carbohydrates of pathogens, leading to aggregation and enhanced uptake by phagocytes. Between the mucous layer and the epithelium lies a thin layer of liquid containing many of the antimicrobial proteins mentioned above, notably lysozyme, lactoferrin, and secretory leuko-proteinase inhibitor (SLPI), which act synergistically, and also numerous low-molecular-weight antimicrobial peptides including defensins, cathelicidin, and

Table 11.2 Numerous infectious organisms enter the body via the respiratory route

Viruses	Adenovirus, rhinovirus, influenza, measles, mumps, rubella, VZV (chickenpox), parvovirus
Bacteria	Staphylococci*, Streptococci*, diphtheria, anthrax, mycobacteria (TB, leprosy)*, *Neisseria meningitidis*, *Haemophilus influenzae**, *Bordetella pertussis* (whooping cough), *Mycoplasma**
Fungi	*Aspergillus, Histoplasma*, Blastomyces*, Cryptococcus**

Most of these organisms cause respiratory disease, but some (*) may spread to other organs. TB, tuberculosis; VZV, varicella zoster virus.

Table 11.3 Several viruses and bacteria can avoid the normal flushing actions of the muco-ciliary escalator

	Viruses	Bacteria
Attachment to respiratory epithelium	Rhinovirus	*Neisseria meningitidis*
	Adenovirus	*Haemophilus*
	Influenza	*Streptococcus pneumoniae*
		Mycoplasma
Inactivation of ciliary function	Influenza	*Haemophilus*
	Measles	*Bordetella pertussis*
		Mycoplasma

various neutrophil-derived peptides. There is some evidence that the level of these antimicrobial molecules may differ from person to person, which may partly explain the very different individual susceptibilities to respiratory infection. The fact that many of these peptides are inhibited at high salt concentrations, such as are found in the lung in cystic fibrosis, may be a further contributory cause of the repeated respiratory infections in this condition. A further point of interest is that some of these peptides may become available for therapeutic purposes.

The highly important part played by the immune system in such infections is described in later chapters, but it is worth mentioning here that respiratory infections are one of the most common consequences of *immunodeficiency*.

■ The intestine

Like the air we breathe, food and water are inevitably contaminated with microbes, although proper cooking and water filtering can reduce this contamination substantially. The first difficulty encountered by microbes on their way to the intestine is the very strong acidity of the stomach contents: about pH 2. The value of this in killing bacteria is illustrated by the fact that swallowing a teaspoonful of sodium bicarbonate is enough to lower the minimum infective dose of cholera or *Salmonella* organisms by a factor of 10 000. The other main mechanisms for ridding the intestinal tract of microbes are vomiting and diarrhoea, though it must be said that these are (1) unpleasant and potentially dangerous to the host, and (2) useful to the pathogen in assisting transmission by what is aptly referred to as the faecal–oral route (Table 11.4). Even normal bowel activity would keep the intestine relatively sterile but for the fact that many viruses, bacteria, protozoa, and worms can bind via specific *receptors* to the gut epithelium. To the surprise of many physicians, it has recently become apparent that one bacterium, *Helicobacter pylori*, adapted to life in the stomach by the production of urease, may be the cause of about 80% of gastric and duodenal ulcers. The detergent action of the

Table 11.4 The faecal–oral route is a major pathway of spread for intestinal pathogens, both human–human and animal–human

Faecal–oral route	Other routes
Enteroviruses	Milk
Polio, Coxsackie, Echo, Hepatitis A	*Listeria*
Rotavirus	*Brucella*
E. coli	Tuberculosis (*Mycobacterium bovis*)
Salmonella	Pets
Shigella	Cats
Cholera	*Toxoplasma*
Amoeba	Dogs
Giardia	*Toxocara*
	Hydatid worm
	Meat and other foods
	Taenia (tapeworm)
	Trichinella
	Ascaris

bile salts is also thought to destroy many bacteria, and there are specialized protective antibodies in the gut which will be described in Chapter 17. As in the respiratory tract, antimicrobial peptides, lysozyme, phospholipases, etc. can be found in the gut, secreted in response to bacteria by the Paneth cells. Like the skin, the intestine is host to huge numbers of *normal flora* (see also Chapter 3); there are estimated to be ten times as many harmless bacteria in the large intestine as there are cells in the body. Their protective value is dramatically highlighted by the effect of over-vigorous antibiotic treatment that kills them and allows dangerous pathogens to proliferate (see Chapter 37 for an example). It is also thought that the normal flora, by constant low-level stimulation of immune defence mechanisms, keeps the immune system in the proper state of preparedness. The possibility that the 'normal' gut flora prevent overgrowth by more virulent bacteria has already been mentioned (see Chapter 3).

■ The urogenital tract

Normally the urine is sterile, and any organisms that make their way in through the urethra are flushed out again. However, because of the shortness of the urethra in females, episodes of bacterial infection in the bladder (cystitis) are fairly common, and the same is true when proper voiding of urine is impeded, for example in males with an enlarged prostate. Ascending infection is limited by the production in the kidney of an antibacterial peptide, β-defensin-1, present in normal urine

(10–100 µg/ml) and increased in response to infection. Similar peptides are produced in the vagina, cervix, and uterus; their concentration fluctuates during the menstrual cycle, suggesting a regulatory role for hormones. One type of bacterium, the gonococcus, possesses specialized structures (pili) that allow it to cling to the urethral wall, which explains why it is mainly transmitted sexually.

■ The eye

Shortly after the First World War, Alexander Fleming noticed that human tears, saliva, and plasma contained something that destroyed the walls of certain bacteria. He had discovered *lysozyme*, an enzyme that cleaves the peptidoglycan of Gram-positive bacteria (see Fig. 3.2) and also the chitin of fungi. Together with the flushing action of the tears, it helps to keep the surface of the eye free of infection, although many bacteria are resistant to it and some of them, particularly the chlamydiae, can persist indefinitely in the cells of the conjunctiva. It is interesting that it was also Fleming who later discovered the first fungal molecule that can attack the bacterial cell wall: penicillin.

■ The maternal–fetal route

A number of diseases can be caught by the baby from the mother, either because the pathogen can cross the placenta during pregnancy (e.g. rubella, HIV, toxoplasmosis) or because they are acquired during the birth process (e.g. herpes simplex virus—HSV, hepatitis B). Table 11.5 gives a list of the most important. In addition, the newborn is particularly vulnerable to staphylococcal and streptococcal infection, tetanus, and trachoma.

■ How pathogens exit

A pathogen that cannot survive free in the environment—a virus, for instance—can only get into its host by getting out of another host. Thus for many pathogens it is vital to find a means of exit. Table 11.6 lists the main escape routes used by pathogens, with some typical examples of each. You will note that the type of spread influences the pattern of disease considerably. Thus an upper respiratory virus that spreads by aerosol (e.g. sneezes) can only maintain its presence where the host population is reasonably dense. Towns are ideal for this, and crowded train carriages are particularly efficient. In very thinly populated or isolated areas, spread by an insect vector is a practical solution (mosquitoes can fly up to 80 km). Urogenital transmission obviously calls for very intimate contact. Perhaps the most unusual form of spread is the eating of the brains of dead ancestors, which transmits the prions that are thought to cause the degenerative central nervous

Table 11.5 The major infections acquired during fetal life or at birth

Disease	How acquired	Possible consequences
Rubella	Via placenta	Fetal malformations
CMV, VZV	Via placenta	Fetal malformations
HIV	Placenta/delivery	Congenital AIDS
HSV	Placenta	Neonatal herpes
Hepatitis B	Placenta	Carrier state
Toxoplasmosis	Placenta	Fetal malformations
Malaria	Placenta (rare)	Neonatal malaria
Syphilis	Placenta	Fetal malformations
Leprosy	Placenta	Congenital leprosy
Listeriosis	Placenta/delivery	Congenital listeriosis
Tetanus	Umbilical infection	Neonatal tetanus
Chlamydia	Delivery	Trachoma

CMV, cytomegalovirus; VZV, varicella zoster virus.

Table 11.6 The principal routes of spread by pathogens

Route	Infection
Contact	Most skin infections
	Epstein–Barr virus (saliva)
Coughing, sneezing	Most respiratory infections
Faecal, diarrhoea	Most intestinal infections
Sexual	Herpesvirus (HSV2)
	HIV
	Neisseria gonorrhoeae
	Treponema pallidum (syphilis)
	Trachoma
Blood and blood products	Hepatitis B, C
	HIV
	Malaria
Insect or animal bites*	See Table 11.1, 11.7

Note the risk of transferring infections by blood transfusion. *see also Chapter 36.

disease *kuru*, an early example of spongiform encephalopthy in humans (see Chapter 8 for the link with bovine spongiform encephalopathy (BSE) and new variant Creutzfeldt–Jakob disease—vCJD).

■ A note on vectors

Vectors, particularly blood-feeding arthropods, have been mentioned in relation to both the entry and exit of pathogens. Their importance can be judged from Table 11.7. Note the slight overlap between *vectors*, which simply transmit pathogens from one host to another, and *intermediate hosts*, in which larval stages develop; strictly speaking, humans are the intermediate host of malaria, mosquito the definitive one!

Table 11.7 The major arthropod-vector-borne infections

Disease	Vector
Viruses	
Dengue	Mosquito
Chikungunya	Mosquito
Yellow fever	Mosquito
Tick-borne encephalitis	Tick
Rickettsiae	
Typhus	Flea, louse
Spotted fevers	Tick
Bacteria	
Plague	Flea
Relapsing fever	Louse
Lyme disease	Tick
Protozoa	
Malaria	Mosquito
Leishmaniasis	Sandfly
Sleeping sickness	Tsetse fly
Chagas' disease	Reduviid bug
Helminths	
Onchocerciasis	Simulium fly
Filariasis	Mosquito
Loasis	Mango fly

SUMMARY

- The skin and mucous membranes of the body constitute efficient barriers against the entry of most pathogens. Each type of surface has components or secretions appropriate to the pathogens likely to be encountered.

- Spread of pathogens from host to host may be by contact, coughing and sneezing, the faecal–oral, urogenital, or maternal–fetal routes, or by vector (e.g. biting insects).

- Certain pathogens may be acquired inadvertently via blood transfusion.

Chapter 12

Innate immunity

The innate immune system comprises all those mechanisms for dealing with infection that are constitutive or 'built in', changing little with age or with experience of infection and, as already mentioned, traceable back to the earliest invertebrate forms of life. It is also known by other names; for example, the synonym *natural* is often used, as a contrast to *adaptive* immunity; another term, *non-specific*, is rather out of date, since specificity in immunity is a relative matter. Although in some ways less sophisticated than adaptive immunity, innate immunity should not be belittled, since it has evidently protected thousands of species of invertebrates sufficiently to survive for up to 2 billion years, compared with the mere 500 million years of vertebrate evolution.

As emphasized in Chapter 10, all immune systems make use of molecular *recognition* elements, *disposal* mechanisms, and a *communication* system. In higher animals, these recognition and communication molecules may be either *cell-bound* or *soluble*. In the case of cell-bound molecules, their function is inseparable from that of the cell itself, and we speak of a 'cellular' type of immunity; an example would be the surface receptors by which phagocytic cells identify their prey (see below). In contrast, molecules that act freely in the extracellular compartment (e.g. complement, see below, or antibody, see Chapter 17) are spoken of as 'humoral'. In the innate immune system, molecules of both types are involved, corresponding to the need to recognize and dispose of different types of pathogen,

Table 12.1 The principal cells and molecules of innate immunity. Note the overlaps between the inflammatory response and the response to infection. +: major role; (+): relatively less important

	Antibacterial/ antifungal	Antiviral	Inflammatory	Interaction with adaptive immunity
Molecules				
Complement	+		+	(+)
Collectins	(+)		+	(+)
Other acute phase proteins	(+)		(+)	(+)
Interferons	(+)	+		+
Other cytokines	(+)		+	+
Cells				
Phagocytes	+	(+)	+	(+)
Dendritic cells			+	+
Mast cells			+	(+)
Natural killer cells	(+)	+		(+)

to promote inflammatory responses, which are of value in all types of infection, and to interact with the adaptive immune system. The principal cells and molecules are contrasted in Table 12.1, with some examples of their function and the appearance of some of the cells shown in Fig. 12.1.

■ Pattern recognition by the innate immune system

One of the key roles of the innate immune system is to distinguish between self and non-self, and where possible between self and *pathogen*. Such a distinction has been required since the evolution of multicellular life forms, which is why inverte-brates, insects, and even plants have well-developed innate recognition systems. Recognition is mediated by the interaction of two sets of complementary mole-cules. Microorganisms possess certain molecular configurations which are either not present in the host or shielded in some way and are therefore known as pathogen-associated molecular patterns or PAMPs. Examples include lipopolysaccharide (Gram-negative bacteria), lipoteichoic acid (Gram-positive bacteria), mannans (fungal cell walls), double-stranded (ds) RNA (viruses), cytidine-phosphate-guanosine (CpG) DNA motifs (bacteria), and many others. These structures have been picked out for recognition because they are characteristic of microorganisms, often essen-tial for their survival, and show minimal variation. Thus a microbe cannot easily evade recognition by simply mutating or eliminating them, although some do achieve this (see Chapter 13). The host structures that recognize them are called pattern-recognition receptors (PRRs); these evolutionarily conserved molecules include many well-studied immune mediators such as complement as well as more

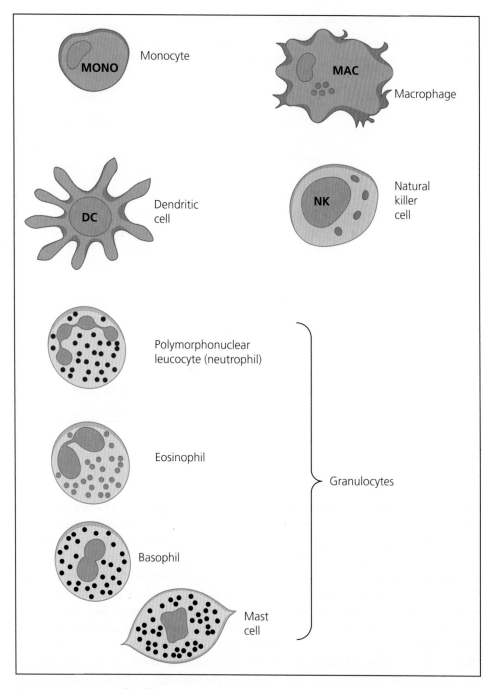

Fig. 12.1 Important cells of the innate immune system. These symbols are used throughout the book.

Table 12.2 The Toll-like receptor family

Location/receptor	Ligands bound	Examples
Cell surface		
TLR1	Triacyl lipopeptides	Bacteria
TLR2	Peptidoglycans	Gram-positive bacteria
	Lipoproteins	Bacteria
	GPI anchors	Trypanosomes
	Lipoarabinomannan	Mycobacteria
	PI dimannoside	Mycobacteria
	Zymosan	Fungi
TLR4	LPS	Gram-negative bacteria
TLR5	Flagellin	Bacteria
TLR6	α1 Acyl lipopeptides	Bacteria
	Zymosan	Fungi
Intracellular		
TLR3	Double-stranded RNA	Viruses
TLR7/8	Single-stranded RNA	Viruses
	Imidazoquinolines	Antiviral drugs
TLR9	CpG DNA	Bacteria, DNA viruses
	Haemozoin	*P. falciparum*

CpG, cytidine-phosphate-guanosine; GPI, glycosyl-phosphatidyl inositol; PI, phosphatidylinositol; TLR, Toll-like receptor.

recently discovered ones such as the Toll-like receptor family (Tables 12.2 and 12.3), identified in mammals by their similarity to the Toll receptors used by the fruit fly *Drosophila* to recognize fungi. PRRs may be either soluble (e.g. in blood) or membrane-bound (e.g. on phagocytes), and they are able to distinguish between, for example, Gram-negative bacteria and yeasts, but without pinpointing the species of either. However, they trigger a sequence of events which not only attack the microorganism but also activate the adaptive immune system (see below and Chapters 16–20). Defined ligands can be identified for individual PRR, but most pathogens express more than one PAMP and most cells express more than one PRR, so the binding of pathogen to cell is usually the result of multiple events. For example the Toll-like receptor TLR2 cooperates with TLR1/6 in the recognition of bacteria, and with Dectin-1 (a receptor for complex carbohydrates) in the recognition of yeasts. This synergy between receptors on cells such as macrophages and dendritic cells might be turned to good use in the design of novel vaccine adjuvants.

Note also that recognition is not restricted to the cell surface, but can occur within intracellular vesicles (e.g. TLR 3,7,8,9) or in the cytoplasm (e.g. the NOD-like receptor family (NLR) for bacteria; RIG-like helicases for viral RNA).

Table 12.3 Other important innate recognition receptors

Location/receptor	Ligands bound	Examples
Soluble		
Complement	Cell-wall components (IgG and IgM antibody)	Bacteria, fungi, etc., antibody-coated material
MBL/Ficolin	Mannose/N-acetyl glucosamine	Bacteria, fungi, etc.
CRP	Phosphatidylcholine, polysaccharide	Pneumococci
SP-A	Lipoarabinomannan, lipid A of LPS	Mycobacteria, *B. pertussis*
SP-D	α1–3-linked fucose	*Cryptococcus neoformans*, schistosome larvae
Cell surface		
Mannose receptor	Mannose, fucose	Fungi, bacteria
DC-SIGN	Mannose cap oligosaccharide	*M. tuberculosis*
	gp120	HIV
	Other glycoproteins	Hepatitis, Marburg, SARS virus
	Lewis X/Y	*H. pylori*
Dectin-1	β glucans	Fungi
Scavenger receptors	Polyanionic ligands	Gram-negative bacteria
Intracellular (cytoplasmic)		
NOD 1	Diaminopimelic acid	Bacteria
NOD 2	Muramyl dipeptide	Bacteria
RIG-like receptors	ssRNA, dsRNA	Viruses

CRP, C-reactive protein; DC-SIGN is a dendritic-cell ICAM-3 receptor; gp, glycoprotein; LPS, lipopolysaccharide; MBL, mannose-binding lectin; NOD, nucleotide oligomerization domain; SARS, severe acute respiratory syndrome; SP, surfactant protein.

Damage-associated recognition

The recognition of pathogen-associated patterns is not the only function of innate immune receptors. Tissue damage can be *sterile*, that is, not caused by infection but by irritant substances such as asbestos, silica, or uric acid deposits in gout. Here the key element is the inflammasome, a multi-protein complex which, via the aspartate-specific protease caspase-1, leads to the release of the inflammatory cytokines IL-1 and IL-18 (Fig. 12.2). Some pathogens also activate the inflammasome pathway and in macrophages this can lead to a novel, pro-inflammatory pathway of host cell death called pyroptosis which contributes to host resistance.

The intracellular responses triggered by pathogen or damage recognition are mediated by a series of cytoplasmic adapter proteins and enzymes (such as MyD88 in the case of most TLRs) which signal into the nucleus to increase the transcription of many genes including pro-inflammatory cytokines such as TNF, IL-12 and

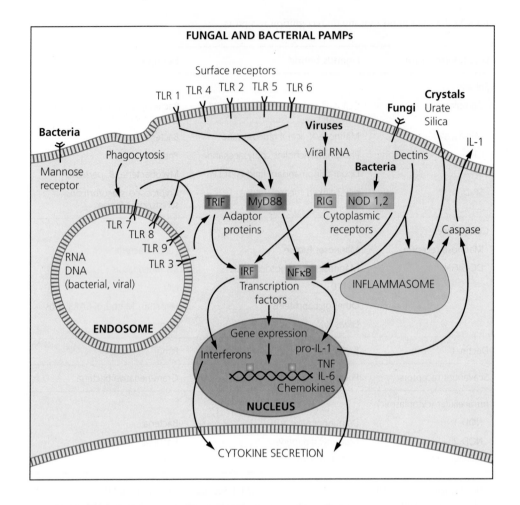

Fig. 12.2 Location and principal signalling pathways involved in pattern recognition and inflammation. TLR: Toll-like receptors; NFκB: nuclear factor κB; IRF: interferon response factor; PAMPS: pathogen associated molecular patterns; TRIF: TIR domain containing adaptor-inducing interferon β.

interferons (summarized in Figure 12.2). As mentioned above, IL-1, IL-18 are unusual in that they are produced as inactive precursors and require cleavage by caspase-1 to become biologically active.

Increased expression of host-derived molecules that signal stress (e.g. the MHC homologues MICA/MICB detected by NK cells) or the release of molecules not normally exposed on living cells (e.g. chromatin-binding proteins such as HMGB1) can also trigger innate immune responses.

At this point it is worth a reminder that, complex and numerous as they are, PRRs are constitutive, germ-line-encoded products identical in all normal individuals. By contrast the B- and T-lymphocyte receptors, to be discussed later under adaptive immunity, are produced following genetic rearrangement, and are unique to each cell.

■ Soluble (humoral) mediators of innate immunity

Complement

Complement is the most striking example of a humoral innate immune mechanism. It is not a single molecule but a 'cascade system' of proteins that activate one another in series, rather like the blood-clotting system (Fig. 12.3). Including the various inhibitors that prevent it getting out of control (see below), there are over 30 plasma and cell-surface complement components, the terminology being complicated by the fact that the full sequence of activation was not understood until quite recently, whereas the existence of the system was known in the 1880s, as soon as it was realized that antibodies needed another serum factor to 'complement' them in some of their functions. Only many years later was it understood that complement activation did not always require antibody, which is why the

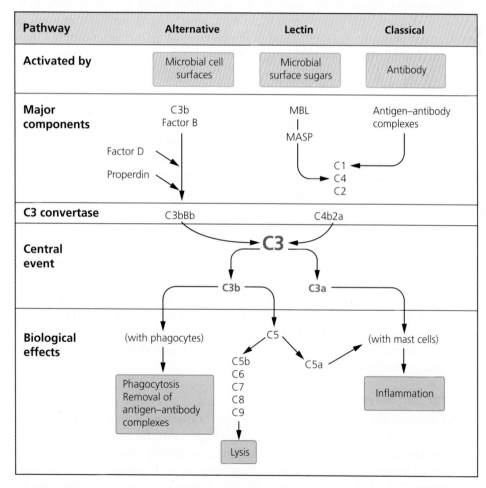

Fig. 12.3 The complement system, showing the three pathways of activation, the central role of C3, and the three biological effects. The many inhibitors by which activation is regulated are not shown.

antibody-requiring pathway (restricted, like antibody, to vertebrates) is confusingly known as *classical*, and the others, found also in higher invertebrates, as *alternative* and *lectin-mediated*.

Although it appears complex, the complement system is actually amazingly economical, since the same central component, a major serum protein known as C3, can be activated in three different ways, and activation can lead to three different useful functions (Fig. 12.3). As always, its real value can be judged by the study of *deficiencies* and from these we learn that it matters most in bacterial infections (the same is true of *phagocytic cells* and *antibody*, as will be seen).

Alternative pathway

The fundamental event in complement activation is the formation of a *C3 convertase* to split C3 into two fragments, C3b (large) and C3a (small), both of which have important functions. The convertase of the alternative pathway, known as C3bBb, involves three other serum proteins, factors B and D and properdin, as well as C3b itself, in a process that 'ticks over' slowly and harmlessly at host cell surfaces but is enormously enhanced at the surfaces of many bacteria, fungi, protozoa, and some viruses, so that large amounts of C3b are deposited there.

Lectin pathway

A second innate pathway of C3 convertase generation involves recognition of microbial surfaces by mannose-binding lectin (MBL) and/or ficolins (see below). These attach to repetitive patterns of mannose and other sugars, which are common in microbial but not mammalian cell surfaces, and activate the proteases MASP-1 and -2, where MASP stands for mannose-binding lectin-associated serine protease, which cleave two complement components C4 and C2, leading to the formation of the C3 convertase C4b2a, which acts similarly to C3bBb.

Classical pathway

The evolution of the antibody molecule (see Chapter 17) allowed a widening of the range of pathogens able to activate C3, through the ability of many antibodies to bind the complement component C1q which, together with C1r and C1s, induces the cleavage of C4 and C2. Thus C1q,r,s acts very much like MBL+MASP, except that not only sugar residues but potentially *any* pathogen-derived molecule can now activate the system. The classical pathway can also be activated by the acute phase protein CRP (see below).

Effector pathways

C3b is responsible for most of the benefits of complement activation. Bound to a pathogen, it can attach to *C3b receptors* on phagocytic cells and lead to *phagocytosis* (see below). C3b bound to a soluble antigen–antibody complex can attach the complex to (mainly) red blood cells and transport it to the phagocytes of the liver and spleen. C3b also cleaves C5 to C5b, which then associates with the complement components C6, C7, C8, and C9 to form the *membrane attack complex* which, by insertion into microbial membranes, particularly those of Gram-negative bacteria, leads to leakage and death by *lysis*. Finally, the small fragment C3a, together with C5-derived C5a, has its own role in promoting *inflammatory* reactions, mainly through binding to mast cells (see below).

Complement receptors

The binding of complement components to cells is mediated by four types of receptor. Types 1, 3, and 4 bind mainly C3b and promote phagocytosis; type 2 binds smaller C3 fragments and enhances B-cell memory; it is also (unfortunately) the receptor for EBV.

Regulation of complement

Almost every stage of complement activation is regulated by inhibitory molecules that bind rapidly to activated components and prevent them damaging host tissue. There are at least seven of these, including the C1 inhibitor, Factors I and H, decay-accelerating factor (DAF), and CD46, which is also the receptor for measles virus.

Collectins and ficolins

MBL and other molecules that recognize sugar patterns unique to pathogens, or normally masked on healthy host cells, for example by sialic acid, are referred to as *collectins*, from their possession of a *coll*agen-like and a *lectin* domain. Other collectins include C1q itself, and the surfactant proteins SP-A and SP-D found in the lung. Ficolins possess an additional fibrinogen-like domain and can activate complement, but their exact role is not clear. Together they form part of a broader group of innate defence molecules called *defence collagens* sharing the property of recognizing pathogens and possibly some tumours (Fig. 12.4).

Acute-phase proteins

One of the earliest detectable reactions to trauma or infection is the *acute phase response*. This is the name given to the inflammatory response leading to *fever* and other symptoms of illness including the appearance in the blood of a variety of 'acute phase' proteins, mostly made in the liver, in turn stimulated by cytokines secreted by phagocytes. From the list of these (Fig. 12.5) you can see that some are obviously useful in removing enzymes and other intracellular material released by tissue damage, but a few appear to have antibacterial properties too. This is especially true of *C-reactive protein* (CRP), a curious pentameric molecule ('pentraxin') that binds to the C polysaccharide of some streptococcal cell walls, activates complement, and promotes phagocytosis, somewhat like a primitive antibody molecule. Other pentraxins that also activate complement are Serum amyloid P protein (SAP) and pentraxin 3.

The acute phase response is generated by a wide range of stimulants, and some of the individual components may not be needed in any one infection, but they flare up at the slightest sign of 'trouble'. For example, a raised level of CRP in the

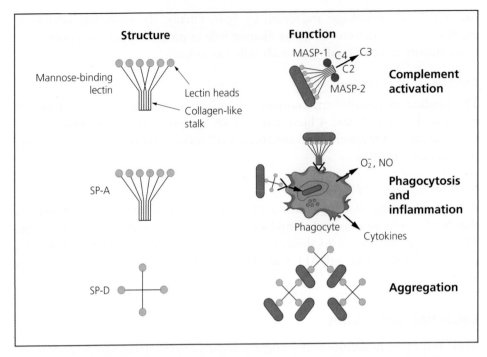

Fig. 12.4 Collectins and inflammation. Binding of pathogens by collectins can result in aggregation, complement activation, phagocytosis, secretion of inflammatory mediators, and recruitment of inflammatory cells. SP-A and SP-D are important mediators of pulmonary inflammation, able to enhance/inhibit production by phagocytes of oxygen radicals, NO, and pro-inflammatory cytokines.

blood can be a useful early sign of an impending relapse in chronic diseases such as rheumatoid arthritis and some infections.

Cytokines

Most of the remaining mediators of innate immunity fall into the category of *cytokines*, already introduced in Chapter 10. As Table 12.4 shows, these have a wide range of activities but are essentially *communication* molecules, lacking in any direct pathogen-recognition or -disposal properties. Their effects overlap considerably, but can be grouped roughly into five categories, namely those involved in the promotion of (1) *inflammatory* responses; (2) cell *differentiation* and *proliferation*; (3) cell *movement*; (4) *inhibition*, and (5) a special group of important antiviral molecules, the *interferons*. Note that cytokines, often the same ones, also play a major role in adaptive immunity; indeed they are responsible for most of the interactions between the two systems.

Interferons

As with most cytokines, the interferon (IFN) terminology is confusing. Two of the three main types of IFN, α and β, are very similar (Type 1) and bind to the same

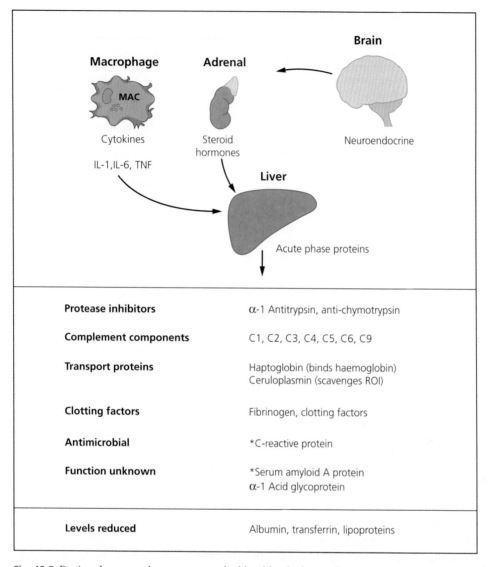

Protease inhibitors	α-1 Antitrypsin, anti-chymotrypsin
Complement components	C1, C2, C3, C4, C5, C6, C9
Transport proteins	Haptoglobin (binds haemoglobin) Ceruloplasmin (scavenges ROI)
Clotting factors	Fibrinogen, clotting factors
Antimicrobial	*C-reactive protein
Function unknown	*Serum amyloid A protein α-1 Acid glycoprotein
Levels reduced	Albumin, transferrin, lipoproteins

Fig. 12.5 During the acute phase response, the blood level of several proteins rises, some (*) by as much as 1000-fold. The response occurs within hours of injury or infection. Note that macrophage-derived cytokines also act on the brain (hypothalamus) to induce fever. IL, interleukin; ROI, reactive oxygen intermediates; TNF, tumour necrosis factor.

receptor, whereas the third, γ (Type 2), is a quite different molecule with many separate properties, notably that of activating macrophages to kill intracellular pathogens and a different receptor. In fact the above is somewhat of an over-simplification, since there are 14 subtypes of IFNα and an ever-increasing number of related molecules (IFNδ,ε,κ,λ,τ,ω,ζ), most of which have been shown to have overlapping properties. However, their antiviral effects are the same: to induce an antiviral state in cells that otherwise might succumb to virus infection. Figure 12.6 illustrates the process by which this is brought about. Together with NK cells,

Table 12.4 Key cytokine groups of the innate immune system

	Cytokine	Cell source	Targets	Function
Inflammation	IL-1, IL-6, TNF	Macrophages, dendritic cells, neutrophils, T cells	Hepatocytes, endothelial cells, hypothalamus, macrophages, T cells and B cells	Induction of acute phase response, recruitment of cells to inflammatory foci, induction of fever, phagocyte activation, proliferation of immunoglobulin-secreting B cells
Differentiation	IL-12, IL-18	Macrophages, dendritic cells, neutrophils	NK cells, T cells	Secretion of IFNγ by NK cells and T cells, increased T cell cytolytic activity, Type 1 T cell differentiation
	IFNγ	NK cells, T cells	Macrophage	Activation
Proliferation	IL-15	Macrophages	NK cells and T cells	Proliferation
Cell movement	Chemokines e.g. CXCL8, CCL3, CCL5, CCL2	Leucocytes, endothelium, epithelium, fibroblasts	Multiple cell types	Recruitment of phagocytes to sites of infection, Leucocyte activation, lymphocyte trafficking, Lymphoid tissue development
Inhibition	IL-10, TGF-β	Macrophages, dendritic cells, T cells	Macrophages, T cells	Inhibitors of macrophage activation, control of excessive inflammation, promote B-cell growth, promote chronic fibrosis
Antiviral	Interferons	IFNα: pDC, macrophages, IFNβ: fibroblasts, IFNγ: NK cells, T cells	All cells	Induces antiviral state, increases MHC class I expression, activates NK cell cytolytic activity

See also Appendix 2. TGF-β, transforming growth factor β.

IFNα and β are probably responsible for inhibiting many acute viral infections, and are also responsible for some of the symptoms, since it has been shown that large therapeutic doses of IFN and other cytokines can induce the fever, muscle pains, and general feeling of illness so typical of virus infections. Nevertheless they have come into use as therapeutic 'drugs' for certain virus infections, such as hepatitis, as well as some tumours.

■ Cells of innate immunity

Phagocytic cells

Phagocytosis is the act of taking particulate matter into a cell, as opposed to taking in small molecules like water (pinocytosis). Many types of cell can phagocytose at times, but the specialized or 'professional' phagocytes of mammals are of two

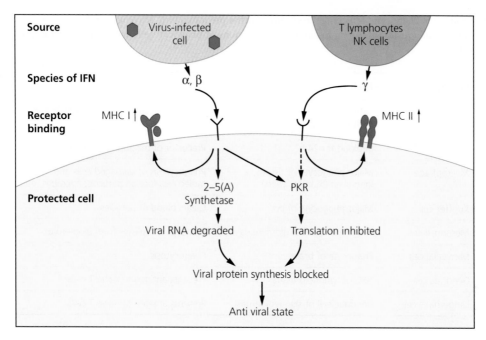

Fig. 12.6 The induction and activity of interferon molecules. The enhancing effects on MHC cell-surface molecule expression are explained in Chapter 8. PKR, RNA-dependent protein kinase.

kinds: the large *macrophages* and the smaller *polymorphonuclear leucocytes* (PMNs). These share many properties, but are designed to deal with different situations (Table 12.5). Cells with the essential features of macrophages may look different and are given different names in different sites (they used to be known collectively as the reticulo-endothelial system, a little-used term nowadays). Macrophages can present antigen to T cells, but there are also more specialized *antigen-presenting cells* (APCs) in which phagocytosis has been reduced to the minimum necessary to induce adaptive responses in lymphocytes; these *dendritic cells* are described below, and will appear again when we consider the immune response in Chapters 18–20.

Phagocytosis

Phagocytosis is a complex, multi-step process by which a particle is 'eaten', prior to being killed and/or digested (Fig. 12.7). Note that a 'particle' may be anything from a speck of inhaled dust to an age-expired red cell or a nucleated cell that has self-destructed from the 'suicide' process known as apoptosis. As regards infectious organisms, phagocytosis is particularly effective against bacteria and fungi, and patients with defective phagocytes suffer from repeated infection with these types of pathogen. Often the phagocyte has to migrate through the tissues to find the pathogen, using *chemotactic* gradients of microbe-derived molecules or signals from other cells such as chemokines. Next, the phagocyte needs to attach the microbe to its membrane—the *recognition* stage—which may be by

Table 12.5 Phagocytic cells range from those with a predominantly scavenging role (top) to those mainly responsible for presenting small portions of phagocytosed material to lymphocytes (APCs)

Cell type	Features	Functions
PMN	Short-lived (2 days), multi-lobed nucleus	Phagocytosis and killing of bacteria and fungi
Monocyte	In blood for 24 h	Precursor of macrophage, some DC
Macrophage	Major phagocyte of tissues, long-lived (months, years)	Phagocytosis of damaged cells and molecules, foreign particles, microbes, etc.
Kupffer cell	Major phagocyte of liver	Clears blood of particles
Mesangial cell	Phagocyte of renal glomerulus	Removes complexes from glomerulus
Microglial cell	Phagocyte of brain	Phagocytosis
Dendritic cell	APC of lymphoid tissue	Presents antigen to naïve T cells
Langerhans cell	Dendritic cell of skin (epidermis)	Presents antigen to naïve T cells

Making contact

1. Movement towards the bacterium (along chemotactic gradient)

2. Attachment to bacterial cell wall (may be assisted by complement or antibody)

Eating

3. Taking the bacterium into a phagosome (requiring membrane movement)

4. Bringing it into contact with lysosomes, to form 'phagolysosome'

Killing and digestion

5. Oxidative and non-oxidative killing mechanisms act

6. Enzymes digest remains

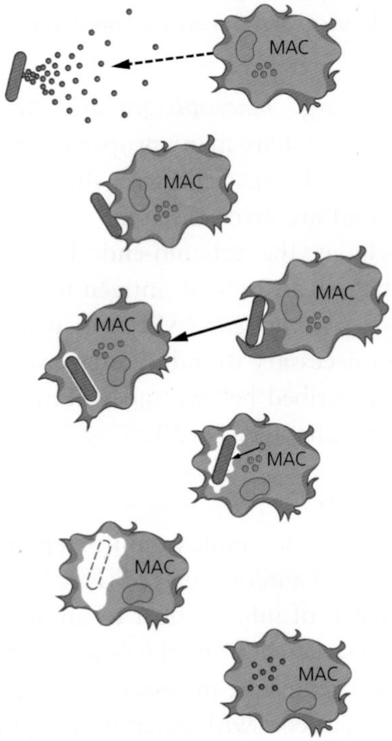

Fig. 12.7 Phagocytosis proceeds in steps, the whole process taking minutes or hours. Macrophages and PMNs operate in much the same way, except that PMNs are somewhat more potent in oxidative killing (see text), and macrophages are more effective in dealing with long-lived parasites.

interaction with components of the microbial surface, often carbohydrate-based such as lipopolysaccharide or mannan (see the section on pattern recognition, above), but which can be rendered more effective by the presence of *complement* or *antibody* on the microbe, because phagocytes also have receptors for these molecules on their surface; this process is known as *opsonization*. From then on, movements of the membrane and of intracellular vesicles guide the particle into the presence of powerful killing and digestive systems, reducing it to its molecular constituents for re-use or, alternatively, for expulsion from the body via sputum or faeces. In addition, small peptides of microbial origin may be transported to the cell surface by MHC molecules, to be 'presented' to T lymphocytes, as described in Chapter 8, and the act of phagocytosis may induce the release of inflammatory cytokines.

Not every phagocytic event proceeds to killing and digestion. Macrophages may need activation by IFNγ. In Chapter 13 you will read about pathogens that allow themselves to be taken into macrophages but not killed: an excellent long-term survival strategy for the pathogen. Some pathogens induce their own uptake by non-phagocytic cells, for example *Salmonella* into enterocytes.

Intracellular killing

Once inside the phagocyte, the majority of microbes are speedily killed. For this purpose, phagocytes have a selection of toxic molecules: some that derive from atmospheric oxygen (oxidative killing) and others that do not require oxygen; the latter are needed where excess oxygen is not available, for example deep in the tissues and in necrotic areas. In addition neutrophils and macrophages are able to increase their activity in response to these reduced oxygen levels via a transcriptional regulator known as HIF (hypoxia inducible factor). Table 12.6 lists some of these non-oxidative molecules, and Fig. 12.8 summarizes the pathways by which the *reactive oxygen intermediates* (ROI) and *nitric oxide* (NO) are formed; some ROI are particularly prominent in PMNs; their toxicity may be either direct or via induction of microbicidal proteases. To protect the phagocyte itself against these toxic compounds, they are packaged into vesicles called *lysosomes*, which can be steered into contact with the vesicles containing ingested material, which are known as *phagosomes* (see Fig. 12.7). Increased production of the oxygen and nitrogen intermediates by IFNγ is often referred to as the 'classical' pathway to distinguish it from the effects of other cytokines such as IL-4, which directs the macrophage into an 'alternative' activation state, shutting down the production of nitric oxide.

Later you will see that some of the most awkward pathogens are those that resist all these killing mechanisms and take up long-term residence in phagocytes. A second possibility, not so well understood, is that macrophages can sometimes stop the growth of microbes without killing them. This process is sometimes seen with intracellular bacteria such as mycobacteria and *Legionella*, and is referred to as bacteriostatic, in contrast to bactericidal; the mechanism is mainly one of starving the microbe of essential nutrients such as iron or tryptophan.

Table 12.6 Cells of the innate immune system contain numerous molecules toxic to parasites

Source	Molecules	Active against
PMN		
(1) in 'primary' granules	Lysozyme	Gram-positive bacteria
	Myeloperoxidase	Bacteria, fungi (with H_2O_2)
(2) in 'specific' granules	Defensins, BPI	Bacteria, fungi
	Lactoferrin	Bacteria (depletes iron)
Macrophage	As PMNs but no myeloperoxidase	Intracellular pathogens
	NO	
Eosinophil	Cationic proteins	Worms (extracellular)
	MBP	Worms (extracellular)
	Peroxidase	Worms (extracellular)
Natural killer cell	Perforins	Virus or bacteria infected cells
	Granzymes	
	Granulysin	Bacteria, fungi

Note that the granules of PMN are of two kinds, with different contents. Note also that the eosinophil granulocyte contains its own highly basic proteins, possibly designed to damage worms. BPI, bacterial permeability-increasing factor, which binds to and inactivates endotoxins; MBP, major basic protein.

Dendritic cells

These cells have only been fully appreciated in the last decade or so but their importance in immunity is immense because they can be regarded as the primary interface between infectious organisms and the adaptive immune system. Their name is due to their shape, which is characterized by numerous long thin processes that project in all directions, giving them an enormous surface area at which to interact with both foreign material and other immunological cells, notably lymphocytes (Fig. 12.1).

Ultimately derived from the bone marrow, dendritic cells show considerable heterogeneity in both appearance and function, and may in fact represent two separate lineages, the majority sharing an origin with monocytes and macrophages (myeloid) and a minority related to NK cells and lymphocytes (plasmacytoid). The latter are an important source of Type I interferons in virus infection. In fact dendritic cells are a very heterogeneous population with many different surface markers and functions. (There is also a separate cell type called follicular dendritic cells which are not related, FDC; see Chapter 9).

Since their main function is in the initial 'presentation' of foreign material to naïve lymphocytes at their surface, dendritic cells (e.g. in lymph nodes but also at many other sites exposed to pathogens, such as skin and mucosa), dendritic cells specialize in recognition rather than phagocytosis. However, dendritic cells do

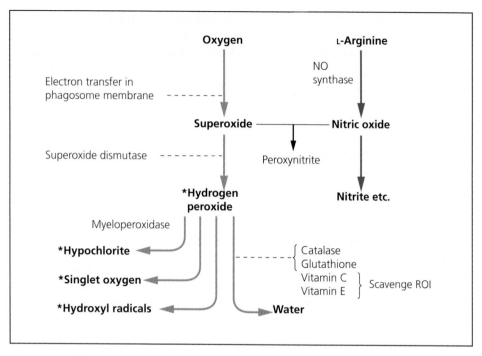

Fig. 12.8 Parallel and interacting metabolic pathways generate reactive oxygen (*ROI) and nitrogen intermediates by phagocytes. Note the presence of 'antioxidant' and scavenging molecules (right) to restrict the toxic activity of the ROI to the target (bacterium, fungus, etc.) without damage to the phagocyte itself.

have some phagocytic activity, particularly when immature in the periphery in order to capture antigens for presentation, and various pathogens are able to enter and survive in them; these include several viruses (measles, influenza, CMV, HIV) and some larger organisms (*Chlamydia, Leishmania*). Recognition by dendritic cells appears to involve much the same pattern-recognizing elements as those used by phagocytes, enabling dendritic cells to respond to a huge range of pathogenic material, from bacterial and protozoal surface molecules to bacterial DNA, viral RNA, and heat-shock proteins. To complete the impressive list of their activities, dendritic cells can secrete a variety of cytokines—interleukin (IL)-6, IL-12, IL-18, tumour necrosis factor (TNF), IFNα, IFNβ, IFNγ—and in some infections, for example leishmaniasis, it is the dendritic cells rather than the macrophages that produce the transient burst of IL-12 which appears to be critical in initiating an effective cell-mediated immune response. In other infections they may be responsible for the IL-10 that *prevents* effective cell-mediated immunity.

Mast cells

Mast cells, prominent in the skin, around blood vessels, and in the gut, and the closely similar basophils in the blood, are of central importance in the *acute inflammatory response*, a series of changes designed to increase the supply of blood and its contents (PMNs, complement, antibody, etc.) at local sites of trauma or infection (see below). Their function is to release the contents of their granules, which include histamine, leukotrienes, and other molecules that increase vascular permeability. This degranulation can be triggered by direct damage or under the influence of a special antibody (IgE); see Chapter 23 for an explanation of how this can lead to distressing *allergies*. Recent work has revealed that mast cells share a number of the features of dendritic cells, being able to some extent to take up foreign material, present antigens to lymphocytes, respond to some cytokines, and secrete others (e.g. TNF). Thus they are not just the 'explosive packages' of allergy but function as part of the innate immune system in a more controlled way to initiate inflammation where required, particularly in response to some bacteria.

■ Lymphoid cells of innate immunity

This may seem a contradictory title, in view of what was said in Chapter 10 about the lymphocyte as the key cell of *adaptive* immunity, but certain cells of lymphocyte-like appearance display features typical of the innate system, most notably the NK cells.

NK cells

These cells, sometimes known as large granular lymphocytes (LGLs), were first identified by their ability to kill tumour cells that the host had not previously encountered: a 'natural' or *innate* type of killing in contrast to the adaptive antigen-specific type displayed by conventional cytotoxic T cells. They carry some of the cell-surface markers of T cells (e.g. CD8) but not the classical T-cell receptor. There is also an intermediate population of 'NK T cells' which do carry a restricted version of the T-cell receptor (see Chapter 18). Unlike cytotoxic T cells they are not stimulated, but actually inhibited, by MHC class I molecules (see below and Fig. 12.8). However they have recently been shown to share some features with CD8 T cells, including some degree of clonal expansion and memory, suggesting that they might be possible targets for vaccines.

The key features of NK cells are that they are much less restricted in their recognition than T cells and they respond rapidly: in hours or days compared with the days or weeks of conventional adaptive T cells. NK cells have been implicated in many immunological processes including tumour surveillance, regulation of haemopoiesis, bone-marrow graft rejection, and the regulation of pregnancy. However, we know most about their role in infection, which is threefold, as follows.

1. NK cells can have a direct effect by binding to the surface of some microorganisms, such as *Cryptococcus neoformans*. They are poorly phagocytic, but it is thought that the lytic machinery by which they kill tumour cells is released at the point of contact. It is fair to say that the evidence for this is derived largely from studies *in vitro*.

2. Better understood are their effects on host cells: *lysis* of cells infected with intra-cellular pathogens, which is carried out by the release of NK granule contents such as the enzymes *perforin* and *granzymes* and the induction of apoptosis, and *killing* of intracellular pathogens by *granulysin*, a peptide with direct anti-microbial activity. The mechanism by which NK cells are triggered to lyse-infected (or cancerous) but not normal host cells depends on a balance between two opposing forces: *activating* receptors that recognize target-cell surface structures, including viral products or stress-related proteins, and give a 'kill' signal, and *inhibitory* receptors that recognize MHC class I molecules and pre-vent killing. Only when MHC molecules are absent or altered (as in virus infec-tion and some tumours) is the kill signal allowed to predominate (Fig. 12.9). The cytotoxic activity of NK cells is rapidly enhanced by Type 1 IFNs and IL-12 induced by viruses and bacteria.

3. NK cells can also be stimulated by cytokines, such as phagocyte-derived IL-12 and IL-18, to release IFNγ which in turn activates the phagocytes to kill inter-nalized pathogens such as bacteria (*Listeria, Salmonella, Mycobacterium*), protozoa (*Leishmania, Toxoplasma*), and some viruses (e.g. CMV) (Fig. 12.10). The key point here is that the NK cells are a potent source of rapid IFNγ pro-duction (and cytotoxic activity), the rapidity being a typical innate immune feature. A recent example is the secretion of IFNγ by human NK cells in response to *Plasmodium falciparum*-infected red blood cells, although it is still not clear exactly how this occurs. NK cells express the Fcγ receptor, enabling them to kill antibody-coated target cells (ADCC). However, the importance of this during infection is also not fully understood.

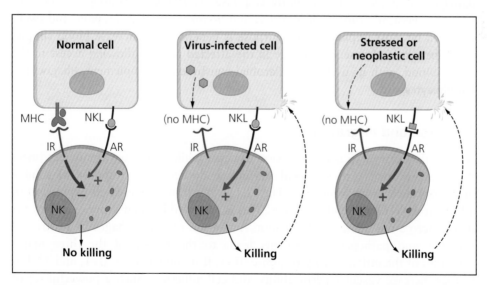

Fig 12.9 Target recognition by NK cells, illustrating the opposing effects of activating receptors (AR) and inhibitory receptors (IR). Under normal conditions, expression of MHC molecules inhibits killing, while their absence in infected or stressed cells allows killing to occur. NKL, NK-cell ligand.

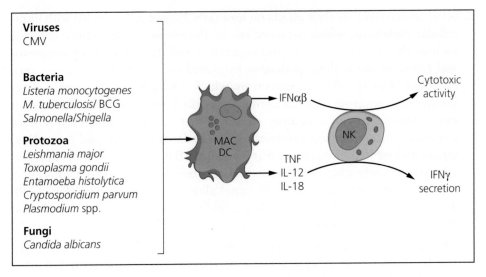

Viruses
CMV

Bacteria
Listeria monocytogenes
M. tuberculosis/ BCG
Salmonella/Shigella

Protozoa
Leishmania major
Toxoplasma gondii
Entamoeba histolytica
Cryptosporidium parvum
Plasmodium spp.

Fungi
Candida albicans

Fig. 12.10 NK cell activation by cytokines. Infections where IFNα/β production is dominant can favour cytotoxic activity (e.g. viruses) whereas IL-12/IL-18 induced by bacteria, protozoa, etc. also promotes IFNγ secretion.

■ Acute inflammation

We have already encountered inflammation in connection with complement, cytokines, and mast cells, but as Fig. 12.11 shows, there is more to it than this. Local inflammation is one of the fundamental responses of the body to almost any kind of injury and a prerequisite for the healing process. Being a response to tissue damage, it is an inevitable part of the response to *pathogens*. Although its outward features, classically *rubor*, *calor*, *dolor*, and *tumor* (redness, heat, pain, and swelling), can be most unpleasant, its purpose is beneficial: to increase blood supply, cell adhesion, and vascular leakage in the affected region, allowing access to the site of blood, with its useful antimicrobial constituents: complement, phagocytes, lymphocytes, etc.

Adhesion and migration

An essential early step is the adhesion of neutrophils, and later monocytes (macrophage precursors), to the local vascular endothelium in response to soluble mediators such as histamine (see Fig 12.11), resulting in increased expression of adhesion molecules and chemokines. This is followed by their movement into the tissues across the 'sticky' endothelium. Activation of macrophages by neutrophil products and pathogen components leads to the release of the three major cytokines of the inflammatory response: IL-1, IL-6, and TNF-α. IL-1, and TNF-α further increase vascular permeability and cell adhesion. Such a powerful set of responses obviously needs regulation, and here the cytokines transforming growth factor β (TGF-β) and IL-10 are important. Systemic effects (fever, etc.) are seen in the acute phase response (see above) but if they become excessive they may be dangerous (see Chapter 14).

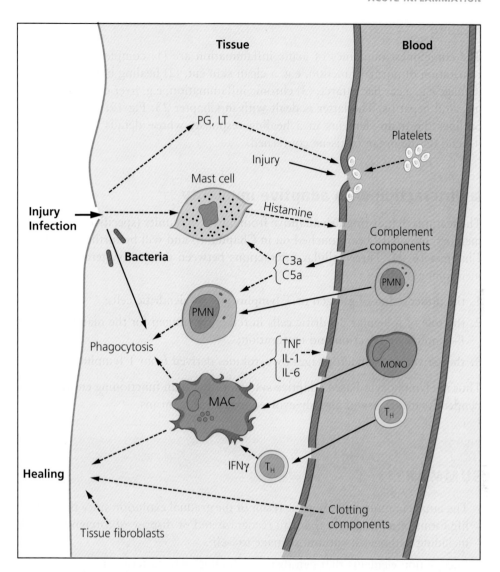

Fig. 12.11 Pathways of acute inflammation, showing the central role of vascular permeability. Solid arrows denote movement of cells/molecules; broken arrows denote effects on (1) blood-vessel permeability: prostaglandins, leukotrienes, TNF, IL-1, IL-6, inflammatory cytokines; (2) mast cell and PMN activity: C3a, C5a, breakdown products of C3 and C5; (3) phagocytosis of bacteria, also enhanced by antibody, not shown; (4) activation of macrophages: T lymphocytes. LT, leukotriene; PG, prostaglandin; T, T lymphocyte. For further details of lipid mediators see Chapter 23.

Once infection is eliminated and damaged tissue removed, healing can begin. Note that Fig. 12.11 represents a great oversimplification; literally dozens of mediators are involved in both the induction and the down-regulation of inflammation, and over 50 genes have been identified which, if deficient or experimentally knocked out, cause inflammation to be prolonged, excessive, or even fatal. In addition, there are pathogens which are not easily eliminated. We shall return to this topic when we consider allergies and chronic inflammation in Chapter 23.

Healing

The commonest outcomes of acute inflammation are (1) complete healing with restoration of normal function, e.g. a clean skin cut, (2) healing but with residual damage e.g. a cardiac infarct, (3) chronic inflammation, e.g. liver cirrhosis following viral hepatitis. The latter is dealt with in Chapter 23. Fig 12.11 (lower part) outlines the main elements in a healing response, whose details will obviously depend on the organ or tissue concerned.

■ Interaction with adaptive immunity

The features that distinguish adaptive from innate immunity (specificity, receptors, memory, etc.) have been touched on in Chapter 10 and will be further detailed in Chapters 16–21. Three cellular interactions between the two systems are worth mentioning here:

1. the presentation of antigen to T lymphocytes by dendritic cells;
2. the role of follicular dendritic cells in retaining antigen for the maintenance of B-lymphocyte selection and maturation;
3. the activation of macrophages by cytokines derived from T lymphocytes.

Thus the lymphocyte-based adaptive system, rather than functioning entirely independently, makes use of already evolved innate mechanisms.

SUMMARY

- The innate immune system is the result of the gradual evolution since the earliest life forms of mechanisms that can recognize and/or dispose of foreign material, including pathogens, without damage to 'self'.

- Recognition elements that can distinguish molecular patterns unique to pathogens include cell-associated 'pattern receptors' and some soluble molecules such as complement.

- Disposal is mainly carried out by phagocytic cells containing molecules, many of them oxygen- or nitrogen-derived, specialized for destroying endocytosed material. There are also NK cells specialized for killing virus-infected cells, some tumour cells, and some other pathogens.

- Communication between the cells of the innate immune system is mediated by small protein molecules called cytokines; examples are the IFNs, which also have antiviral activity.

- An important element of the immediate response to infection is inflammation, a complex series of changes resulting in the local enhancement of blood supply and increased availability of immune components.

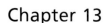

Chapter 13

How pathogens escape innate immunity

Just as any parasite wishing to get into the body has to overcome the external defences (see Chapter 11), for a pathogen to survive in the body for more than a few hours, it will have to escape the powerful defence mechanisms of innate immunity, described in the previous chapter: phagocytes, complement, etc. A pathogen that fails to do so will probably not survive long enough to spread to another host. The principal ways in which pathogens achieve this are summarized in Table 13.1, in which they are classified according to the immune component they are designed to avoid. Another way to look at them is by analogy with an agent operating in enemy territory, and from *his* point of view. He has four main choices: to conceal his presence, to camouflage his appearance, to wear protective clothing, or to destroy the enemy agents hunting him down.

1. In the case of pathogens, *concealment* includes getting inside host cells, as all viruses and many bacteria, fungi, and protozoa do, secreting impermeable barriers (some fungi), or inducing the host to form *cysts* or *granulomas* around the still-living pathogen (some bacteria and worms).
2. 'Camouflage' strategies are usually aimed at preventing recognition, a particularly vital point where the lymphocytes of adaptive immunity are concerned (see Chapter 22) but also effective against recognition by complement and/or phagocytes, for example, the *capsules* that cover the cell wall of many of the most virulent bacteria (see below), and devices for avoiding pattern recognition, for example by Toll-like receptors (TLRs).
3. 'Protective clothing' would correspond to the many devices pathogens have evolved to block or neutralize host attack, such as scavengers or inactivators of reactive oxygen intermediates.

Table 13.1 Some examples of pathogen strategies for escaping the defence mechanisms of the innate immune system

Strategy	Examples
Intracellular habitat	Viruses: HIV, measles
	Bacteria: mycobacteria, *Brucella*
	Fungi: *Cryptococcus*
	Protozoa: *Leishmania, Toxoplasma*
Avoiding pattern recognition via TLR	
Reduced activation by LPS	*Salmonella, Yersinia, Coxiella*
Signalling blocked	Vaccinia
Avoiding complement	
Capsules block activation	*Staphylococcus, Haemophilus, Neisseria meningitidis*
LPS side chains block complement	Gram-negative bacteria
Enzymes destroy complement components	*Pseudomonas*
Mimicry of receptors for complement	HSV
Expulsion of membrane attack complex	*Leishmania*
Avoiding phagocytosis	
Killing of phagocytic cell	*Staphyloccocus, Streptococcus, Listeria, Yersinia, Entamoeba*
Production of capsules	*S. pneumoniae, Haemophilus, N. meningitidis*
Prevention of opsonization by antibody	Staphylococci (protein A)
Paralysis of uptake	*Yersinia*
Inhibition of chemotaxis	*Clostridia*, streptococci
Avoiding being killed in phagocyte	
Entry without activation	*Leishmania*
Inhibition of phagosome–lysosome fusion and/or acidification	Mycobacteria, *Toxoplasma*
Inhibition of reactive oxygen intermediates	Staphylococci (catalase)
Resistance to killing mechanisms	Mycobacteria, *Salmonella, Brucella*
Escape into cytoplasm	*Listeria, Shigella*
Inhibition of dendritic cells	HIV, CMV, *Leishmania*, filaria
Interference with cytokine network	
Mimicry of cytokine receptors	Pox viruses
Mimicry of inhibitory cytokines	EBV
Inhibition of interferon	Adenovirus, vaccinia
Failure to induce interferon	Hepatitis B
Suppression of macrophage-derived cytokines	*Leishmania*, measles
Induction of inhibitory cytokines	*Yersinia* (IL-10)

4. Finally, some pathogens attack host defences directly, bacterial toxins that destroy phagocytes and complement-splitting enzymes being good examples of this.

The actual protective value of an individual escape mechanism is not always obvious, but if experimental deletion (e.g. by knocking out the gene concerned) leads to a reduction in virulence, one can be fairly sure of its importance to the pathogen. Note that many of the most successful survivors use more than one escape mechanism (e.g. *Leishmania*; see Table 13.1).

■ Avoiding pattern recognition

The importance of TLR and other cell-surface receptors in the initial recognition of microbial surfaces is described in Chapter 12. Pathogens can circumvent this in several ways (see Table 13.1). Particularly interesting examples are modifications of the LPS molecule to reduce or prevent TLR4 activation, the presence of viral proteins (such as A52R in vaccinia) which block signalling, the anthrax toxin which destroys some of the key signal transduction enzymes, and the modulation by *Listeria* of intracellular nucleotide oligomerization domain (NOD)-mediated detection. Some organisms such as *Yersinia* and *B. pertussis*, preferentially induce a strong IL-10 response as a result of TLR engagement which impairs innate immunity.

■ Avoiding complement

As well as blocking recognition by phagocytes, capsules can prevent activation of the alternative complement pathway. The thick peptidoglycan of Gram-positive membranes prevents the insertion of the C56789 complex, while *Leishmania* can expel the whole C56789 complex from its membrane, which then re-seals. Other anti-complement strategies include direct attack on the complement molecules themselves, by binding, cleaving, or expelling them. Examples include the elastase of *Pseudomonas* which destroys C3b and C5a, and the proteins of some viruses, bacteria, fungi, and protozoa which successfully mimic the inhibitors by which complement activation is normally regulated. Organisms that are usually exposed to the blood need to have multiple evasion strategies—*Staph. aureus* for example encodes at least 5 different molecules all targeting the mammalian complement system.

■ Avoiding phagocytosis

For bacteria, fungi, and protozoa, the phagocytic cell is their deadliest enemy, particularly when it is assisted by complement and/or antibody. Here pathogen survival strategies fall into three main categories: (1) prevent uptake; (2) if taken up, avoid being killed; (3) damage or destroy the phagocyte.

Preventing uptake

This can be further subdivided into the prevention of *recognition* and the *paralysis* of the *uptake* mechanism. The most striking example of the former is the bacterial *capsule*, usually polysaccharide, which covers up structures on the cell wall which the phagocyte would otherwise recognize (see TLR, above). The protective effect of a capsule is illustrated by experiments in mice. Whereas about 10 capsulated pneumococci can kill a mouse, it takes 10 000 if the capsules are removed; in other words the capsulated bacterium is 1000 times more virulent. There is a fascinating molecule secreted by staphylococci, *protein A*, which inhibits IgG antibody from attaching to receptors and enhancing phagocytosis (see Chapter 17 for the molecular basis of this), and there are complement decoy proteins too (see above). Paralysis of the cytoskeletal reorganization required for the membrane movements of phagocytosis represents a most sophisticated approach; *Yersinia* (the plague bacterium) can do this, via injection of its own enzymes across the phagocyte membrane (so-called Type III secretion), which can inhibit the assembly of host actin into microfilaments.

Survival in the phagocyte

Some pathogens take a quite different approach, namely to let themselves be phagocytosed but resist the killing process. Often they are so successful that they are able to live unmolested within macrophages for months or years and thus establish chronic infection. Mycobacteria (the tubercle and leprosy bacilli) are the classic example, but there are many others. Again, the mechanisms can be further subdivided, viz: (1) 'peaceful' entry into the phagocyte without triggering killing mechanisms (e.g. *Leishmania*); (2) escape from the phagosome into the cytoplasm, where killing mechanisms do not operate (e.g. *Listeria*); (3) inhibition of phagosome–lysosome fusion, notably by mycobacteria, the fungal pathogen *Histoplasma*, and the protozoan *Toxoplasma*; and (4) mopping up of microbicidal molecules, for example by the phenolic glycolipids of *Mycobacterium leprae*, the catalase of *Staph. aureus*, and the lipophosphoglycan of *Leishmania*, all of which counteract the respiratory burst and its toxic products. Bacteria can also evade antimicrobial peptides such as defensins by changing their surface structures and charge to reduce insertion of the peptide into their membranes or by actively removing or destroying the peptides via proteases. Note that in general, PMN have too short a lifespan to be suitable long-term hosts, but they can still aid pathogen survival (e.g. of phagocytosed *Leishmania*) by being themselves killed and then phagocytosed by macrophages—the 'Trojan Horse' strategy. Note also that intracellular survival is not just a matter of avoiding killing mechanisms but also of getting access to essential nutrients not freely available within cells. Thus, for example, mycobacteria prefer to live in endosomes where host iron stores are more plentiful. Finally, intracellular survival is a useful way for pathogens to travel to distant sites; the spread of staphylococci, *Toxoplasma* (to the brain), and HIV (in dendritic cells) being examples.

When we consider adaptive immunity (Chapter 20) you will see that these persistent intracellular pathogens constitute a real problem for the immune system. Activation of macrophages to overcome some of these inhibitory effects is one of the major roles of the T cell.

Damage to the phagocyte

The tendency of staphylococci and streptococci to cause cell necrosis is due to their *toxins*, the typical pus that fills a staphylococcal abscess being mainly composed of dead PMNs and destroyed tissue cells. A more subtle approach is the induction of macrophage apoptosis ('cell suicide') as practised by *Yersinia*. Interestingly, some pathogens (e.g. *Chlamydia* and some viruses) *inhibit* apoptosis to ensure longevity of their host cell, while some *Salmonella* and *Shigella* species promote inflammation in the intestine, possibly to provide more cells to invade.

■ Avoiding NK cells

Look back to Chapter 12 to be reminded that NK cells are inhibited by the presence of MHC class I molecules on the target cell. Some viruses (e.g. CMV) respond to this ingeniously by encoding an MHC class I homologue which tricks the NK cell into inactivity while not engaging the attention of cytotoxic T cells, which respond to real MHC molecules (see Chapter 18). Other viruses (e.g. HIV, HSV) are able to infect and destroy NK cells, block the production of activating cytokines (e.g. Type 1 IFNs), or interfere with the NK cells' cytolytic machinery.

■ Interference with dendritic cell function

Dendritic cells play a vital role in T-cell activation, and some pathogens can inhibit this by directly infecting dendritic cells, leading to reduced maturation and cytokine release. In the case of HIV, infection of dendritic cells via a surface C-type lectin (DC-SIGN) leads in turn to increased infection of T cells.

■ Interference with the cytokine network

Given the importance of cytokines in both natural and adaptive immunity, it is not surprising that pathogens have found ways to interfere with their function. There are now many different examples of how viruses specifically interfere with the immune system by encoding their own cytokines or cytokine inhibitors/decoys. Among the most remarkable are the possession by the EBV of a gene that codes for a molecule virtually identical to IL-10, a cytokine that inhibits the production of several other cytokines (an example of *mimicry*), and the possession by pox viruses of a molecule similar to the soluble TNF receptor, which can 'mop up' the natural cytokine (see Table 22.2). Virally encoded chemokine antagonists can block chemokine binding to receptors on migrating cells or interfere with chemokine display on the endothelial surface of blood vessels, in either case impairing the migration of cells to sites of inflammation. Inhibition of interferon induction or activity is another obviously useful strategy for viruses. In other cases the same result is achieved by stimulating the over-production by the host itself of inhibitory cytokines such as TGF-β and IL-10.

■ The role of vectors

Biting insects are an important means of transmission for several tropical pathogens (malaria, leishmaniasis, dengue, etc.; see Chapter 11) and may also help them survive. For example, the saliva of sandflies (the vector of *Leishmania*) inhibits macrophages and T cells, and can induce inhibitory host factors such as prostaglandin E_2 and IL-10. While not actually pathogen-derived, this local immunosuppression protects the pathogen in the earliest stages of infection (see Chapter 36).

Taking all these evasion strategies into consideration, one can appreciate that, powerful as innate immunity is, the battle does not always go its way. It is generally assumed that the success of these ingenious pathogens was the driving force for the evolution of adaptive immunity, to be described in Chapters 16–20.

SUMMARY

- Many of the most important pathogen virulence factors are aimed at escaping the effects of the innate immune system (and there are others for the adaptive system).
- Pathogens can conceal their presence inside cells, granulomas, or cysts.
- Various structures, such as capsules, can interfere with recognition by phagocytes or complement.
- Others can inactivate or decoy immune molecules, including complement and cytokines.
- Some pathogens destroy immune cells directly, neutrophils being especially vulnerable.

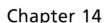

Chapter 14

Disease due to innate immunity

Referring back to Chapter 9, you will be reminded that disease—that is, pathology—is sometimes due to the pathogen alone (e.g. cytopathic viruses, toxins), but can also be produced by the immune system. Here we will discuss the ways in which innate immune mechanisms can lead to pathology; the much more diverse ways in which adaptive immunity can do this are described in Chapters 23 and 24.

■ Sepsis and septic shock

Both the phagocytic cells and the complement system have tremendous potential for damaging host cells, but fortunately they are normally only triggered by foreign materials, and usually most of their destructive effects are focused on the surface of these, or in the safe environment of the phagolysosome. However, there is a group of microbial molecules which can cause havoc in the immune system by overstimulating macrophages to release their cytokines. The best known is *endotoxin*, the cell-wall LPS of some but not all Gram-negative bacteria (see below and Table 14.1), which is responsible for many cases of *sepsis*. Gram-positive bacteria lack endotoxin, but their cell-wall peptidoglycans can have similar though not identical effects. They also release toxins (e.g. the TSST-1 of *Staph. aureus*) whose effects depend on over-stimulation of T lymphocytes (see Chapter 18).

Table 14.1 The major endotoxin-containing bacteria

E. coli	Klebsiella
Proteus	Neisseria
Bordetella	Salmonella
Pseudomonas	Shigella
Haemophilus	

Three related terms need to be distinguished: *septicaemia* denotes the presence of bacteria in the blood; *sepsis* refers to the failure of one or more organs caused by over-reaction to infection; *septic shock* describes the most severe situation with vascular collapse, which carries a mortality of up to 50%. For example, septicaemia, leading to septic shock, is one of the feared complications of *meningococcal meningitis*.

■ Endotoxin, cytokines, and disease

The number of systems affected by LPS, an innocuous-looking molecule (Fig. 14.1), is quite remarkable (Table 14.2). Some of these, for example the clotting system, are

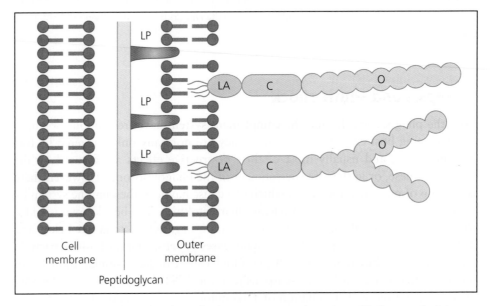

Fig. 14.1 Two LPS molecules in the wall of a Gram-negative bacterium. LP, lipoprotein; LA, lipid A; C, core polysaccharide; O, O polysaccharide side chains (O antigens).

Table 14.2 Pathological consequences of endotoxin and similar microbial molecules

Stages	Examples
Microbial components	Endotoxin (lipopolysaccharide)
	Exotoxins
	LTA, peptidoglycans
	Glycolipids
Recognition structures:	
Soluble	Complement
Cell-bound	TLR on endothelium, neutrophils, monocytes
Soluble mediators	Tissue factor, PAI-1
	Superoxide, NO, etc.
	Lysosomal enzymes
	Lipids (PAF, PGs)
	Cytokines (TNF, IL-1, IL-6, etc.)
	Chemokines (IL-8, MCP-1, MIP)
Pathological processes	Microvascular coagulation
	Capillary leakage
	Vasodilatation
	Hypo/hyperglycaemia
Clinical effects	Fever
	ARDS
	Shock
	Multiple-organ failure
	Death

ARDS, adult/acute respiratory distress syndrome; LTA, lipotechoic acid; MCP, monocyte chemotactic protein; MIP, macrophage-inflammatory protein; PAF, platelet-activation factor; PAI-1, plasminogen-activator inhibitor; PG, prostaglandin.

not strictly immunological, but the comment of a famous American immunologist that 'when we sense lipopolysaccharide, we are likely to turn on every defence at our disposal' makes the point.

The effects of LPS, particularly those on the vascular system, appear to be due mainly to the induction of excessive cytokine secretion by macrophages, mediated by complex signalling systems particularly involving TLR4 (Fig. 14.2). TNFα, IL-1, IL-6, IL-12 (and subsequently IFNγ) are the major cytokines involved. In some cases measuring levels of TNF in the blood of patients can predict their clinical outcome and risk of death. In a classic experiment it was shown that a neutralizing antibody against the cytokine TNFα was all that was needed to protect baboons from the otherwise lethal drop in blood pressure ('endotoxin shock')

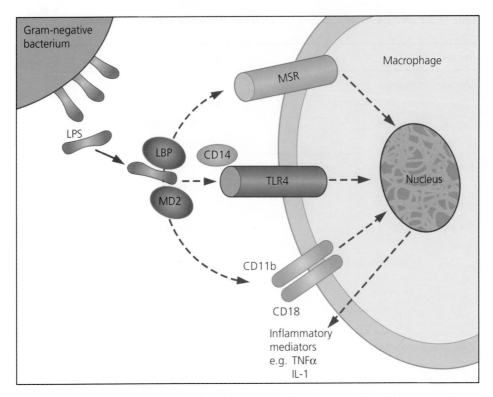

Fig. 14.2 Recognition of LPS occurs primarily via interaction of LPS and LPS-binding protein (LBP) with CD14–TLR4–MD2 but other receptors such as macrophage scavenger receptor (MSR) and CD11b/CD18 can also be involved. CD14, LPS receptor; MD2, TLR4 co-factor.

following a large injection of *E. coli*, and the same approach has been tried in patients with septic shock. This seemed to offer an alternative to the use of antibodies against endotoxin itself, which have proved very hard to produce. However, by its very nature, septic shock is a complex and multi-component syndrome, and the effects of cytokine-based intervention have been generally poor, although some selected patients have in fact responded. Usually when patients present to the physician they are already well into the cascade of cytokine production and at this stage blocking a single cytokine is too late. This is supported by the preclinical studies in experimental animals where such treatments need to be given at or before the time of infection in order to have a significant effect. However, there is evidence that some degree of self-regulation occurs naturally, in the form of cytokine inhibitors (e.g. TNF and IL-1 receptor antagonists), inhibitory cytokines (e.g. IL-10), complement inhibitors, anti-inflammatory corticosteroids, etc. Note that pathogens other than bacteria share the property of inducing high levels of inflammatory cytokines; these include mycobacteria, yeasts, and the malaria parasite.

Another target of endotoxin is the complement system (alternative pathway, see Fig. 12.3). Massive complement activation, with the consequent inflammation, can damage small blood vessels and this, together with the accumulation of PMNs and perhaps the direct effects of TNF, can lead to leakage of fluid into the lung alveoli, a condition known as *adult respiratory distress syndrome* (ARDS), one of the most dreaded complications of severe injury and/or infection. Widespread blood clotting (*disseminated intravascular coagulation*, DIC) and overactivation of the fibrinolytic pathway, coupled to the lowered blood pressure and decreased oxygen supply, lead to the vital organ failure of *septic shock*.

At a more benign level, many people have experienced the effects of small doses of endotoxin following injection of killed *Salmonella typhi* organisms—the original typhoid vaccine—and with a little practice one can distinguish for oneself the feeling of illness due to TNF and/or IL-1 (e.g. Gram-negative intestinal infections) from that due to interferon (e.g. severe influenza). It is suspected that the endotoxin of *Bordetella pertussis* may be to blame for the neurological complications attributed to the whooping-cough vaccine, although this whole field is controversial (see Chapter 28). There may also be a transient inflammatory response following treatment with antibiotics that disrupt large numbers of bacteria and release endotoxin, although other similar reactions may be allergic in nature, for example the Mazzotti reaction that can follow the killing of some worms.

Other cytokine-mediated diseases

There is evidence, mainly derived from experiments with mice one or more of whose cytokine genes have been knocked out, that several *inflammatory bowel diseases*, notably ulcerative colitis and Crohn's disease, may be due to excessive local cytokine secretion. In rheumatoid arthritis, raised levels of TNFα are found in joint fluid. The additional roles of infection and of adaptive (e.g. T cell) responses in these conditions has yet to be fully worked out. The role of cytokines in the *acute phase response*, including the fever often associated with infection, has been referred to in Chapter 12.

Attempts to control sepsis

Considering the number of steps in the sepsis pathway (see Fig 14.3 for some of these) and the number of factors involved, it might have been expected that various inhibitors might be effective in therapy. Unfortunately the results to-date have been disappointing. Inhibition of TNF and IL-1, of the coagulation pathway, and of TLR activation, have all been introduced with high hopes, but failed to influence survival significantly. Part of the problem is that when first detected, sepsis is often already far advanced. Another is that improved antimicrobial and intensive care strategies have themselves reduced mortality considerably.

Despite the disappointing results in septic shock (see above) inhibition of cytokines has proved of value in some clinical inflammatory conditions. Most strikingly, inhibiting TNFα over-production benefits many rheumatoid arthritis, Crohn's disease, and psoriasis patients. Thalidomide, a drug with a tragic clinical history, turns out to be a potent and relatively selective inhibitor of TNF production and is being tested for preventing TNF-mediated pathology and wasting in

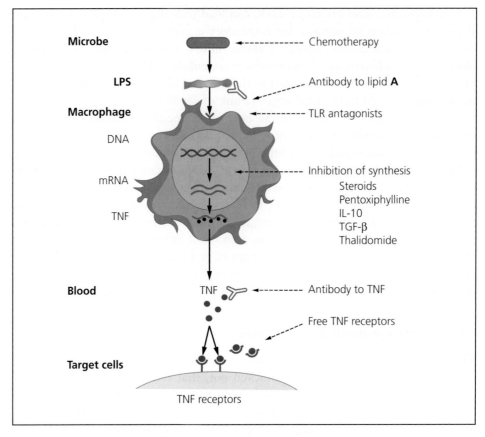

Fig. 14.3 The induction of excessive amounts of TNF by bacterial LPS could be inhibited at several levels. Similar strategies can be designed for other cytokines.

leprosy and HIV, respectively. One should remember, however, that there are dangers in interfering too drastically in pathways that have presumably been selected for their overall benefit. A few patients receiving these antibodies now show an increased risk of reactivating latent *M. tuberculosis*, reminding us that TNF is also an essential component of the protective innate response. Nevertheless the remarkable effect of anti-TNF drugs in rheumatoid arthritis (over a million patients treated to date) stands out as a rare example of useful intervention in the cytokine network. Figure 14.3 illustrates some possible approaches to these problems.

■ Complement and disease

The activation of complement, normally restricted to the vicinity of pathogens by inhibitors (see Chapter 12), may also lead to tissue damage in extreme cases; examples are endotoxin shock (see above) and *immune complex disease*, although the latter is initiated by antibody (see Chapter 23). Complement activation may also cause damage when one of the natural inhibitors is absent, as in the disease

CASE STUDY 14.1 Meningococcal meningitis and septicaemia

Presentation

A 17-year-old girl living with a school friend was visited by her mother, saying she thought she was going down with flu. She had been up late at a party two days earlier, where she admitted there had been 'a bit of contact'. Her mother had been a nurse and noticed that she had a temperature, had the light turned down low, and was reluctant to move her head because of a stiff neck. She had no obvious rash, but her mother took her to hospital, where the casualty officer detected faint petechial spots on her arms and legs, which did not fade when a glass slide was pressed on the skin. Meningitis was the probable diagnosis, and she was admitted to the ward.

Diagnosis

Because the most likely cause of the symptoms was *Neisseria meningitidis* infection (the patient had received the vaccine against *Haemophilus influenzae*, the other common cause, as a child), a lumbar puncture was performed. At this point it was noted that her pulse was rapid and blood pressure low. The rash was now obvious and widespread. Septicaemia was diagnosed. It was realized that due to error she had not been given the usual benzylpenicillin injection on admission. Intravenous ceftriaxone was begun immediately. She made an uneventful recovery, but was referred for testing for some possible residual deafness.

Treatment and prevention

About 20% of individuals carry *N. meningitidis* in their nose and throat without symptoms, yet it is the cause of 60% of bacterial meningitis infections, 90% of which are with type B (there are effective vaccines against types A and C). A vaccine against type B, based on protein rather than polysaccharide antigens, is still on trial. Since most of the pathology in meningococcal septicaemia appears to be due to the release by monocytes of high levels of the cytokines TNFα, Il-1, Il-8, and GCSF, in response to the bacterial endotoxin, future management may include anti-cytokine therapy, but at present antibiotics are the mainstay of treatment.

hereditary angioedema (see Chapter 15), in which C1 inhibitor levels are reduced and excessive activation of C2 and C4 leads to oedema of the face and airways. The effects of *complement deficiencies* are discussed in Chapter 15.

■ Polymorphs, mast cells, and disease

As mentioned in Chapter 12, much of the destructive power of phagocytes—particularly polymorphs—is due to the intracellular production of ROI derived from atmospheric oxygen. Unfortunately, whenever large numbers of polymorphs are activated, there is the risk of ROI escaping and damaging the surrounding tissues. It is thought that in some degenerative diseases, especially of blood vessels, the damage is caused by ROI, which is why chemists' shops are full of pills containing 'antioxidants' such as vitamin C, vitamin E, selenium, etc. Whether these really do any good has never been critically established, but certain lipids found in fish oil do appear to have mild anti-inflammatory activity.

For completeness we should mention the curious phenomenon of *anaphylactoid* reactions, in which mast cells are triggered by chemical means (e.g. some radiological contrast media) rather than as usual by antibody, and discharge their contents (histamine, etc.) resulting in violent and dangerous local inflammation.

SUMMARY

- Excessive stimulation of innate immune mechanisms can lead to dangerous and even fatal symptoms.

- Endotoxins (LPS from Gram-negative bacteria) and related molecules can over-activate the complement, clotting, and cytokine systems, leading to the vascular collapse of septic shock.

- Cytokine over-production, mainly by macrophages, may underlie the pathology of several chronic inflammatory diseases, including rheumatoid arthritis and psoriasis.

- Inhibitors of particular cytokines may have a role in therapy, though hitherto unsuccessful in sepsis.

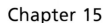

Chapter 15

Immunodeficiency I: primary defects of innate immunity

It would be surprising if such a complex collection of cells and molecules as the immune system did not occasionally malfunction. In fact, serious *immunodeficiency* is fairly rare (about three per 100 000 of the UK population, rising to one in 1500 if the most minor defects are included) but remains an important cause of increased susceptibility to infection. Almost any part of the immune system may be affected. Two main kinds of defect are recognized:

1. it may be faulty from the start because of a congenital defect (*primary immunodeficiency*);
2. it may be damaged later in life for a variety of reasons (*secondary immunodeficiency*).

In this chapter we will concentrate mainly on immunodeficiency affecting the innate immune system; defects of adaptive immunity, which are considerably more common (see Fig. 15.1), are dealt with in Chapter 25.

Genetics of primary immunodeficiency

Primary defects are *genetic* abnormalities, usually single recessive mutations, that affect the proper development of some component: currently some 120 of these have been defined. They may be *inherited* if the mutation is in a gene present in

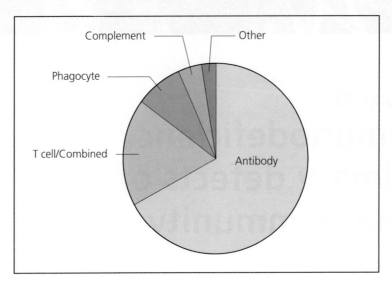

Fig. 15.1 Comparative frequencies of the major immune deficiency syndromes.

the germ-line; if not, they are *somatic* and will only affect one individual. Two patterns of inheritance can be distinguished, depending on which chromosome is affected.

1. X-linked. The gene lies on the X chromosome, but being recessive it does not cause symptoms in females, because they will also have a normal gene on the other X chromosome except in the rare *homozygous* situation where both their parents carry the defect. However, 50% of male offspring, which have only one X chromosome, will be affected. This is the same 'sex-linked' inheritance as seen in haemophilia: mother to male offspring.

2. Autosomal recessive. The gene lies on some other chromosome. Heterozygotes are likely to be normal *carriers*, but homozygotes (both parents being carriers) will be affected.

Since more than one mutation per gene is possible, and sometimes two or more versions of the same gene can coexist in the population (polymorphism), the results can vary from severe losses of some important immune function to quite mild deviations from the normal. Correspondingly some patients are dramatically prone to infection from birth or a few months later when maternal antibody has waned, whereas other defects pass unnoticed except in special circumstances, and even patients with the same defect may display varying levels of susceptibility to infection. Infections in immunodeficient patients include not only the common pathogens but also organisms that are not pathogenic at all in normal individuals: the so-called *opportunistic* infections (for some examples see Tables 15.1 and 26.7). In addition, there is often a significantly increased risk of malignancy and autoimmunity.

Ironically, the study of immunology has benefited greatly from immune deficiencies, which are often the best guide to the real role of a particular immune

Table 15.1 Common infections in defects of innate immunity

Defect	Most frequent infections			
	Viruses	Bacteria	Fungi	Protozoa and worms
Complement				
C3		Staphylococci, streptococci, Pseudomonas, Neisseria		
C5–C9		Neisseria		
Cytokines				
Interferon, IL-12	Respiratory	Mycobacteria		
Phagocytic cells		Staphylococci, streptococci, Pseudomonas	Candida, Aspergillus	
CGD		Staphylococci, E. coli		
MPO			Candida	
NK cells	Herpes			
Other				
Cystic fibrosis		Staphylococci, Haemophilus, Pseudomonas		
Splenectomy*		S. pneumoniae, N. meningitidis		Babesia

CGD, chronic granulomatous disease; MPO, myeloperoxidase.
*Probably includes an element of adaptive (antibody) deficiency.

component. Further knowledge has come from animals, either from naturally occurring defects or, most informative of all, from the deliberately engineered elimination of particular genes by the so-called knock-out technology. In general, it has been found that the absence of most immune components affects only resistance to infection (and some tumours), although it is of course possible that some of the defects we do *not* see are in fact incompatible with normal fetal development for other reasons.

Immunodeficiency versus susceptibility

In Chapter 9 we reviewed the evidence that individual genetic differences can increase host susceptibility to a single pathogen. Clearly this could be considered a form of very restricted immunodeficiency. However, the same genetic difference might affect different pathogens in different ways. A good example is the chemokine receptor deletion CCR5Δ32 which in double dose protects significantly against HIV-1, but also appears to increase susceptibility to West Nile virus. Whether this deletion is beneficial or harmful therefore depends on the individual environment. Indeed the mounting evidence for effects of HLA alleles on suscep-tibility/resistance suggest that almost every HLA phenotype could ultimately be regarded as 'immunodeficient' in some respect, yet it obviously makes no sense to call all HLA phenotypes 'abnormal'.

■ Primary defects of innate immunity

The most common primary defects affecting the innate system are those involving complement and phagocytic cells, which give rise to quite characteristic patterns of infection (Table 15.1).

Complement defects

Four main patterns of complement deficiency can be distinguished.

1. Reduced levels of C1s esterase inhibitor, resulting in overactivity of the 'classi-cal' pathway and reduction in levels of C2 and C4, with recurrent inflamma-tory attacks and swelling of mucosal tissue which may lead to laryngeal or intestinal obstruction. This condition, the commonest defect involving comple-ment, is known as *hereditary angioedema*. Other regulatory proteins may more rarely be deficient.

2. Low or absent levels of C1, C2, or C4, which lead to difficulty in clearing anti-gen–antibody complexes from the circulation, and are a frequent feature of the disease systemic lupus erythematosus, in which the kidney and other organs are damaged by the deposition of immune complexes (see Chapter 23); a defect in the maintenance of self-tolerance in B lymphocytes may also contribute.

3. Low or absent levels of C5–C9, which predispose to serious infections with bacteria of the *Neisseria* class such as disseminated gonorrhoea and meningo-coccal meningitis. This increased susceptibility suggests that in this group of infections, the formation of a lytic membrane-attack complex (see Chapter 12) is of real importance in clearing the infection. It is surprising that the great majority of bacterial infections are *not* worsened by these defects, emphasizing the importance of phagocytosis rather than lysis in most infections.

4. In the absence of the central component C3 survival is, as one might expect, extremely rare, though it has been reported.

Other soluble molecules

Deficiency of the mannose-binding lectin, MBL, can lead to severe infections in children. MBL is a member of the collectin family (see Chapter 12) with a role in complement activation, phagocytosis, and inflammation, and considerable indi-vidual variations exist in MBL levels, reflected in different susceptibility to infection, particularly in young children. In addition there are mutations that affect the structure of the molecule, or that lead to its complete absence; such children are at increased risk of severe recurrent bacterial and fungal infections. Low MBL levels in adults are less serious except when adaptive immunity is also defective, as for example in AIDS (see Chapter 26).

Other deficiencies in innate recognition

Children with defects in molecules involved in the early or late stages of TLR signalling do have increased susceptibility to bacterial infections, particularly with *S. pneumoniae*. Mutations affecting TLR3 predispose to encephalitis caused by HSV-1 but apparently not to disease in other tissues or to infection with other viruses. Interestingly the incidence of infection decreases in children with some defects (e.g. the signalling molecule IRAK-4) as they get older.

Cytokines

The most commonly reported defects in innate cytokines relate to the IL-12, IL-23, and IFNγ axis. Defects in either chain of the IFNγ receptor, IL-12p40 (shared in both IL-12 and IL-23) or the IL-12 receptor β chain (used to respond to both IL-12 and IL-23) predispose to serious infection with intracellular bacteria such as atypical mycobacteria, *Salmonella*, *Listeria*, and unfortunately even the BCG vaccine. Deficiencies in the signal transduction molecule STAT-1 also impair responses to IFNα and IFNγ, and cause additional susceptibility to repeated viral infections. Children with defects in IFNγ receptors are most severely affected and often die before the age of 10. This group of cytokine deficiencies is now called Mendelian susceptibility to mycobacterial disease, to reflect the greater risk from otherwise attenuated mycobacteria, but it may also be responsible for increased susceptibility to virulent *M. tuberculosis* too. Interestingly, absence of the chemokine receptor CCR5 causes significant *resistance* to HIV infection (see above), this molecule being also the macrophage 'second receptor' for the virus.

Cellular defects

Defects in myeloid cell development

1. In reticular dysgenesis there is bone-marrow stem-cell failure with an almost complete absence of blood monocytes and neutrophils plus reduced numbers of lymphocytes and a rapidly fatal outcome.

2. Congenital neutropenia (low or absent neutrophil numbers) may be constant or cyclical, leading to severe bacterial and fungal infections. In the cyclical type, blood neutrophils oscillate periodically with often a 3-week cycle and recurring bouts of oropharyngeal and/or skin infection.

Defects in myeloid cell function

Phagocytic cells

1. Inability to respond to chemotactic stimuli and move through the tissues towards an inflammatory site due to defects in integrin activation, the actin cytoskeleton, or proteolytic enzyme function.

2. Leucocyte adhesion deficiency. Inability to attach to vascular endothelium as a prelude to migrating from blood to tissue. Two different defects have been identified, both affecting molecules involved in leucocyte–endothelial cell interaction. As a result blood leucocyte levels are abnormally raised but functions such as chemotaxis and phagocytosis may be reduced. Bacterial and fungal infections are therefore common. Killing by T and NK cells may also be impaired.

3. Chediak–Higashi syndrome. Failure of phagosomes to fuse with lysosomes (see also NK cells, below).

4. Chronic granulomatous disease.

Chronic granulomatous disease

A defect in one of the four components of NADPH oxidase involved in the oxidative killing pathway (see Chapter 12, Fig. 12.8), leading to prolonged infection and abscess and granuloma formation with bacteria and fungi that would normally be killed by the oxidative burst. Catalase-positive organisms are the most dangerous because they produce catalase which destroys hydrogen peroxide, while catalase-negative organisms such as *S. pneumoniae* produce their own hydrogen peroxide

---

CASE STUDY 15.1 Chronic granulomatous disease

Presentation
A 7-month old boy was brought to the doctor with an open abscess on one leg. On examination the lymph nodes in both groins were enlarged and one appeared to be suppurating. He had a history of recurrent ill-health with episodes of productive cough and was just below normal weight for his age. He was referred to hospital with a suspected diagnosis of an immune defect.

Diagnosis
Microscopy of the ulcer revealed a massive infection with the filamentous fungus *Aspergillus fumigatus*. Culture of pus from the groin lymph node showed strong growth of *Staphylococcus aureus*. His blood count was within normal limits but an NBT test on a drop of blood was negative (PMN did not reduce formazan to a blue product) and this was confirmed by flow cytometry with DHR-rhodamine. A diagnosis of chronic granulomatous disease (CGD) was made and treatment was started at once with antifungals.

Management
After complete evaluation he was maintained on long-term antibiotics, interferon gamma, and prednisone.

which to some extent overrides the cell's defect. Thus the dominant bacterial infections are with staphylococci, *Pseudomonas*, *Burkholderia*, *Serratia marcescens*, in addition to fungi such as *Aspergillus* and *Candida*. Many mutations can give rise to the disease, about 90% of which are X-linked; roughly 2-5 per million births are affected.

NK cells

In the Chediak–Higashi syndrome, the intracellular movement of lysosomes is abnormal, resulting in giant non-functional lysosomes. NK cell and neutrophil-mediated killing is affected (and in some cases that of cytotoxic T cells too, see Chapter 20).

Total absence of NK cells is very rare and is associated with repeated infection with the herpes viruses HSV and CMV.

Cystic fibrosis

In this recessive but common condition, which is due to defects in the transmembrane molecule cystic fibrosis transmembrane conductance regulator (CFTR), required to transport chloride ions across epithelia, abnormally sticky mucus prevents the normal functioning of the muco-ciliary escalator (see Chapter 11) and other organs, notably the gut and pancreas. Over 1000 different mutations can cause the disease, which affects one in 4000 to 30 000 births, depending on the country. The lung infections are similar to those in CGD (see above). Although not strictly an immune defect, cystic fibrosis is one of the commonest causes of repeated bacterial lung infections in children.

Treatment

The treatment of both innate and adaptive immunodeficiency syndromes is discussed in Chapter 25. In the case of the innate defects, replacement therapy is usually not practicable and management usually relies on treatment of infection with antibiotics. However long-term administration of the cytokines G-CSF in neutropenia and IFNγ in CGD can substantially reduce the severity of infection.

■ Secondary immunodeficiency

Most adult immunodeficiencies fall into this category, and taken together they are far more common than the primary deficiencies discussed above. The causes range from malnutrition (the commonest worldwide) to infections such as HIV, tumours, drugs, X-irradiation, trauma, and diseases such as diabetes. It is not always possible to identify which immune component is affected, but since there is usually an element of lymphocyte (adaptive) involvement, they will be discussed in more detail in Chapter 26.

SUMMARY

- Immunodeficiencies are classified as primary (genetic) and secondary (due to external causes).

- Primary defects can be autosomal or sex-linked. The commonest sex-linked ones are X-chromosome-linked (inherited from mother to son).

- In the innate immune system, complement, MBL, cytokines, and NK and myeloid cells may display deficiencies.

- Phagocytic cells may be deficient in movement, attachment to vessel walls, phagocytosis, or intracellular killing.

- Secondary immunodeficiency is discussed in Chapter 26.

Tutorial 2

You have now learned something about the immune system, and quite a lot about innate immunity. Write specimen sets of headings for the following essay questions, concentrating as before on presenting them in a logical and interesting sequence. Some comments and ideas for you to consider in response to these questions are given in the section at the back of the book (p. 371).

1.   *'Because the phagocytes have retained the primitive property of taking up food, they can act as destroyers of parasites. They seem, therefore, as the bearers of Nature's healing power . . .' (Metchnikoff, 1884).* Was Metchnikoff right?

2.   *'. . . the mixture becomes clear and red within minutes . . . the corpuscles of this rabbit have thus become sensitive to their own alexine under the influence of a foreign clumping substance from a guinea pig treated with injections of the blood' (Bordet, 1898).* What did Bordet mean by alexine? What was the clumping substance? Discuss the significance of Bordet's finding.

3. Cytokines are the hormones of the immune system. Discuss.

4. Recognition of foreignness; the more specific the better. Discuss.

5. Oxygen is the cell's best friend and worst enemy. Discuss.

6. What is 'natural' about natural killer (NK) cells?

Chapter 16

Adaptive immunity: introduction

Compared to the numerous components of the innate immune system just described, adaptive immunity, which evolved around the time of the first vertebrates (see Box 10.2) merely added one new element, a small round cell called the *lymphocyte*. But the possibilities inherent in this cell are so extraordinary and apparently endless that the adaptive immune system ranks second only to the brain in scope and flexibility. It is called 'adaptive' because of the way it allows both species and individuals to 'tailor-make' their own set of recognition molecules, adapted to the microbes they actually encounter, rather than simply relying on a fixed set and hoping that one or other of them will succeed. The analogy has already been made of the immune system as a kind of army, but another good parallel is with the *police*: if innate immunity is like the policeman on the street, watching out for obvious villains of whatever kind, adaptive immunity is like the detective branch, trained to spot each individual criminal, however elusive, track him down, and keep him on file for the future. In immunological language, the system displays *high specificity* and *memory*.

■ The lymphocyte

Besides specificity and memory, two other properties distinguish lymphocytes from other immunological cells: the ability to *recirculate* throughout the body and the ability to *proliferate* and *differentiate* (that is, to *respond*) on demand. Table 16.1 brings out the essential differences between lymphocytes and phagocytic cells.

Table 16.1 Lymphocytes differ from phagocytic cells such as macrophages in four main respects, which together maintain the flexibility of the adaptive immune system

1. They *recirculate* through the blood, tissues, and lymphoid organs, waiting to encounter foreign molecules (or *antigens*).

2. They are individually *specific* for the antigens they recognize. This is due to the possession of antigen-specific surface receptors.

3. When they recognize 'their' antigen, they *respond* by proliferating and switching on a particular function (e.g. cytotoxicity; secretion of antibody or cytokines).

4. Once they have functioned, some of them remain for years as *memory* cells, with the capacity for faster and larger future responses.

Table 16.2 B and T lymphocytes differ in several important respects

	B lymphocytes	T lymphocytes
Origin	Bone marrow (in the liver in fetal life, in the bursa in birds)	Thymus (stem cells from bone marrow)
Recognition molecules	Antibody (immunoglobulin)	T-cell receptor
Secreted product(s)	Antibody	Cytokines
Disposal mechanisms	Antibody (leading to phagocytosis, lysis)	Some T cells are cytotoxic, others activate phagocytes
Mainly effective against	Extracellular infection	Intracellular infection

There are two major classes of lymphocyte, known as B and T because of their origin from the *bone marrow* and *thymus*, respectively (by a lucky chance, the B cells of birds are derived from an organ near the cloaca called the *bursa* of Fabricius). Put very simply, B lymphocytes (or B cells as they are often called) are responsible for 'policing' the extracellular body spaces—blood, tissue fluids, etc.— whereas T cells monitor the intracellular compartments, a more difficult task. However, as you will see (Chapters 19 and 20) they frequently interact with each other and with components of the innate immune system. Furthermore, once lymphocytes have carried out their recognition step, phagocytic cells, complement, etc. are still responsible for much of the disposal of the foreign material. Table 16.2 sums up the main differences between B and T cells.

■ The lymphoid system

This term is used to describe the total mass of lymphocytes in the body, some of which are at any given time recirculating through the blood, while others are in scattered solid organs such as the lymph nodes, spleen, tonsils, etc. (Fig. 16.1). It is

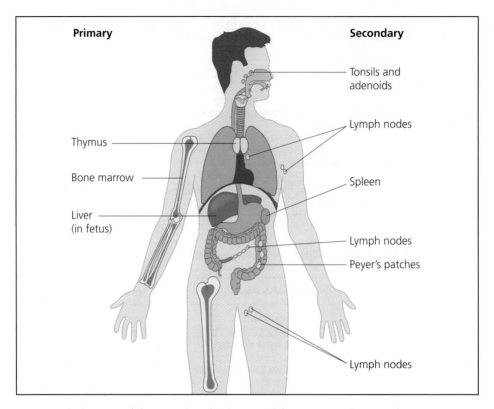

Fig. 16.1 The location of the major lymphoid organs: left, primary; right, secondary.

estimated that, if put together, the lymphocytes of a normal adult would occupy a space about the size of a football. Lymphoid organs are conventionally classified as *primary* or *secondary*, the former being the sites of lymphocyte formation and the latter the sites in which they carry out their function of recognizing and responding to foreign material. Secondary lymphoid organs are situated in strategic positions where infectious organisms are likely to be found: lymph nodes for the tissues; the spleen for the blood; tonsils and adenoids for the nose and throat; Peyer's patches and other lymphoid collections for the gut. A simple test for the difference between primary and secondary lymphoid organs is that if a primary organ fails to develop or is removed very early in life, the corresponding population of lymphocytes is permanently missing; this does occasionally happen (see primary immunodeficiency, Chapter 25).

Within the lymphoid organs, B and T lymphocytes are concentrated in particular sites, mainly determined by the resident antigen-presenting cells (APCs) and chemokines in the different microenvironments. Different cells 'present' foreign molecules (the word *antigen* is used for molecules that lymphocytes recognize, as will be explained in Chapters 17 and 18), and the flow of lymphocytes through the lymphoid organs is arranged so that each type encounters the right APC as well as other lymphocytes with which it needs to interact. Figure 16.2 illustrates

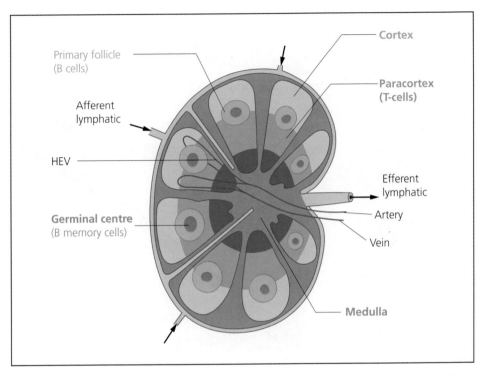

Fig. 16.2 The structure of a typical lymph node, showing the compartmentalization of B and T lymphocytes. Only one vascular loop is shown. HEV is a high endothelial venule, the site of lymphocyte emigration from blood to lymph node.

the general design of a lymph node, and Figure 16.3 shows the different arrangement in the spleen.

■ Recirculation

The ability to recirculate through the tissues, the lymphoid organs, and the blood is a fundamental part of lymphocyte function, enabling any lymphocyte eventually to make contact with an antigen, no matter where it is. Recirculation follows two patterns: (1) a constant 'tick-over' that goes on all the time, from blood to tissues to lymph and back to blood, even in the absence of infection, and (2) an enhanced and focused attraction of lymphocytes to where an antigen actually is; for example, the site of an infection. These processes are mediated by various adhesion molecules on both lymphocytes and blood vessels and by special cytokines known as *chemokines*, as shown in Table 16.3. Note that T and B lymphocytes are not identical in their homing characteristics, and also that the circulation of lymphocytes is quite distinct from that of cells of the myeloid lineage. Neutrophils circulate only through the bloodstream and do not enter the tissues except at local sites of inflammation or infection, from which they do not return.

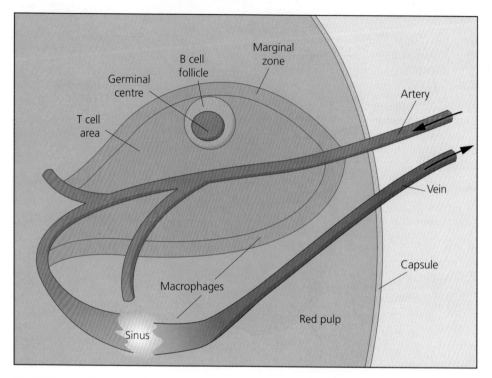

Fig. 16.3 A small portion of the spleen, showing a central arteriole surrounded by the periarteri-olar T cell zone, and one B cell follicle containing a germinal centre. Most of the organ is made up of red pulp containing red cells and macrophages; this is where old red cells and other parti-cles are removed from the circulation.

Monocytes show an intermediate pattern, with a high baseline rate of entry into the tissues (up to 50% of blood monocytes per day) which is further increased in response to inflammation.

■ Antigen and antigen-recognition molecules

As already mentioned, it is in recognition that lymphocytes excel. The surface molecules used by B and T cells are not the same, but they share one absolutely vital feature. They are put together from several genes in a huge number of pos-sible combinations, in such a way that each lymphocyte carries a different combi-nation and, as a result, recognizes a different shaped molecule, or, in immunological jargon, displays a different *specificity*. Molecules recognized in this way are referred to as *antigens;* the word originally meant substances that induced anti-body (see Chapter 17) but the definition has been widened to include any molecule specifically recognized by a B or T cell recognition unit or *receptor*. The word *immunogen* is sometimes used to describe molecules that induce a specific immune response (see Chapters 19, 20). The basic plan is shown in Fig. 16.4, and further details will be given in later chapters. The T-cell antigen-recognizing molecule is

Table 16.3 Adhesion molecules involved in leucocyte migration, adhesion, and activation

Molecule/expressed on	Target cell	Effect
I. Selectins		
L-Selectin/leucocytes	HEV, endo	Bind carbohydrates,
P-Selectin/platelets, act endo	Platelets, endo, PMN	initial binding,
E-Selectin/act endo	Leucocytes	lymphocyte recirculation
II. Integrins		
LFA-1/leucocyte subsets	endo, APC	Adhesion and arrest,
MAC-1 (CR3)/mono; PMN; mac	endo, C3b on pathogens	leucocyte extravasation
VLA-1/PMN; T; mono.	endo	via HEV or inflammation,
LPAM-1/lymphocytes; mono	endo	T cell–APC interactions, phagocytosis, homing to gut
III. Immunoglobulin superfamily		
ICAM-1/DC; act endo	T cells, phagocytes	Ligands for integrins,
VCAM-1/act endo	PMN, T, mono	leucocyte migration,
ICAM-3/naïve T cells	DC	T cell–APC interaction
Other		
CD44/memory T cells	endo/extracellular matrix	Adhesion

act, activated; APC, antigen-presenting cell; DC, dendritic cell; endo, endothelium; HEV, high endothelial venule; ICAM, intercellular adhesion molecule; LFA, leucocyte function antigen; LPAM, lymphocyte Peyer's patch adhesion molecule; mac, macrophage; mono, monocyte; VCAM, vascular cell adhesion molecule; VLA, very late activation (antigen).

known, logically, as the *T-cell receptor* (TCR). That on the B cell is known as *immunoglobulin* or *antibody*, being structurally similar to the antibody secreted by the B cell when triggered.

■ Clonal selection and memory

An individual lymphocyte that recognizes selectively 'its own' antigen (plus various signals from cytokines) will respond by proliferating into a population of lymphocytes with identical specificity. This population is referred to as a *clone*, and the sequence of (1) selection of one lymphocyte to respond and (2) expansion into a clone is known as *clonal selection*. The enlargement of lymph nodes during infection reflects the trapping of antigen-specific lymphocytes and their clonal expansion. Note that this would be very inefficient in the absence of recirculation; thus clonal selection and recirculation are interdependent. Some of the members of the clone will then differentiate and carry out their function (the actual functions of B and T cells are different; see Chapters 17–20) while others stay behind as *memory cells*. Thus any subsequent (secondary) response to the same antigen will start from a larger number of lymphocytes of the right specificity, and the

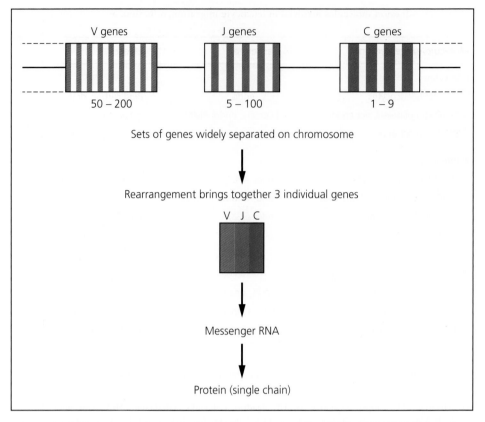

Fig. 16.4 The basic pattern of lymphocyte receptor generation. V, variable genes; J, joining genes; C, constant genes. In some cases there are also one or more D (diversity) genes between V and J. Since both the B-cell receptor (antibody) and the T-cell receptor are made up of two different chains, the possible combinations (the B- and T-cell 'repertoires') run into millions. This process of rearrangement occurs only in lymphocytes. In all other cells the genes remain in their original separated (and therefore non-functional) locations.

response will be faster and bigger, with changes in antibody affinity (B cells) and triggering requirements (T cells) (Fig. 16.5). The host is now said to display memory for that particular antigen, and if the antigen is potentially dangerous—a bacterial toxin, for example—the difference between a secondary and a primary response may be the difference between life and death.

■ Regulation of adaptive immunity

Given this ability to proliferate and accelerate their response, lymphocytes clearly need fairly tight regulation, otherwise a single response would be in danger of occupying the entire system. In fact both B and T cells are under several types of control, involving both the inhibition of their proliferation and their actual death (see Chapter 21 for further details), with the result that responses usually die down when they have achieved their purpose of eliminating the infection. But if elimination fails or regulation is faulty, *immunopathology* and *autoimmunity* may result, as you will see in Chapters 23 and 24.

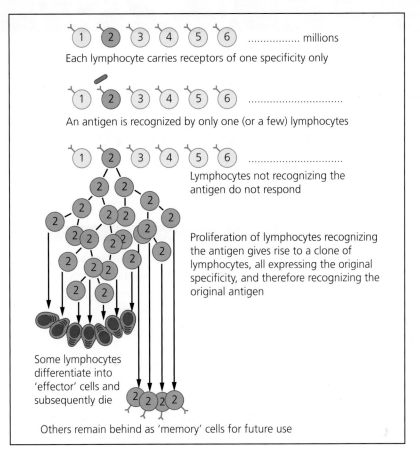

Fig. 16.5 Adaptive immunity operates on the principle of clonal selection. Since individual lymphocytes rearrange their receptor genes differently (see Fig. 16.4), they express only one of the millions of possible specificities in the 'repertoire'. A lymphocyte recognizing a particular antigen is selected for expansion into a clone of plasma cells (as shown) or effector T lymphocytes large enough to mount an effective response. Both B and T lymphocytes undergo clonal selection, although with slight differences in the later stages.

SUMMARY

- Adaptive immunity makes use of the special properties of lymphocytes. These are recirculating cells, each specifically able to recognize a particular antigen through the possession of restricted surface-recognition molecules.

- The two main types of lymphocyte have different origins (B cells, bone marrow; T cells, thymus) and use different recognition molecules (B cells, antibody; T cells, T-cell receptor, TCR).

- Antibody and TCR specificity is achieved by rearrangement of genes (V, J, and C) in the germ-line to produce a unique sequence of DNA, mRNA, and protein.

- When stimulated, lymphocytes proliferate into clones of identical daughter cells, some of which mature into effector cells, while others remain as memory cells.

Chapter 17

B cells and antibody

B lymphocytes (or B cells) are essentially little antibody factories, able to switch on high-rate synthesis and secretion of antibody molecules when stimulated by recognition of the 'right' antigen (the word *antigen* strictly implies a molecule that stimulates antibody production, but it is loosely used for any molecule recognized by a lymphocyte). When this happens the cell changes its appearance from the rather dull-looking lymphocyte, which is almost all nucleus, to the large plasma cell, with its cytoplasm full of rough endoplasmic reticulum (Fig. 17.1). High-rate antibody synthesis (up to 100 000 molecules per minute) can be kept up for 4–5 days, after which the plasma cell normally dies.

Recognition and response in B cells are perfectly coordinated, because their surface antigen receptor is the *same molecule* (antibody) as they will secrete when stimulated. Thus only those antibody molecules are made that can bind to the stimulating antigen and help in its disposal, and production of unwanted antibodies is avoided. Having said this, it must be added that recognition is a relative matter (see below) and some of the antibody made during an infection probably binds too weakly—or in immunological jargon, is of too low *affinity*—to be of great use. However, the affinity of some antibodies is very high indeed, up to 10^{-11} molar, which is above the range of most enzyme–substrate interactions, and when thousands of antibody molecules bind to the surface of a virus or a bacteria, the microbe is doomed unless it takes evasive action (which many do, see Chapter 22). The diversity of the antibody repertoire is so enormous (look back to Chapter 16 to be reminded of the genetic recombination events that allow this) that it is very rare to find a microbial molecule, or even a totally synthetic one, against which antibody cannot be made.

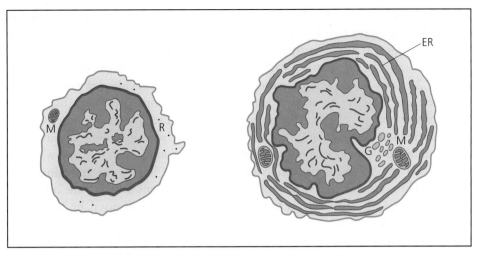

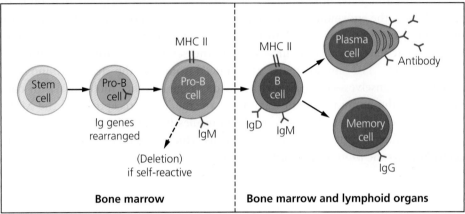

Fig. 17.1 Top: the resting B lymphocyte (left) has a small amount of cytoplasm, containing few organelles and only occasional ribosomes (R). The plasma cell (right) has more cytoplasm, mainly occupied by ribosome-rich rough endoplasmic reticulum (ER) which, together with the Golgi apparatus (G) is the site of high-rate antibody synthesis. Mitochondria (M) are more prominent in the metabolically active plasma cell (×8000). Bottom: B cells are produced by a series of maturation steps from precursors in the bone marrow.

■ The antibody molecule

Antibodies are globular proteins, which explains their alternative name *immunoglobulins* (sometimes abbreviated to Ig). They are found predominantly in the gamma region on electrophoresis (but also in the beta and alpha 2 regions), and the name *gammaglobulin* is sometimes applied to crudely purified antibody preparations, for example, as used in treatment of antibody-deficient patients (see Chapters 25 and 28).

Antibodies are made up of four polypeptide chains: two long or *heavy* chains and two short or *light* chains. The two heavy chains are identical and so are the two light chains, and each chain is coded for by genes rearranged as described in the previous chapter (see Fig. 16.4). The result is a Y-shaped molecule with the variable regions at the two tips of the Y and as its stem the constant region, to which only heavy chains, with their larger constant portions, contribute (Fig. 17.2). Even the constant regions of all antibody molecules are not identical, because there are nine different C genes and an individual B cell can use one or other of these, often switching C genes in mid-response. This is because different constant regions can mediate different biological effects, including activation of innate immune elements such as phagocytic cells or complement (see below). Thus the antibody molecule can be seen as a focusing device linking the individual antigen, bound to one end, to a variety of disposal mechanisms to which the other end binds. In effect, the antibody is marking the antigen for disposal by the innate immune system.

Note that there are many other soluble molecules with the ability to bind to and dispose of pathogens, notably the collectins (see Chapter 12), but that none of these display the enormous discriminating power of antibody since their genes are not subject to recombination. A further interesting point about the antibody molecule is that its general structure—that is, the sequence of *domains* containing approximately 110 amino acids, and indeed some of the actual amino acid sequences themselves—is shared with a wide range of other molecules with connections to the immune system. Examples are the T-cell receptor and the MHC molecules (see Chapter 18) and various molecules involved in adhesion, lymphocyte activation, and binding antibody to cells which, together with antibody, are referred to as the *immunoglobulin superfamily*.

■ Antibody classes and subclasses

All antibody molecules using a particular heavy-chain constant-region gene, whatever their specificity for antigen, are defined as belonging to the same *class*. The differences between different classes are fairly major, but there are smaller differences within classes, which are referred to as *subclasses*. In evolutionary terms, the class differences go back to the earliest vertebrates, whereas subclasses have evolved more recently. Thus fishes, birds, and mammals all have the IgG class, but their subclasses (IgG1, IgG2, etc.) evolved independently and are quite different for each species. The term *isotype* is used to cover both classes and subclasses.

The five classes—M, D, G, E, and A—differ considerably in their biological effects (Table 17.1). In general, IgG is the most useful and constitutes about 75% of the serum immunoglobulins. It is active both in the blood and in the tissues, can activate both complement and phagocytosis, and can cross the placenta, giving the fetus and newborn a protective level of maternal antibodies against many common infections. However, its half-life is only a few weeks, so after about 6 months maternal IgG is essentially all gone and the baby must make its own. IgM, which was probably the first antibody to evolve, also activates complement, and owing

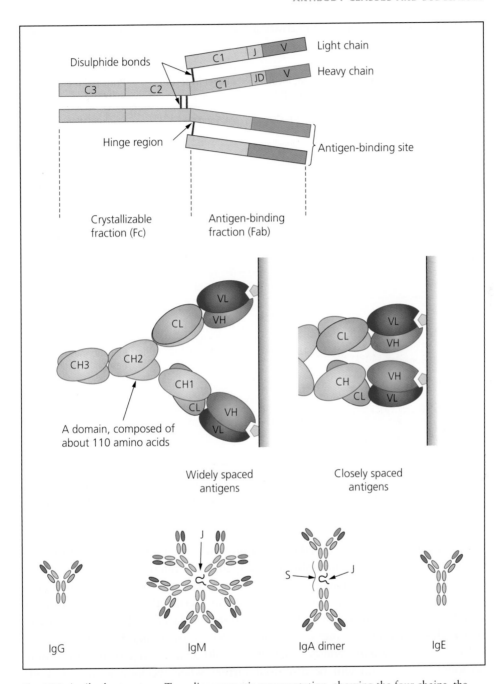

Fig. 17.2 Antibody structure. Top: diagrammatic representation, showing the four chains, the products of the rearranged genes (V, C, and J), and some of the terminology. Centre: how the molecule folds, emphasizing the repeating 'domain' structure and the value of the hinge region in adapting to differently spaced antigens. Both illustrations are of the IgG molecule. Bottom: the other classes differ in the number of C regions and disulphide bonds, and the total number of chains (Table 17.1). C, constant region; J, joining chain; S, secretory piece; V, variable region; dark, variable domains; light, constant domains.

Table 17.1 Antibodies are divided into classes and subclasses according to the C genes used for their heavy chains

Class and subclass	Number of C domains	Molecular weight (Da)	Level in serum	Principal biological activities
IgM	4 (×5) (pentameric structure)	970 000	1.5 mg ml^{-1}	Agglutination; complement activation
IgD	3	184 000	30 μg ml^{-1}	B cell triggering
IgG1	3	146 000	9 mg ml^{-1}	Complement activation; opsonization for phagocytosis; reaches extravascular spaces; transfer across placenta
IgG2	3	146 000	3 mg ml^{-1}	As IgG1 but less
IgG3	3	170 000	1 mg ml^{-1}	As IgG1
IgG4	3	146 000	0.5 mg ml^{-1}	As IgG1, but does not activate complement
IgE	4	188 000	50 mg ml^{-1}	Binds to mast cells and basophils; involved in allergies
IgA1 and 2				
Serum	3	160 000	3.5 mg ml^{-1}	
Secretory	3 (×2) (dimeric structure)	380 000	–	Active in secretions

Here the essential characteristics and properties are shown for human antibodies. Note that activities not involving the Fc region (such as neutralization of toxins) can be performed by all classes of antibody.

to its size (almost 1 million Da, the largest protein in the blood) and its 10 antigen-binding sites, it is able to immobilize and agglutinate microbes very efficiently. It cannot, however, get out of the circulation or across the placenta. In its mono-meric form it serves as the receptor molecule on B cells, although after they have switched to IgG production (see Chapter 19) it is replaced by IgG. This ability to *switch* classes without changing specificity—that is, to change Fc while retaining Fab—is another valuable consequence of the multi-gene arrangement of the immu-noglobulin locus, and will be discussed further when we look at the antibody response (Chapter 19).

IgA is specially adapted to function at mucosal surfaces such as those in the intestine, lungs, urogenital system, and breast, and has additional components to protect it from proteolysis, which are acquired during its secretion into these sites. IgA accounts for about two-thirds of all immunoglobulin present in the body. IgE, present in only trace amounts, comes into prominence as the cause of allergies (see Chapter 23), but it is probably useful in setting off inflammatory responses; some believe its main function is in worm infections. IgD is found mainly on B cells rather than in serum, and is part of their activation pathway.

In addition to these heavy-chain variants, there are two completely separate types of *light chain*, named lambda (λ) and kappa (κ), each with its own V, J, and C genes. A given antibody molecule has either both λ or both κ light chains (if it had one of each, the antigen-recognizing sites at the two ends of the Y would be different!). This choice of light chains doubles the already enormous number of possible antibody specificities. Yet another genetic variation is seen in the *allotypes*, which are small inherited differences, mainly in the C regions of the immunoglobulin molecule, somewhat analogous to the blood groups on red blood cells; like blood groups, their influence seems relatively minor but they can serve as useful genetic markers.

■ The antigen-binding site and antigenic determinants

What exactly do antibodies recognize? As Fig. 17.2 implies, only a very small part of the V domain is actually involved in binding the antigen—about 15–20 amino acids in fact, representing the tips of six *hypervariable* loops, three from the light chain and three from the heavy chain, coded for by those regions of the V gene where sequence variability is at its highest. Since these determine what shapes on the antigen the antibody will bind to, they are referred to as *complementarity determining regions* (CDRs). The two domains fold in such a way that these six loops form a shallow patch or cavity about 700 Å^2 in size, large enough to make contact with, for example, 15–20 amino acids from a protein or six sugar residues from a polysaccharide (Fig. 17.3). The closer the molecules can approach, the tighter the fit (see *affinity*, below). Since this small portion of the antigen may be a unique shape, it follows that the binding site that fits it is also a unique shape, possibly found on only antibody molecules from that particular clone of B cells. This unique region of the antibody molecule is called the *idiotype* and has fascinating properties: for instance it can itself stimulate and bind to another antibody with a binding site complementary to it, which would then resemble the original antigen! This ability to mimic an antigen using an idiotype has found applications in experimental vaccination.

Thus we see that antibodies recognize three-dimensional shape, but not the shape of a whole bacterium or even virus, rather the shape of just a small portion of one of its surface molecules (also known as an antigenic *determinant* or *epitope*). So even the smallest virus can be recognized by a large number of different antibodies; as it were, 'looking at it' from different directions and 'seeing' different determinants. One slightly surprising consequence of the smallness of the antigenic site is that similar shapes occasionally occur by chance on completely different microbial or animal cells, so that an individual antibody stimulated by, for example, a bacterium, may be found to 'cross-react' with a completely unrelated microbe or even the cells of some foreign species of animal. Since microbial and animal cells are made up of essentially the same amino acids, sugars, etc., such

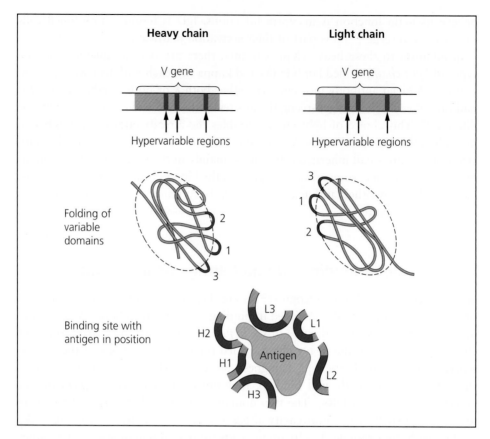

Fig. 17.3 The antigen-binding site, showing the location of the hypervariable regions in the V genes (top), their position in the folded variable immunoglobulin domain (centre), and how they make up the binding site (bottom: seen from 'end on' as the antigen molecule sees it). Note that the amino acid sequences that make up the binding site are discontinuous; the same may be true of the amino acids or sugars making up the antigenic site.

cross-reactions are in fact quite common, and this may account for the unfortunate production of antibodies against 'self' molecules which occurs in some *auto-immune* diseases (see Chapter 24).

■ Antibody affinity

As already mentioned, the affinity of the antibody–antigen bond can be very high, ranging from 10^{-7} to 10^{-11} M. Nevertheless, it must be stressed that it is a noncovalent bond, capable of coming apart, the affinity being merely the expression of this probability. The forces that hold antibody and antigen together are the usual intermolecular ones: hydrophobic, hydrogen bonding, electrostatic, and van der Waals. During the antibody response (see Chapter 19) the average affinity of all the antibody in the serum rises, owing partly to selection of the highest-affinity

B cells and partly to small random improvements in the antibody-combining site by mutation, so that antibody formed later in the response, and in subsequent responses, is even better adapted to the antigen in question. These unusually frequent mutations in the CDR genes of individual B cells, inherited by the progeny of that cell, are an example of *somatic hypermutation*. Note that the term *affinity* applies to the binding of one antibody-combining site–antigen bond; in practice, since antibodies are at least divalent it is the total strength or *avidity* that matters.

■ What antibodies do

Antibody functions in three main ways: on its own to *neutralize* threatening molecules or pathogens; in conjunction with cells to promote *phagocytosis*; and to activate the powerful effects of *complement* (see Fig. 17.4).

Neutralization and blocking

One of the first properties of antibody to be discovered, in 1890, was its ability to neutralize bacterial toxins, such as those of tetanus, diphtheria, etc., which forms the basis of vaccines against these diseases, and of the ability of injected antibody to save life in an acute infection ('passive immunization'). This is simply a matter of the immunoglobulin molecule blocking the binding of the toxin to the cell receptor via which it enters and damages cells.

A similar process can effectively prevent the entry of viruses into their intended target cells and is the basis for many, though not all, virus vaccines (see Chapters 28

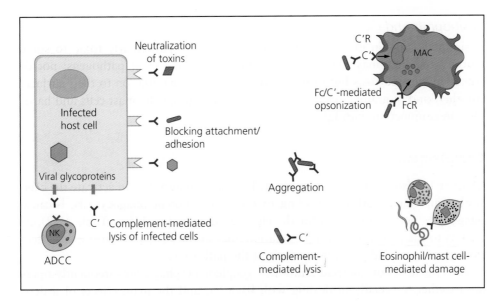

Fig. 17.4 A summary of the protective effects of antibody.

and 31). Where pathogens enter via the gut or the respiratory system, as so many do, it is the IgA class of antibody which is most important although IgG can be effective here too.

A more subtle form of neutralization is the effect of antibody, especially the large IgM molecule, in preventing the movement of bacteria that use flagellae. Antibody is also effective in agglutinating bacteria, as can easily be shown *in vitro*, but the role of this *in vivo* is hard to evaluate.

Opsonization, phagocytosis, and degranulation

In Chapter 12 we described how phagocytic cells such as macrophages and neutrophils can bind to many pathogens through 'pattern recognition' of their surface features. The presence of antibody bound to the pathogen extends this recognition to potentially *any* pathogen, because now the cell can recognize the antibody molecule itself by virtue of the presence of 'Fc receptors' into which the end of the molecule opposite to that binding the pathogen can dock (see Fig. 17.2). This 'opsonic' effect is critical in overcoming the anti-phagocytic activity of bacterial capsules (see Fig 3.1) and allows bacteria such as the meningococcus, pneumococcus, and Haemophilus to be phagocytosed in the presence of high levels of antibody such as are found after vaccination. Other Fc receptor-dependent mechanisms of interest in e.g. HIV infection include the lysis of infected cells (Antibody Dependent Cell-mediated Cytotoxicity; ADCC), as well as intracellular destruction of virus-antibody complexes, and viral inhibition via the release of chemokines (Antibody Dependent Cell-mediated Viral Inhibition; ADCVI). As Table 17.2 shows, there are numerous types of Fc receptor, located on different cell types, binding different antibody isotypes, and mediating different functions, both stimulatory and inhibitory.

Eosinophils and mast cells

Eosinophils contain granules with contents that are particularly toxic to some worms, and they may play a part in destroying these large pathogens: not of course by phagocytosis but rather by releasing toxic material on to their surface. Another kind of granule release, important in allergies, is by mast cells and basophils in conjunction with IgE.

Complement

Chapter 12 also describes how antibody bound to an antigen can activate the classical complement pathway, leading to even more potent phagocytosis, because phagocytes possess receptors for the cleavage fragment C3b (see Table 17.2), as well as to the promotion of inflammation and, in the case of the neisserial infections meningitis and gonorrhoea, lysis of the pathogen.

Thus members of the triad antibody+complement+phagocytes frequently operate together, especially in dealing with bacteria, and the main effects of a deficiency of any one of the triad are much the same—an increased incidence of

Table 17.2 Summary of Fc and complement receptors

Receptor	Expressed by (induced*)	Binds to	Effect on cell function
FcγRI (CD64)	Macrophages, dendritic cells neutrophils*, eosinophils*	IgG1=IgG3>G4>G2	Uptake, activation, respiratory burst/ microbicidal activity, antigen presentation
FcγRII A (CD32)	Macrophages, neutrophils, eosinophils, Langerhans cells, platelets	IgG1>G3=G2>G4	Uptake, eosinophil degranulation
FcγRII B1 (CD32)	B cells, mast cells	IgG1=G3>G4>G2	No uptake, inhibition
FcγRII B2 (CD32)	Macrophages, neutrophils, eosinophils	IgG1=G3>G4>G2	Uptake, inhibition
FcγRIII A (CD16)	NK cells	IgG1=G3	Killing, cytokine secretion
FcγRIII B (CD16)	Eosinophils, macrophages, neutrophils, mast cells	IgG1=G3	Uptake, activation
FcεRI	Mast cells, basophils, eosinophils*	IgE (high affinity)	Degranulation
FcεRII (CD23)	B cells, macrophages, eosinophils	IgE (low affinity)	Activation
FcαRI (CD89)	Monocytes*, neutrophils*, eosinophils	IgA (low affinity)	Uptake, activation, respiratory burst, antigen presentation
CR1 (CD35)	Follicular dendritic cells, B cells, monocytes, macrophages, erythrocytes, neutrophils, eosinophils, some T cells	C3b, C4b	Binds immune complexes, phagocytosis (with C5a)
CR2 (CD21)	B cells, follicular dendritic cells, some T cells	C3d, C3dg, iC3b	Binds EBV, B-cell activation (component of B-cell receptor complex)
CR3 (CD11b/18)	Monocytes, macrophages, neutrophils, NK cells, some T cells	iC3b	Phagocytosis, cell adhesion
CR4 (CD11c/18)	As above	iC3b	As above
C3a/4aR	Mast cells, basophils	C3a, 4a	Degranulation
C5aR	Mast cells, basophils, monocytes, macrophages, neutrophils, platelets, endothelial cells	C5a	Degranulation, migration, and adhesion of phagocytes to endothelium

bacterial infection. The added power contributed by antibody is illustrated by the inability of innate immunity (i.e. complement+phagocytes) to control many infections until sufficient antibody has been made, one of the best examples being streptococcal ('pneumococcal') pneumonia, where the patient is desperately ill until about a week after infection: the time it takes for a significant amount of IgG to be synthesized (see Chapter 13).

■ The antibody industry

Another useful role of antibody (not anticipated by Nature!) is as a *targeting* device for toxic drugs, radioactive molecules, etc., in the monitoring and treatment of disease, including tumours. Antibodies are also invaluable in the laboratory for *typing* cells (e.g. red cells for blood transfusion) because they can identify the small differences carried on the molecules of different blood groups, and for identifying pathogens in *diagnosis*. For such purposes the purer the antibody the better, and as a result of steady technical improvements, the production of pure antibody has progressed to the point where virtually unlimited amounts of antibody of any specificity can be synthesized. So important was the invention of *monoclonal antibody* technology that it earned the 1984 Nobel Prize for Köhler and Milstein. How monoclonal antibodies are made is described in Box 17.1 and Table 17.3, but it is worth remarking here that their value in infection therapy has been disappointing, with the exception of one virus: respiratory syncytial virus (RSV).

BOX 17.1 Exploring the antibody molecule

From antitoxin to antibody

French and German scientists, in quick succession, laid the foundations of the understanding of the antibody molecule. Roux and Yersin in Paris had showed (1888) that diphtheria caused disease via a soluble molecule: toxin. Von Behring and Kitasato in Berlin (1890) showed that such toxins could induce immunity, which was mediated by another soluble molecule present in serum after infection. This was baptized antitoxin and later renamed *antibody*. Antibodies were soon shown to be able to agglutinate, precipitate, and (with complement) lyse microorganisms.

First steps towards a structure

By 1938 it had been shown (Tiselius, Kabat) that antibodies resided in the gammaglobulin region of the serum, but further significant chemical analysis had to wait for the work of Porter and Edelman (1959), using enzymes to cleave the molecule into Fab and Fc portions and to build up the well-known Y-shaped structure. The study of whether different antibody molecules actually had different amino acid sequences required antibodies of a single specificity, and was limited by the need to use 'monoclonal' myeloma (B-cell tumour) proteins, which were only available in small quantities.

The monoclonal breakthrough

Köhler and Milstein (1975) solved the problem by devising a method for producing unlimited amounts of antibody of a single specificity. The trick was to fuse single B lymphocytes to myeloma cells with a gene defect preventing them growing in the medium used. Thus only B cells that had successfully fused were capable of long-term growth. Subsequent cloning led to single immortal antibody-producing cell lines. It is safe to say that this technique has revolutionized immunology. Not only have large amounts of single-specificity antibody become readily available for further detailed molecular analysis, but a reagent can now be prepared for identifying virtually any molecule, which has proved particularly useful in classifying cell *surface markers* (e.g. the CD classification), infectious organisms, and tumours. In addition, monoclonal antibodies can be used therapeutically to stimulate or inhibit cells or molecules. Monoclonal antibodies are usually prepared from mouse cells, but the genetic technique of 'humanization', by which the antigen-binding portion of the monoclonal antibody can be spliced into an otherwise human molecule, has minimized the problem of rejection. A number of other sophisticated methods are increasingly available that make use of portions of the antibody molecule or portions of the corresponding DNA.

Table 17.3 Some examples of monoclonal antibodies to illustrate manufacture and terminology

How made	Nomenclature	Example	Specificity	Clinical use
Mouse hybridoma (plus radio-isotope)	-omab	ibritumomab	CD20	B cell lymphoma
Mouse V region human C region	-ximab	rituximab	CD20	B cell lymphoma
Mouse hypervariable otherwise human	-zumab	trastuzumab	HER2 receptor	Breast cancer
Transgenic mouse, with human Ig genes	-mumab	adalimumab	TNF	Rheumatoid arthritis

Monoclonal antibodies against other viruses such as hepatitis B, EBV, and HIV are still at the experimental stage. On the other hand monoclonal antibodies against particular immune-cell-surface molecules or soluble mediators have proved very useful; examples are anti-CD3 for removing T cells from bone marrow before grafting, anti-CD20 for B-cell lymphoma, and anti-TNF to reduce inflammation, notably in rheumatoid arthritis (three of today's six top-selling monoclonal antibodies are against TNF). The production of monoclonal antibodies is now a multi-billion dollar business and nomenclature is standardized by using the last four or five letters as a code to specify which of the four main methods of manufacture has been employed in each case (Table 17.3).

SUMMARY

- The basic antibody molecule is composed of two heavy and two light chains, in the form of a Y, with an approximate molecular weight of 150 000 Da.

- The two arms of the Y (Fab region) carry the hypervariable regions that determine the specificity for antigen; the stem (Fc region) determines the class of the molecule: IgM, G, A, E, or D. IgM contains five units of the basic molecule, some IgAs contain two.

- Phagocytic and other cells display receptors for the Fc region of IgG; some inflammatory cells carry receptors for IgE.

- Each class is specialized for a particular function; for example IgG for crossing the placenta and binding antigens to phagocytes, IgA for action in secretions, IgE for inducing inflammation, and IgM and IgG for the activation of complement.

- The degree of fit between a portion ('determinant') of antigen and the hypervariable portion of an antibody molecule is reflected in the strength of binding, referred to as affinity.

Chapter 18
T cells and the MHC

Resting T lymphocytes look very much like resting B lymphocytes, but when they respond the difference becomes apparent: instead of turning into plasma cells and secreting antibody, they enlarge slightly, proliferate, and secrete *cytokines* and/or *toxic molecules* with effects on other cells, but with no specificity towards particular antigens. As the effects of these molecules are usually fairly short range, it is the cell to which the T cell responds (the 'target' cell) that receives the main impact, so that T cell responses essentially operate at close quarters. Depending on the type of T lymphocyte, this effect can result in the target cell being activated or killed (Table 18.1), the common feature being that the T cell is responding to changes detected on the surface of the target cell but reflecting the presence of foreign material *inside* it: the 'internal environment'. In a typical situation such as a virus infection, the T cell makes use of the ability of target cells to convey small bits of viral protein (i.e. peptides) from inside the cell to the cell surface, using a special set of molecules known as MHC proteins (for *major histocompatibility complex*; see later for an explanation of this strange name). Since these peptides are derived from a foreign microbe (in this case a virus) there will be, among the repertoire of T cells, a few whose receptors recognize that combination of MHC and peptide and only these T cells will respond. Thus although the effects of T cells are non-specific, their recognition of antigen is highly specific. But T cells do not only recognize protein fragments; glycolipid antigens are recognized too, although here another set of antigen-presenting molecules known as CD1 are involved, as will be explained later.

Table 18.1 The main types of T lymphocytes and their functions

Common name	Receptor chains	Characteristic surface marker	Main secreted product	Target cells	Main effect
Cytotoxic (CTL)	α/β	CD8	Perforins, granzymes, cytokines (IFNγ)	Any nucleated cell	Killing (especially viruses)
Helper					
(T_H1)	α/β	CD4	Cytokines (especially IFNγ)	Macrophages	Activation
(T_H2)	α/β	CD4	Cytokines (especially IL-4, 5, 13)	B lymphocytes	Proliferation, antibody secretion
(T_H17)	α/β	CD4	Cytokines (especially IL-17)	Stromal cells, endothelium	Neutrophil production and recruitment
Regulatory	α/β	CD4	IL-10, TGF-β	T, B lymphocytes, macrophages	Inhibition
Gamma/delta	γ/δ		IFNγ	Macrophages	Activation, regulation
NKT	α/β	NK1.1	IFNγ, IL-4	NK cells	Activation, regulation

CD, cluster of differentiation, a terminology used for cell-surface molecules, of which at least 160 are now recognized.

■ Subpopulations of T cells

Not all T cells have the same range of functions (see Table 18.1). The major distinction is between *cytotoxic* and *helper* cells. Cytotoxic T cells are predominantly equipped to kill cells harbouring intracellular pathogens such as viruses, while helper cells are designed to switch on or enhance the activity of B lymphocytes, macrophages, and other cells involved in defence, as described in the following two chapters. Helper T cells are further subdivided into T_H1 and T_H2 and, recently, T_H17 cells (see Chapters 19 and 20). The process by which antigens reach the surface of these cells is described below.

It is vital for the two quite different functional effects of cytotoxicity and help to be applied to the right target cell. This is ensured by another set of surface molecules on the T cells. One, known as CD4, is found mainly on helper T cells, and recognizes one set of MHC molecules (class II, see below); thus helper T cells will only help cells bearing MHC class II, which normally means B cells, macrophages, and dendritic cells. Another, known as CD8, is found mainly on cytotoxic cells, and recognizes MHC class I molecules, which are carried by all nucleated cells

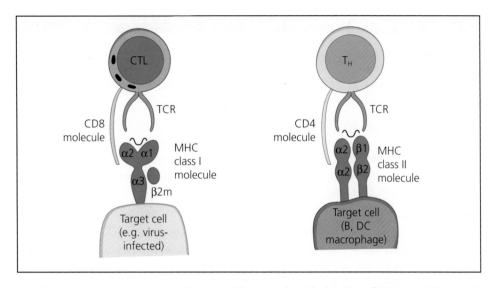

Fig. 18.1 Interactions between T cells and MHC molecules. The binding of CD8 to MHC class I, and of CD4 to class II, ensures that cytotoxic and helper T cells only interact with an appropriate target cell. ∿ represents a peptide antigen; CTL, cytotoxic T lymphocyte; T_H, T helper.

(i.e. all but red blood cells). The biological sense is excellent, because only B cells, macrophages, and dendritic cells can benefit from 'help', whereas any cell may pick up a virus and will then need to be killed. Thus the two functional T-cell subpopulations are often described simply as 'CD4' and 'CD8' cells. By contrast, both types of T cell carry the CD3 molecule, which is commonly used as a marker for T cells in general.

A further distinction can be made between T cells with receptors composed of α and β chains, or with γ and δ chains (see below). Figure 18.1 illustrates these distinctions and the processes are described further in Chapter 20. There are also T cells whose main function appears to be to *regulate* other cells, sometimes switching them off, a process vital to all adaptive immune responses (see Chapter 21). Finally we should mention the NKT cell, a cell with both natural killer and T cell features (see below).

■ What T cells recognize

Proteins: the MHC

One cannot discuss the T cell receptor, or TCR, without also discussing MHC molecules, since they usually act together in protein recognition; that is, the most commonly expressed TCR (α/β) will not respond to a peptide unless it is bound to an MHC molecule (see Box 18.1). This again makes excellent biological sense because MHC molecules are found on cell surfaces and T cells can only act usefully on a cell; their secreted products in the majority of cases cannot affect microbes directly. Thus the presence of MHC molecules advertises the presence

Box 18.1 Bringing T cells and the MHC together

B cells need T cells

The separate origin of B and T lymphocytes was established for birds in 1956 (Glick) and for mice in the early 1960s (Miller). By 1966 it was evident that most antibody responses by B cells required 'cooperation' by T cells (Claman, Mitchison *et al.*).

Genetics of immunity (1)

The role of genetics in tissue-graft rejection had been known for some time (Gorer, 1936; Medawar, 1944). Genetic control of antibody responses then became evident and it was unexpectedly shown that the same genes (MHC/HLA) were involved: T cells would only cooperate with B cells of the right MHC type (McDevitt, Benacerraf, 1969).

Processing and recognition

During the 1970s it became clear that antigens, to stimulate a response, had to be processed; that is, taken in and modified by specialized cells. At the same time, studies with cytotoxic T cells revealed that they recognized not only fragments of antigen (in this case virus) but also MHC molecules (Zinkernagel, Doherty, 1975). A decade later it was shown that processing was again involved, the MHC molecules being of a different type (class I for cytotoxicity, class II for antibody). The term 'MHC restriction' was coined to describe this general phenomenon.

The T-cell receptor

This last element in the T–B interaction pathway defied analysis until 1984, when it was shown (Marrack, Davis) to be a two-chain molecule analogous, but not identical, to the B-cell receptor (antibody). The distinction between CD8 (cytotoxic) and CD4 (helper) T cells was established, and in 1986 the further subdivision of CD4 cells into T-helper 1 and 2 types, broadly responsible for different classes of antibody response and macrophage activation.

Genetics of immunity (2)

With the widespread availability of MHC typing facilities, it emerged that some diseases were commoner (or rarer) in people of certain MHC types. The most striking association is that between the ankylosing spondylitis group of rheumatic diseases and HLA B27, but many infectious diseases show a degree of susceptibility or resistance depending on HLA type. When fully analysed, this will have implications for monitoring, treatment, and vaccine design.

---

of a *cell*, and the presence of a foreign peptide bound to it advertises the presence of a *foreign* microbe inside the cell: an ingenious way for one cell to 'look inside' another! MHC molecules are two-chain structures, composed of either two two-domain chains (class II) or one three-domain chain stabilized by the smaller β2 microglobulin chain (class I; see Table 18.2). In both cases they express a peptide binding groove which opens outward in order to bind the peptide and display it to the T cell. The groove only contains one peptide at a time but has the ability to bind a wide but finite range of different peptides, which differs for each MHC allele. The peptide is 'anchored' into the groove by interactions of just a few of the amino acids with pockets in the floor (plus some interactions with the side walls). Other amino acids face outward and are more involved in binding to the

Table 18. 2 MHC and CD1 molecules compared

	MHC class I	MHC class II	CD1 group 1	CD1 group 2
Genes	HLA A,B,C	HLA DP, DQ, DR	CD1a,b,c	CD1d
Chains	α, β2M	α, β	α, β2M	α, β2M
Polymorphism	++	++	–	–
Ligands	Peptides (8–11 aa)	Peptides (10–30 aa)	(Glyco)lipids e.g. mycobacteria	(Glyco)lipids, α-galactosyl ceramide, mycobacteria (PIM), protozoa
Antigen processing	+	+	+	+
Expressed on	All nucleated cells	DCs, mac, B cells	DCs, B cells	Mono, mac
Responding cells	CD8 T (TCR α/β)	CD4 T (TCR α/β)	CD4–/8– T, CD8 T,CD4 T (TcR α/β, γ/δ)	NKT, iNKT

aa, amino acids; DC, dendritic cell; iNKT, invariant NKT cells; mac, macrophage; mono, monocyte; PIM, phosphatidylmyoinositol mannoside.

T cell receptor. The preference for each MHC allele to bind only peptides which share a common motif can be used to predict which peptides of a pathogen might be recognized by the T cell system. The binding of MHC to peptide is much weaker than that of antibodies to their antigen but nevertheless holds the peptide for several hours to days, long enough for a specific T cell to make contact and be activated.

TCRs are highly heterogeneous, such that an individual T cell will preferentially recognize one unique combination of MHC molecule and microbial peptide, although this restriction is not absolute (see Chapter 24). The peptide, lying in the long narrow binding cleft on the MHC molecule, will no longer be in the three-dimensional form in which it occurred in the larger protein it was derived from. So the TCR recognizes *continuous linear* protein fragments, unlike antibody which recognizes three-dimensional shapes that may be discontinuous parts of protein or sugar (look back to Fig. 17.3). And since it only recognizes a peptide bound to the right MHC molecule, such a response is referred to as 'MHC restricted'. Figure 18.2 illustrates these basic principles.

Interestingly, MHC restriction is involved in T-cell development even before any contact with foreign antigens, because in the thymus, where T cells mature, they are exposed to the combination of self-MHC and self-peptides in a complex process that ensures that the minimum of self-reactive T cells and the maximum of foreign-reactive ones reach the peripheral lymphoid organs. These events are referred to as *negative* and *positive* selection, respectively.

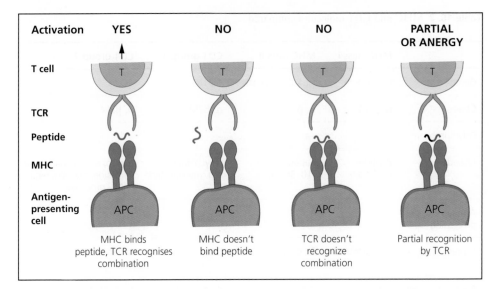

Fig. 18.2 MHC restriction of T-cell recognition. The T cell shown here recognizes only one combination of MHC and bound peptide. Other T cells will recognize other combinations. Note that a given peptide may bind to several (though not all) MHC molecules. T-cell activation will not occur if the peptide fails to bind both MHC and TCR. Subtle modifications in amino acids of otherwise immunogenic peptides (so-called altered peptide ligands) may lead to partial T-cell activation or anergy.

Glycolipids and carbohydrates: CD1

To present non-protein molecules a completely different set of presenting structures is used, the CD1 molecules which bind lipid-containing molecules via their hydrophobic lipid portions (see below and Table 18.2). There is apparently no specialized molecule for presenting a pure carbohydrate; as mentioned in Chapter 19, many carbohydrates do not need T cells in order to induce antibody.

■ Antigen-presenting molecules

The MHC and its molecules

At this point, a digression is required to explain the MHC in more detail. As mentioned above, the initials stand for *major histocompatibility complex*, which is the name given to a large genetic region containing the genes that determine the success or failure of graft rejection. If two individuals have the same set of MHC molecules (as identical twins do) they will not reject each other's grafts; if they differ (as unrelated people do) there will be some degree of rejection. Although this is historically the way in which the MHC was discovered, it is, of course, not its real function, which as stated above is to transport and 'present' foreign peptides to T cells. The MHC is extraordinarily polymorphic, some loci having up to 150 allelic variants, and as they are heterodimers (made up of two different chains)

Table 18.3 T- and B-cell receptors compared

	T-cell receptor	Antibody molecule
Recombination of V–J–C genes	In T cells only	In B cells only
Junctional diversity	Yes	Yes
Subsequent mutation	No	Yes
Chains	α and β, or γ and δ	2 heavy (M, G, D, A, or E) and 2 light (κ or λ)
Molecular weight (Da)	95 000	146 000–970 000
Recognizes	(1) Small linear peptides (9–15 amino acids) plus MHC molecule (2) Glycolipids plus CD1 molecules	Three-dimensional shape of proteins and sugars
Secreted into blood	No	Yes

there are an estimated 10^{13} different possible combinations, so that identity between two individuals (other than identical twins) is virtually impossible.

There is no obvious reason why everybody's MHC antigens should differ in this way, but it is generally assumed to be something to do with ensuring that everybody does not respond identically to every infection; if they did, the argument goes, a new one might wipe out the entire species. Be that as it may, differences in MHC type are undoubtedly responsible for some of the differences in the responses of individuals to the same infection (see Chapter 9 for a further discussion of this point). Evolutionists speculate that the MHC and the TCR developed together, in invertebrates, as a recognition pair involved in normal cell adhesion. Interestingly, both of them, together with antibody and many other molecules, share considerable DNA homology, including the all-important *domain* pattern. This suggests that they originated from the same primordial gene, and they are collectively known as the *immunoglobulin superfamily*.

Human MHC molecules (in humans, the MHC is referred to as HLA, for 'human leucocyte antigen') are of two types, known as class I and class II, with slightly different structure and function (Fig. 18.3). There are three kinds of class I molecule (A, B, and C) and three of class II (DP, DQ, and DR). Since they are *co-dominantly* expressed (i.e. both parental chromosomes are used), each cell carries two sets of molecules of each kind, 12 in all. Class I molecules are found on all nucleated cells, class II only on some; this is part of the process of selecting the right type of T cell for the job (e.g. killing or help). The MHC is a large locus, and the class I and II genes are separated by a number of other genes of immunological interest, including those for several cytokines and complement components as well as for the proteasomes and transporter proteins used for antigen processing (see below).

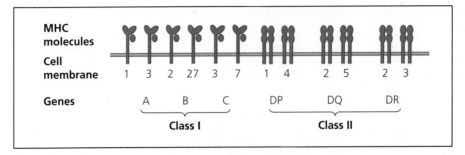

Fig. 18.3 MHC (HLA) genes and the corresponding molecules in the membrane of a human cell. Because there are many alleles at each locus, the number of combinations is astronomical (about 10^{13}). The cells of this individual would be typed as A 1,3; B 2,27; C 3,7; DP 1,4; DQ 2,5; DR 2,3. The small circles represent β2 microglobulin, a quite separate molecule that stabilizes class I molecules.

CD1 molecules

These are not part of the MHC, but they do have some structural resemblance to MHC class I molecules and like them are physically associated with a smaller molecule called β2 *microglobulin*. However, they lack the enormous polymorphism of MHC molecules, there being just four types: CD1 a, b, and c (group 1), and d (group 2). As Table 18.2 shows, group 1 CD molecules follow trafficking pathways within the APC, enabling them to pick up glycolipids from either endogenous or exogenous pathogens for presentation to T cells (see *antigen processing*, below) while those of group 2 are specialized for presenting to NKT cells. As one might predict, the best-established microbial ligands for group 1 molecules are glycolipids from mycobacteria: intracellular organisms renowned for their almost impenetrable waxy cell wall, the lipid portion being held in the CD1 binding groove and the hydrophilic sugar residues presented to the TCR (Fig. 18.2). The originally described ligand for group 2 is α-galactosyl ceramide, a glycolipid first found in sea sponges. More recently ligands have been identified in bacteria and protozoa, including *M. tuberculosis* and *Leishmania donovani* (see Table 18.2).

■ The T-cell receptor

The antigen receptor on the T cell (TCR) has similarities to the antibody molecule, but with important differences (Table 18.3, Figs 18.1 and 18.4). Unlike the antibody on the B cell, which can be thought of as a sample of what that cell can produce, like the goods in a shop window, the TCR can be thought of rather like a hand reaching out to feel the surface of neighbouring cells, with some fingers devoted to contacting MHC molecules and others probing for the peptide bound to them (Fig. 18.1). Thus the TCR is not a secreted molecule with a separate function as antibody is.

Taking the α/β receptor as an example, it can be seen that the TCR somewhat resembles the antibody molecule minus most of its constant region, being composed of one V and one C region on each of the two chains. As with antibody, the antigen-binding region is at the tips of the V regions, where the three hypervariable regions of each chain come together. TCR molecules are associated in the membrane of T cells with CD3 molecules, themselves composed of γ, δ, ε, and ζ chains, important in signal transduction and activation of the T cell.

Unlike antibody genes, TCR genes do not undergo mutation, with the result that the changes in affinity seen during antibody responses do not occur within the T-cell population. This greatly diminishes the chance of a T cell acquiring self-reactivity.

■ Antigen processing and presentation

Processing

An intracellular virus or other pathogen is, in immunological terms, a large complex structure, and to convert it into a series of small peptides in the groove of the MHC molecules on the cell surface, quite complicated processes must occur. These take place in the *antigen-presenting cells* (APCs), which may be dendritic cells (the most important for activating resting T cells), macrophages, or B lymphocytes. A pathogen or its molecules can be intracellular for two reasons: (1) *exogenously*, that is, actively taken into the presenting cell by phagocytosis, of which bacteria are typical examples, for presentation by MHC class II molecules to CD4 T cells; and (2) *endogenously*, that is, already growing in the APC—particularly viruses—and presented via MHC class I molecules to CD8 T cells. Each type is handled by a different set of intracellular processes (Fig. 18.4).

The exogenous (class II) pathway

Like all phagocytosed material (see Chapter 12), an engulfed bacterium will normally end up in an endosome (phagolysosome) where it is digested at acid pH by proteases into short peptides of up to about 20 amino acids. These endosomes fuse with Golgi-derived vesicles containing MHC class II molecules whose groove is temporarily blocked by a molecule called invariant chain; this is now exchanged for the bacterial peptide. The new MHC–peptide complex is then transported to the cell surface to be recognized by CD4 T cells (see below). Not surprisingly, some successful pathogens can interfere with this process, for example by inhibiting endosomal proteases (e.g. the roundworm *Brugia*) or blocking phagosome–lysosome fusion (e.g. *M. tuberculosis*).

The endogenous (class I) pathway

Here it is a question of getting peptides newly synthesized in the cytoplasm of the host cell onto the cell membrane bound to MHC class I molecules. This involves specialized structures called *proteasomes* that chop proteins into peptides of rather precise length (8–10 amino acids) which just fit the MHC class I groove, and

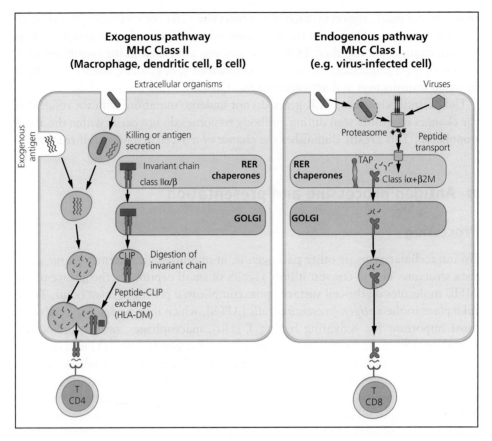

Fig. 18.4 Pathways of antigen processing. RER, rough endoplasmic reticulum; TAP, transporter associated with antigen processing; CLIP, class II-associated invariant chain peptide; DM, a non-polymorphic MHC class-II-like molecule which acts as a peptide exchanger.

transporter proteins (TAP) that carry them across the membranes of the endoplasmic reticulum. Here they meet MHC molecules in the course of assembly. Golgi vesicles then bud off from the endoplasmic reticulum and carry the MHC–peptide complex to the cell surface to be recognized by CD8 T cells. Note that neither pathway incorporates any mechanism for distinguishing foreign from 'self' proteins, and in fact even during a virus infection only a small proportion of MHC class I molecules will carry viral peptides, most of them being loaded with self peptides.

Note also that the two pathways are not in practice quite so rigidly separate, since dendritic cells can acquire viral proteins by phagocytizing material from virus-lysed cells which then proceed through both the exogenous and endogenous pathways to CD4 and CD8 T cells respectively. The latter is called 'cross priming' or 'cross presentation' and occurs when these endosome-derived peptides cross over to the cytoplasm via the endoplasmic reticulum by as yet poorly understood mechanisms, resulting in loading of the class I MHC. Conversely, proteins in the cytoplasm can cross over to the exogenous pathway by a process known as autophagy. Autophagy is a basic intracellular process for recycling cytoplasmic cellular components and in addition is used by the immune system to deliver proteins from this site to the class II processing pathway. In practice most pathogens elicit both CD4 and CD8 responses to some degree.

Presentation and co-stimulation

It is not sufficient merely to display MHC–peptide complexes on the APC surface to activate T cells. Even when the TCR binds to the peptide, several *co-stimulatory* non-antigen specific molecular interactions are also required. Two have already been mentioned: the binding of CD4 on the T cell to MHC class II on the APC, and the binding of CD8 to MHC class I; these ensure that the appropriate type of T cell is activated, for example CD4 helpers for a macrophage struggling to eliminate mycobacteria compared with CD8 killers for a virally infected cell. Other essential interactions involve molecules induced on the APC by contact with the pathogen itself; these help to ensure that T cells concentrate their attention on infected rather than normal cells and that the initial contact between T cell and APC proceeds to firmer, more prolonged binding and optimal activation (Fig. 18.5).

In general, infection improves T cell activation by antigens. Interferons up regulate MHC class I and II expression and the processing and TAP transporter systems. Ligation of pattern-recognition receptors on DCs also increases co-stimulator

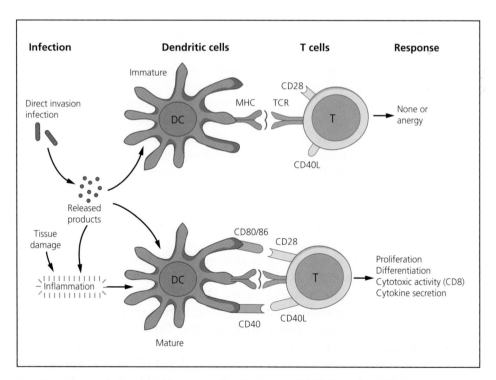

Fig. 18.5 Antigen presentation and co-stimulation. Immature dendritic cells (DCs) do not generate T-cell responses unless stimulated by pathogen-derived or inflammatory products.

expression (e.g. CD80/86, which binds to CD28 on T cells) and converts DCs from the antigen-uptake to the antigen-presentation mode.

Thus there are important quantitative and temporal elements to antigen presentation. To summarize this whole complex process, its outcome depends on (1) properties of the antigen, which proteases generate which peptides, (2) the available MHC molecules, since these have a broad but not infinite range of peptide-binding capacities, and (3) the repertoire of TCRs for the MHC–peptide complexes produced. The result is inevitably a hierarchy of antigens from each pathogen, some being more effective ('immunodominant') than others while some components of the pathogens may not function as antigens at all.

■ Superantigens

There is one exception to the normal 'MHC-restricted' pattern of T-cell responses to proteins described above. Some microbial proteins, notably the enterotoxins of staphylococci, have the ability to stimulate a substantial number of T cells, for example up to 20%, instead of the one per million or so expected if the recognition were receptor-specific. These responses do require class II MHC molecules, but are not restricted to a single MHC type. The explanation is thought to be that these 'superantigens' bind to parts of the MHC and the TCR (always the same one of the two variable domains known as Vβ), *outside* the usual polymorphic peptide-binding site, although some may also interact with the peptide. The stimulation of so many T cells at once and the release of huge amounts of pro-inflammatory cytokines such as IL-2 and TNFα and β, together with IL-1 from activated macrophages, contributes to the toxicity of these antigens, which can be terrifying. For example, *Staph. aureus* and *Streptococcus pyogenes*, which together have no less than 21 different superantigens, can cause massive fatal food poisoning and the toxic shock syndrome (rash, vomiting, and multi-organ failure associated with infected tampons). There are also mycobacterial, clostridial, and viral superantigens. Exactly what role these bizarre responses play, and even whether they are of use to the pathogen or the host, or neither, is still a mystery.

■ γδ T cells

Yet another exception to 'classical' presentation as described earlier are the γδ T cells, which constitute a minor (1–5%) fraction of all T cells but are enriched in epithelial tissues such as the intestinal mucosa (Table 18.1). These cells can recognize phosphate containing molecules and lipids (e.g. on mycobacteria) by a process involving their TCR but not classical MHC or CD1. They also respond to stress and tissue damage via TLRs and NKG2D, a molecule used by NK cells for the same purpose. Their role in infection is complicated and still somewhat mysterious; they have immediate effector functions, they can produce IFNγ and are cytotoxic, and can be a major source of IL-17 for rapid recruitment of neutrophils to mucosal sites. However they may later serve to down-regulate immune responses to limit tissue damage, such as via release of TGFβ and IL-10, and help to initiate tissue repair.

■ NKT cells

NKT cells (see Chapter 12) carry TCR molecules, but do not show MHC restriction and specialize in recognizing lipids associated with CD1 (see above). They can respond rapidly by secreting cytokines such as IL-4 and IFNγ, and are also able to activate classical NK cells. Thus NKT cells have been implicated in innate resistance to bacteria (such as *M. tuberculosis*) and protozoa and, more recently, in allergic asthma.

SUMMARY

- There are several subpopulations of T lymphocytes, referred to either by function (cytotoxic, helper), surface molecular markers (CD8, CD4), or TCR chain structure (α/β, γ/δ).

- Helper (CD4) T cells are further divided into T_H1, T_H2, and T_H17 cells, depending on the cytokines they secrete.

- T cells do not respond to antigens unless they are processed and presented. Processing follows one of two pathways in phagocytic or B cells, depending on the source of the antigen and leading to presentation of small peptides at the cell surface by MHC class I or class II molecules.

- Peptides associated with class I MHC molecules (HLA A, B, or C) are recognized by CD8 T cells, those associated with class II MHC (DP, DQ, DR) are recognized by CD4 T cells. This allows the appropriate type of T-cell response to be generated.

- Some antigens bypass the above by binding directly to TCR molecules. These are called superantigens and may generate excessive T-cell responses.

Chapter 19

The antibody response

Lymphocytes do not just *function*; they *respond* by proliferating into clones, changing their size and shape, and secreting important molecules. As emphasized in Chapters 16–18, B and T lymphocytes differ in many respects, and this includes the way they respond. In this chapter we will consider how B cells and T cells, acting together, give rise to the production of antibody molecules: the *antibody response*.

The antibody response illustrates perfectly the principles of adaptive immunity. Consider the life story of a typical individual with respect to *Streptococcus pneumoniae* (the pneumococcus) in the days before antibiotics. At birth, if the mother has previously had pneumonia, the baby will acquire some antibody specific for the bacterium across the placenta (see Chapter 17), so he or she is protected against infection. By about 6–9 months most of this is gone, and the baby is now susceptible to infection, although pneumonia with this organism is in fact more common at older ages. If it does develop, the patient is severely ill for about a week, during which time innate immune mechanisms (mainly phagocytes and complement) struggle to control the rapidly growing organisms. But *antibody* production has begun, and after a week the IgG antibody in the blood reaches a level sufficient to opsonize all the bacteria, the *phagocytes* home in, and a few hours later the patient is miraculously better. This illustrates the time lag characteristic of primary antibody responses.

A second infection with the same strain of pneumococcus will be met by a secondary antibody response so rapid that the patient will be unaware of the infection. This illustrates *memory*. However, infection with a different strain (there are over 90) will require production of a different antibody, because of the very high specificity of antibody for the antigens of the bacterium; meanwhile the patient will again develop serious pneumonia (Fig. 19.1). You can now be *vaccinated* against this disease, but a complete vaccine would have to contain over 90 different antigens! (In practice, about

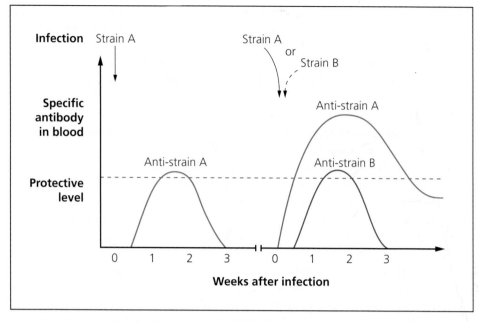

Fig. 19.1 Primary and secondary antibody responses, illustrating the slow appearance of antibody in the primary response, and the faster and greater response to a second contact with the same antigen. If the first contact with strain A had been in the form of a non-pathogenic vaccine, subsequent infection would lead directly to a secondary response. For details of the difference between primary and secondary antibody, see Table 19.2.

20 are enough to protect most people.) Patients who for some reason are *deficient* in producing antibody are extremely susceptible to this type of infection, but they can be kept healthy by monthly injections of immunoglobulin pooled from large numbers of normal people, showing that (1) it really is antibody that protects, and (2) normal people have protective levels of it.

For the production of a typical IgG antibody response such as that described above, four events must take place: activation of B cells; presentation of antigen to T cells; activation of T cells; and 'help' for the B cells by T cells.

■ Activation of B cells

Activation of B cells occurs mainly in the lymphoid organs, the site depending on the route by which antigen arrives. It occurs in the mucosal lymphoid tissue for inhaled and ingested antigens, in the spleen for blood-borne antigens, and in lymph nodes for antigens entering the tissues through the skin.

T-dependent and T-independent antigens

Different sorts of antigen activate B cells in different ways. Some do not in fact require T-cell help, and are known as *T-independent* (Ti antigens). This may be because they have intrinsic *mitogenic* activity (Ti I antigens such as LPS); that is, they induce mitosis, or cell division, in many B cells, followed by antibody secretion (Fig. 19.2a). Others (Ti II), consisting of *repeated identical antigenic determinants*, can stimulate specific B cells to divide and secrete antibody, by binding to and linking together several of their surface immunoglobulin receptors (Fig. 19.2b). Ti II antigens include many of the polysaccharides in the capsules of dangerous bacteria such as the Meningococcus, *Haemophilus*, and *S. pneumoniae*, and the antibody they induce, although it may be life-saving, lacks some of the features of T-dependent responses, with only limited class switching and no affinity maturation (see below). In adults, polysaccharide antigens induce some IgG responses and robust immunological memory for many years. However, Ti II antigens do not induce immunity in very young children, who therefore are susceptible to infection with *Haemophilus influenzae* and *Neisseria meningitidis* and *S. pneumoniae*, and cannot be vaccinated with polysaccharides of these organisms unless they are combined with a protein carrier, as they are in protein–polysaccharide–conjugate vaccines. Note that the original definition of a T-independent antigen was that it induced antibody in animals lacking thymuses and *most* T cells, as some bacterial polysaccharides can; however, this does not mean that some T cells cannot recognize and provide help for polysaccharides and some lipids, and in fact Ti II antigens can derive help from the Tγδ subpopulation of T cells (see Chapter 18).

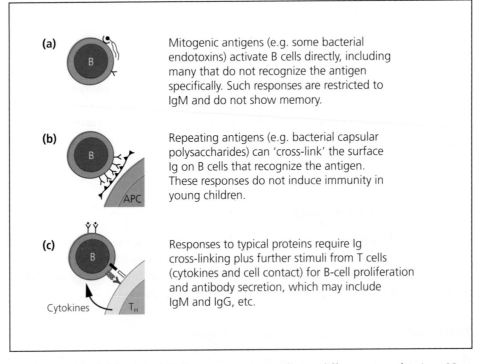

Fig. 19.2 B cells can be activated in three ways, corresponding to different types of antigen. Note that (a) and (b) illustrate 'T-cell-independent' responses and (c) illustrates a 'T-cell-dependent' response. B, B lymphocyte; Th, CD4 T-helper cell.

Mitogenic and repeating antigens are relatively uncommon and most pathogen-derived molecules, particularly proteins such as toxins, have neither of these two properties; for them to activate B cells, several molecules need to be 'presented' to the B cell simultaneously, and this is done by special *antigen-presenting cells* (APCs), found mainly in the lymphoid organs. This type of response also requires further 'help' from T cells (see below), and for this reason it is referred to as *T-dependent* (TD). The ability of protein antigens to enlist T help is made use of in the improvement of polysaccharide vaccines by conjugating them to proteins (see Chapter 28).

Activation through the B-cell antigen–receptor complex

The immunoglobulin molecule in the surface of the B cell, although it does penetrate the membrane, has no intrinsic enzymatic activity: so how does it switch on the intracellular mechanisms that lead to antibody formation? The answer is that it is associated in the membrane with other molecules that can transduce signals from outside the cell to the nucleus; these together form the B-cell receptor (BCR) complex. Without the BCR, a B cell cannot respond, and interestingly there are B-cell-infecting viruses, such as EBV and HHV8, which can inhibit BCR function, presumably to evade recognition and promote their own survival. Signal transduction via the BCR is not 'all or nothing'; it depends on the extent and duration of interaction and is influenced by such factors as antigen valency, state of aggregation, and persistence. In fact, under certain conditions it can induce not responsiveness but unresponsiveness, and even death of the B cell! In addition to the BCR other *co-stimulatory* molecules play a part in B-cell activation, particularly CD21 (CR2) in association with CD19 and CD81. The involvement of CR2 (the receptor for the complement factor C3d) explains why depletion of C3, for example by cobra venom factor, inhibits antibody responses in mice, and also why conjugation of C3d with an antigen makes it a more powerful inducer of antibody: a potentially useful adjunct to vaccination.

During normal activation by a multivalent antigen, clusters or 'arrays' of these BCR and co-stimulatory molecules are drawn together into so-called *lipid rafts*: areas of altered lipid composition floating in the plasma membrane phospholipid bilayer, which selectively promote molecular interactions and signal transduction. It is thought that the inhibitory effect of EBV mentioned above is partly due to blocking the formation of lipid rafts. This 'cross-linking' of the BCR in turn improves the ability of the B cell to present antigen to T cells by increasing the levels of co-stimulatory molecules and cytokine receptors to receive T-cell help in return (see below). When we consider the activation of T cells, you will see many similarities to B-cell activation, particularly in the existence of co-stimulatory molecules, although there are important differences too.

Consequences of activation: proliferation and differentiation

Whatever the route of activation, B cells need to proliferate into a large enough population to make the enormous numbers of antibody molecules required for a useful response. Note that in the examples shown in Figs 19.2b and c this prolif-eration only occurs in antigen-specific B cells—that is, it is *clonal*—whereas in Fig. 19.2a the proliferation would be *polyclonal* and much of the antibody would not react with the inducing antigen. This is because Ti I antigens do not act through the highly specific BCR complex whereas Ti II and TD antigens do.

Proliferation involves entry into cell cycle and cell division; differentiation refers to enlargement of the cell and its organelles, with a visible change from lympho-cyte to *plasma cell* morphology, immunoglobulin synthesis, and the increased expression of anti-apoptotic molecules that prolong survival as well as molecules that facilitate interaction with T cells. Further differentiation steps include the switch from secreting IgM to IgG, IgA, etc. (see below) and the generation of cells involved in memory—long-lived plasma cells and memory B cells (see Chapter 21).

■ Presentation of antigen to T cells

In Chapter 18 it was stressed that, although T cells can undoubtedly respond to some glycolipids, the responses to proteins are the most fully understood. Here what the T cells actually recognize are *small peptides* bound to MHC *molecules*, so for them to be activated a presenting cell is needed, and it must display MHC molecules of the appropriate class, associated with a peptide derived from the interior of the cell. These presenting cells are of three types: antigen-specific B cells, macrophages, and specialized antigen-presenting *dendritic cells*. In general, the dendritic cells are more important in primary responses, when there are rela-tively few B cells of the right specificity available; in secondary responses and at sites of infection, B cells and macrophages become major sources of antigen presentation. One of the functions of lymphoid organs is to facilitate close con-tact between B and T cells. These cells, initially segregated in different areas of the lymph node (see Fig. 16.2) move towards each other following contact with antigen, to meet and interact at the border between the B-cell follicle and the T-cell zone.

Let us consider B cells first (Fig. 19.3, steps 1–4). Following activation of a B cell as in Fig. 19.2c, the complex of antigen plus BCR is taken into the cell, and the antigen is 'processed', i.e. digested by enzymes so that its constituent peptides can be picked up by the newly synthesized MHC class II molecules, which are then transported to the cell surface. This processing into peptides is not in itself restricted to foreign antigens, but is tremendously more efficient (up to a million times) with foreign antigens because of their association with the BCR, which is where the specificity lies. (Note that in a primary response it will be predominantly dendritic cells that carry out the initial presentation to T cells, but the mechanism is similar; see below). Any CD4-bearing T cell that recognizes this combination of MHC and peptide will be activated to proliferate into a clone of helper T cells capable of helping any B cell carrying the same combination of MHC+peptide. This means that B cells whose own Ig receptor binds one part of an antigen can be helped by T cells that recognize another part. Thus the B and T cells do not

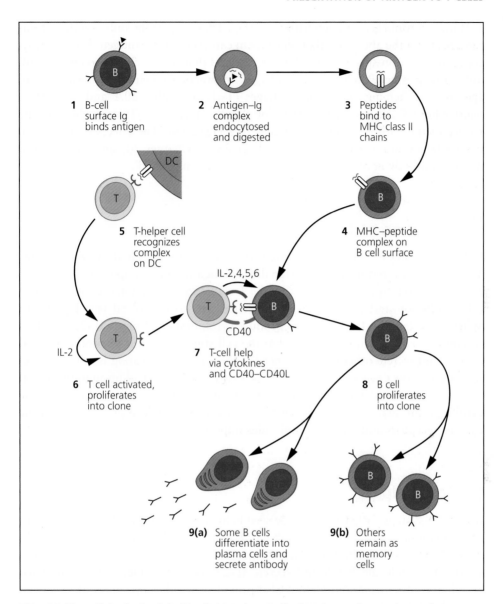

Fig. 19.3 The cellular basis of the T-cell-dependent antibody response. In practice, antigen-presenting dendritic cells (DC) would predominate in the primary response, and B cells in secondary responses.

have to recognize the same portion of the antigen: indeed almost invariably they do not, and the terms *B epitope* and *T epitope* are used to describe parts of the antigen 'seen' by B and T cells, respectively. Historically this distinction was worked out using small chemical groups conjugated to proteins—*haptens* and *carriers*—a situation that can occur naturally, e.g. in allergic responses to penicillin. Normally the result is a beautifully integrated process by which only B cells of the right specificity receive help, although in practice there is some 'leakiness' in the system because cytokines can affect bystander B cells too.

With macrophages and dendritic cells (Fig. 19.3, step 5) the only significant differences from the above are that all of them can take up the antigen (because their recognition is non-specific; see Chapter 12), and that the T-cell clone is then available to help either B cells or macrophages. In practice T helper (T_H) cells tend to specialize in helping either macrophages (T_H1; see Table 20.1 and Fig. 20.6), neutrophils (T_H17; see Table 20.1), or B cells (T_H1 or T_H2) depending on the nature of the pathogen and its antigens (see Fig. 20.6). The effects of T cells on macrophages and neutrophils will be described in Chapter 20; since they do not involve antibody at all, they are referred to as 'cell-mediated'.

■ Activation of T cells

In Fig. 19.3, steps 5 and 6, T cells are shown becoming activated. As with B cells, T-cell activation requires several signals, of which the most important is recognition of the MHC–peptide complex by the T-cell receptor, but interactions between other adhesion and co-stimulatory molecules are also involved (see Fig. 19.4). When activated, the T cell starts to produce cytokines, particularly IL-2, as well as receptors for IL-2, with the result that the cell stimulates itself to proliferate into a clone and secrete other cytokines needed for, in turn, activating B cells (or macrophages). Note once again the economical way in which, in addition to the actual T–B cell contact-dependent helper mechanisms, non-specific molecules (the cytokines) are made to act only on the right cell by the close proximity that the various receptors and adhesion molecules impose.

■ T-cell help

In Fig. 19.3, steps 7–9, T cells can be seen helping B cells to proliferate into clones and differentiate into antibody-secreting plasma cells. This involves a distinct subset of CD4 T cells called follicular helper T cells (T_{FH}), which express the co-stimulatory molecule ICOS and secrete IL-21, both of which are essential for germinal centre formation. Help is also provided by other *cytokines*, IL-2, -4, -5, -6, and IFNγ being some of the most important secreted T-cell products in this case. Some of these cause proliferation, others differentiation, while others again dictate the switch of antibody class (IgM to IgG, IgA, etc.; see Table 19.1), and the generation of memory cells (see below). In the absence of T-cell help, all the B cells of a clone will become short-lived plasma cells, which as terminally differentiated cells live only days or weeks. However, plasma cells generated in germinal centres under the influence of T cells can migrate to the gut or bone marrow and survive for years, keeping up the level of antibody long after exposure. Other B cells do not differentiate into plasma cells but remain as memory cells, ready to generate a faster and better antibody response on re-exposure (see Fig. 19.1 and Table 19.2

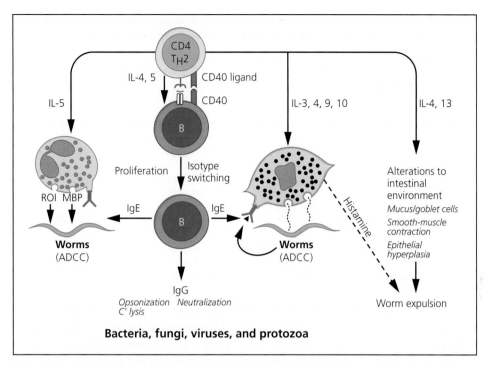

Fig. 19.4 Anti-microbial actions of type 2 CD4 T cells and B cells. MBP, major basic protein; ROI, reactive oxygen intermediates.

Table 19.1 Cytokines involved in B-cell development and function

Cytokine	Source	Effect
IL-2	T cells	Proliferation, IgM secretion
IL-4	T_H2 cells, NKT cells	Proliferation, switch to IgE, IgG
IL-5	T_H2 cells	Proliferation, IgM, IgA
IL-6	T cells, macrophages	Differentiation to plasma cells
IL-7	Bone-marrow stromal cells	Early maturation and proliferation
IL-10	T_H2 cells	Proliferation, differentiation
IL-13	T_H2 cells	Switch to IgE
IL-21	T_{FH} cells	Germinal centre formation
IFNγ	T_H1, CTL, NK, NKT cells	Switch to IgG
TGF-β	T cells	Switch to IgA

Table 19.2 The antibody produced during secondary and subsequent responses differs from primary antibody in several ways, all of which make it more biologically effective

	Primary response	Secondary response
Speed	Slow (days–weeks)	Rapid (1 day)
Duration	Fairly brief (weeks)	Longer (weeks–months)
Amount	Relatively low	High
Ig classes	Mainly IgM at first, with later switch to IgG	Mainly IgG
Affinity*	Variable, medium (but avidity of IgM may be high, owing to multivalency)	High, increases progressively owing to selection of high-affinity B cells and mutation of V genes

*Note the distinction between *affinity* (the strength of binding between a single antigenic determinant and a single antibody-combining site) and *avidity* (the strength of the bond between the two whole molecules).

for the differences between primary and secondary antibody). Actual contact between B and T cell is needed for effective help through the interaction of molecules such as CD40 and its ligand on the T cell (CD154); absence of the latter gives rise to the X-linked hyper-IgM syndrome in which B cells fail to switch from IgM to IgG (see Chapter 25).

Thus we see that T-cell–B-cell interaction is a two-way process: B cells activate T cells to become cells that can help the B cells. Two separate portions of the antigen have to be recognized, with the result that antibody is normally only made against genuinely foreign material. The effect of all these interactions on the fate of pathogens is summarized in Fig. 19.4.

■ B-cell memory

Memory in the immune system compares well with that in the brain; for instance Faroe Islanders were still immune to measles 65 years after their last known contact with the virus, and similarly, in a US trial, antibody to yellow fever virus was still present in the serum nearly 70 years after vaccination. Indeed, long-lasting memory is the basis of all successful vaccines. The way in which long-term B-cell memory is maintained is discussed in Chapter 21.

The germinal centre

Following initial T–B cell contact at the follicle boundary, the remaining processes described in this chapter (B-cell activation, class switching, affinity maturation, formation of memory cells) occur in special regions of lymphoid tissue known as germinal centres (one is shown diagrammatically in Fig. 16.2). Germinal centres are common in lymph nodes, but can develop wherever there are accumulations of lymphoid tissue. It is the resident *follicular dendritic cells* in germinal centres, specialized for trapping and retaining antigen in the form of complexes with antibody and complement (and not identical to the DCs that activate T cells), that regulate B-cell activation and the development of memory.

■ Antibody responses at mucosal surfaces

Although pathogens may enter the tissues through wounds, insect bites, etc. (see Chapter 11), the great majority gain entry across the mucous membranes of the respiratory and gastrointestinal system. Therefore it is not surprising that the *mucosal immune system* comprises over 50% of all the lymphocytes in the body and two-thirds of all B lymphocytes secrete IgA, the antibody class specialized for protection of mucous surfaces. *Mucosa-associated lymphoid tissue* (MALT) is found in the *gut* (GALT), *bronchi* (BALT), nasopharynx, and genitourinary system. The most thoroughly studied is the GALT, which also has the most complex task: to mount responses that prevent entry of intestinal pathogens without making responses against the normal gut flora or against food antigens, and without inducing excessive inflammation. How this is managed is still not fully understood; probably pattern recognition by macrophages and dendritic cells as well as suppressive T-cell-derived cytokines such as IL-10 and TGF-β are involved. The essential components of GALT are (1) *lymphoid aggregates* such as the Peyer's patches, where T and B lymphocytes encounter antigens transported across the epithelial layer by microfold cells and dendritic cells, and (2) the *diffuse lymphoid regions* of the villous lamina propria to which these lymphocytes 'home' after entering the circulation (Fig. 19.5). Lamina propria lymphocytes are mainly memory T cells (see Chapter 20) and B cells secreting IgA under the influence of the cytokines TGF-β and IL-5. Secreted IgA has the advantage of (1) surviving in the proteolytic environment of the gut lumen, and (2) not promoting inflammation,

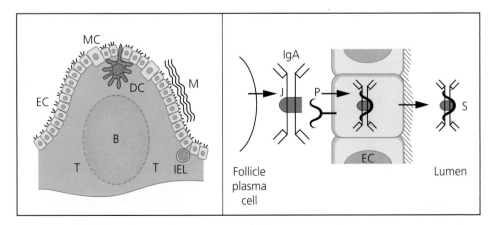

Fig. 19.5 Gut-associated lymphoid tissue, showing (left) a subepithelial 'dome' of lymphoid tissue and (right) how IgA is transported into the gut lumen. DC, dendritic cell; EC, epithelial cell; IEL, intraepithelial lymphocyte; J, joining piece; M, layer of mucus; MC, microfold cell; P, polyimmunoglobulin receptor; S, secretory piece.

since it does not activate complement or mast cells; its role is to block attachment of pathogens to the epithelium and to export those that penetrate the epithelial barrier.

SUMMARY

- Antigens stimulate B cells either directly (T-independent, Ti) or only with the help of T cells (T-dependent, TD).
- For T-cell–B-cell interaction, processed antigen-derived peptides, MHC class II molecules, and CD4 are required, as described in Chapter 18.
- T-cell help for B cells is provided by the secretion of cytokines, particularly IL-2, -4, -5, -6, -21, and IFNγ together with surface molecular interactions, e.g. CD40 with its ligand.
- Once triggered, B cells divide and proliferate into either antibody-secreting plasma cells or memory cells.
- Stimulated B cells start by making IgM, then may switch to IgG, IgA, or IgE. Over half the B cells in the body make IgA for use in the intestine, eye, or respiratory and urinary tract.

Chapter 20
Cell-mediated responses

In this chapter we look at those T-cell responses that do not involve B cells and antibody. As Table 18.1 indicated, they are of two distinct kinds, which will need to be considered separately. One type, the activation of macrophages by CD4 (helper) T cells, has many points of resemblance to the activation of B cells, and will be dealt with first. The other, the CD8 (cytotoxic) T-cell response, is very different (see below). They do, however, have features in common. Both involve the selection and expansion of *clones* of effector cells from a tiny number of precursors and both result in the long-term survival of a population of *memory* cells that ensure a more vigorous secondary response to the same pathogen, just as B cells do. First we will consider how T cells become activated for these responses. Note that they are referred to as 'cell-mediated' purely for convenience to distinguish them from 'antibody-mediated' B-cell responses; in fact, of course, all immune responses originate in *cells*.

■ T-cell activation

There is one important difference between T-cell and B-cell responses, in that while the B-cell product (the antibody molecule) can travel anywhere in the body and has a lifespan of weeks, T cells and their cytokines (see Table 20.1) act transiently and primarily at very short range; thus T cells themselves need to travel to where the pathogen is, or at least close enough to encounter its antigens. This is most likely to be at one of the major sites of pathogen entry: the epithelium of skin and the mucous membranes of the gut, lungs, etc. Here specialized dendritic cells take up the pathogen or its antigens and migrate to the local lymph nodes. In the

Table 20.1 Cytokines involved in T-cell development and function

Cytokine	Source	Effect
IL-2	T cells	T-cell proliferation, enhances cytokine production; NK cell activation and growth; B-cell proliferation
IL-3	CD4 T cells	Promotes haemopoiesis; mast cell growth and development
IL-4	T_H2 CD4 T cells, Mast cells	Promotes T_H2 differentiation/proliferation; B-cell IgE, macrophage inhibition
IL-5	T_H2 CD4 T cells	Eosinophil production and activation, B-cell growth, IgM, IgA
IL-7	Bone-marrow stroma	Maturation/proliferation of precursor lymphocytes; proliferation of naïve T cells
IL-10	CD4 T cells (T_{reg} and $T_H2 > T_H1$), macrophages, DCs	Inhibition of macrophage and DC activation (e.g. IL-12 secretion, induction of MHC class II)
IL-12	Macrophages, DCs, neutrophils	Promotes T_H1 CD4 T-cell differentiation and NK cell/T-cell IFNγ secretion and cytotoxic activity
IL-13	T_H2 CD4 T cells	Mucus production by epithelium, B-cell IgE, macrophage inhibition
IL-15	Macrophages, etc.	NK cell and CD8 T-cell proliferation (maintenance of memory T cells)
IL-17	T_H17 CD4 T cells	Induces production of chemokines, TNF and IL-1; indirectly promotes neutrophil responses
IL-18	Macrophages, DCs	Promotes T_H2 (alone) but T_H1 T cells with IL-12; secretion of IFNγ by NK, T_H1 and memory CD8 T cells (with IL-12)
IL-22	T_H17 CD4 T cells, γ/δ T cells	Inflammation, activation of epithelial cells, maintenance of epithelial barriers
IL-23	Macrophages, DCs	Inflammation, proliferation of memory CD4 T cells, IFNγ production/T_H1 differentiation
IL-27	Macrophage, DCs	Proliferation of naïve T cells, IFNγ secretion
IFNγ	T_H1 CD4 T cells, CD8 T cells, NK, NKT, and γδ T cells	Macrophage activation; B-cell class switching (e.g. IgG2a); T_H1 differentiation; APC activation (e.g. class II expression)
TGF-β	T cells, macrophages, etc.	Inhibits T-cell proliferation and function; promotes IgA; inhibits macrophages
Lymphotoxin	T cells	Neutrophil recruitment/activation; lymphoid organ development

skin it is the Langerhans cells that do this, detaching from the skin during inflammatory responses, migrating via lymphatics to settle in the paracortex of the node where they will eventually encounter, among the ceaselessly passing T cells, those with the appropriate receptor.

The migration of T cells out of the blood vessels to a site of infection is in turn promoted by inflammatory products ('chemokines') and increased expression of adhesion molecules on the vascular endothelium at the site of infection. Local inflammation is also responsible for switching the dendritic cells to an active state capable of full antigen processing and presentation by the time they reach the draining lymph node (see Fig. 18.5). The precise mixture of pro-inflammatory mediators released by dendritic cells is a major influence on which type of T-cell response is initiated, which is a good example of the subtle interplay between innate and adaptive immunity. The key involvement of local inflammation helps to restrict T-cell activity to the site of infection, and in particular to minimize the activation of any T cells that might recognize 'self' peptides.

Note that the above emphasis on dendritic cells applies particularly to primary responses; in subsequent responses involving mainly memory T cells, macrophages and B cells also become important sources of T-cell activation (Fig. 20.1).

■ Effector functions 1: activation of macrophages and other cells

Here the macrophage plays a role analogous to that of the B cell in the previous chapter, conveying antigenic peptides from inside the cell to the surface via MHC class II molecules (Fig. 20.2). However, the aim is not to stimulate it to make antibody (which only B cells can do) but to *kill*, or least *control*, the intracellular microbe from which the peptides are derived. As in the case of B cells, 'help' from the CD4 T cell (T_H1 variety) consists of various cytokines, the most important here being IFNγ. The need for this help arises because so many microbes are able to survive and grow inside the macrophage (see Chapter 13 to be reminded that these include some important bacterial and protozoal infections), whereas it would be dangerous for macrophages, unlike B cells, to be permanently activated in the absence of any microbial stimulus.

A vivid example of how valuable T-cell help can be to macrophages is the effect of IFNγ on the protozoon *Leishmania in vitro*. Normal macrophages are unable to stop this pathogen growing, but a few drops of pure IFNγ, followed by the microbial trigger, are sufficient to tip the balance in favour of the macrophage, with complete killing of the parasite. Translated into real-life terms, this would suggest that patients with defective T cells would suffer worse leishmaniasis than their neighbours, which is exactly what is observed. The same goes for tuberculosis (TB), leprosy, toxoplasmosis, and many other intracellular infections. The explosion of TB in the tropics in recent years is largely associated with immunosuppression of CD4 T cells by the AIDS virus HIV. The well-known BCG vaccine, which causes no more than a transient skin lesion in healthy people,

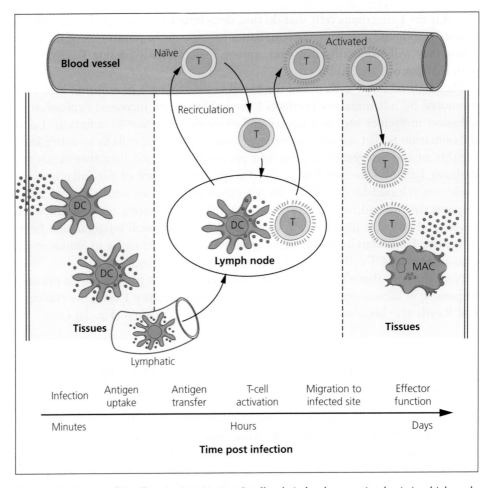

Fig. 20.1 Pathways of T-cell activation *in vivo*. Small red circles denote microbes/microbial products. Note that free antigen is also delivered to the lymph node via the lymphatics where it interacts with dendritic cells resident at this site.

can lead to disseminated infection and even death in someone with deficient T-cell immunity.

While IFNγ remains the major macrophage-activating cytokine, direct T-cell contact involving CD40–CD40L is also important, just as it is for T–B cell cooperation. The consequences of this 'classical' macrophage activation are increased release of pro-inflammatory mediators such as TNF, IL-12, chemokines, etc., increased expression of MHC II and co-stimulators for further T-cell activation and, most importantly, improved killing of ingested microbes via increased generation of ROI and of NO via the induction of NO synthase (NOS2). In contrast, exposure of macrophages to other cytokines or signals (such as IL-4 and IL-13 from T_H2 cells) leads to an 'alternative' or 'deactivation' state with increased expression of the mannose receptor, reduced NO-mediated killing, and distinct immunological functions such as promoting tissue fibrosis.

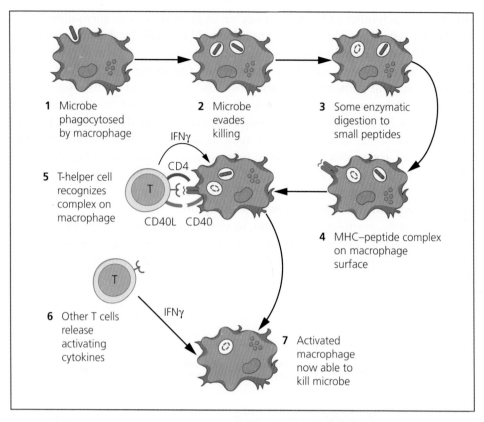

Fig. 20.2 Activation of macrophages by T cells. The same general mechanism operates for intracellular bacteria (e.g. *M. tuberculosis*), fungi (e.g. *Histoplasma*), and protozoa (e.g. *Leishmania*). Note the similarity to the B-cell activation pathway (Fig. 19.3).

The ability of a macrophage, however strongly stimulated, to kill an intracellular microbe or one it has phagocytosed depends on the possession of the appropriate killing machinery. Fortunately, activated macrophages are well armed with both oxidative and non-oxidative mechanisms (see Chapter 12), but many pathogens can resist one or other of these (Chapter 13 and Table 13.1), and even when there is some degree of control of the pathogen the balance is often quite precarious. A good example is the tendency of long-healed TB lesions to break down and cause a flare-up in people who become run-down from malnutrition, drugs, diabetes, HIV, etc.

Granulomas and chronic inflammation

The mechanisms described so far refer to the activation of individual cells. But in real life there is likely to be extensive recruitment of macrophage precursors (monocytes) as well as PMNs to the site of infection, where they mature and become activated. Unless the pathogen is eliminated quickly these will develop into an organized mass of tissue with macrophages at its centre, some of which may fuse to each other to form multi-nucleated giant cells, with surrounding CD4 and CD8 T cells. This is known as a *granuloma*. The T cells, by secreting cytokines, will recruit further cells to the lesion. In the absence of T cells (e.g. in T-cell-deprived mice) some macrophage recruitment can occur via NK cell-derived cytokines, but true granulomas do not form. TB, syphilis, and the liver stage of the blood fluke *Schistosoma* are examples where either killing or 'walling off' of the pathogen is achieved in this way, although granulomas can also be caused by non-microbial but indigestible substances such as asbestos, silica, metals, etc. The mechanism of granuloma formation in tuberculosis is illustrated in Fig. 20.3. Not all granulomas are identical, for example, in tuberculosis IFNγ and activated macrophages predominate, whereas in the schistosome egg granuloma, a mainly T_H2-mediated response, there are also many eosinophils.

Unfortunately, granuloma formation, as well as being beneficial to the host, can also be dangerous. For example, the granulomas surrounding schistosome eggs can coalesce and block off the circulation of portal blood through the liver, with disastrous results. This is an example of *immunopathology*, which will be dealt with in more detail in Chapter 23.

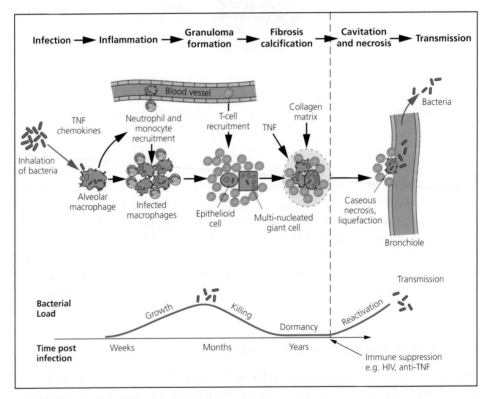

Fig. 20.3 Mechanism of granuloma formation in tuberculosis. In most individuals, small numbers of bacteria can remain for decades under active control by the immune response; immunosuppression leads to reactivation and transmission of the bacterium. Some infected individuals go directly to acute, necrotic disease.

Activation of other cells by T cells

As well as macrophages, other cells can benefit from T-cell-derived cytokines. These include eosinophils, PMNs, NK cells, and the haemopoietic cells in the bone marrow. Indeed, so important are T-helper cells in regulating the function of other cells that they are sometimes regarded as the 'brains' of the immune system, although this does not do justice to the dendritic cells from which T cells in their turn receive important 'instructions'.

■ Effector functions 2: cytotoxicity

Viruses differ from most bacteria and higher microorganisms in that they infect and replicate in cells of almost every kind, including many where T-cell help would be of no value. For example, a liver cell infected with hepatitis B virus could not kill the virus even if helped, since liver cells lack virus-killing mechanisms. One solution is for a neighbouring cell to make the antiviral cytokine interferon (see Chapter 12). Another somewhat more drastic approach is to kill both the virus and its host cell. Cytotoxic T lymphocytes (CTLs) are specialized for this purpose. They are predominantly CD8 T cells designed to recognize viral peptides bound to MHC class I antigens (see Fig. 20.4) and to destroy all cells carrying that combination. This is made possible by the fact that (1) all nucleated cells carry MHC class I molecules, and (2) CTLs carry CD8 molecules, which recognize MHC class I molecules. Generation of functional CTLs can also be dependent on CD4 helper T cells: indirectly via their effect on antigen-presenting cells or directly by the secretion of cytokines (e.g. IL-2) that promote proliferation and differentiation of CTLs.

Proof that this occurs in any given virus infection is quite hard to obtain, but one clear example is the killing of B lymphocytes infected with EBV during glandular fever; the CTLs that do this were once thought to be 'atypical monocytes', hence the alternative name 'infectious mononucleosis'. Note that T-cell-mediated cytotoxicity is the only exception to the rule that T cells work by influencing the 'effector' functions of other cells.

CTLs kill in two related ways: (1) the transfer of granule-derived enzymes ('granzymes') via the actions of perforin into the target cell cytoplasm where they activate the caspase enzymes that in turn induce *apoptosis* or 'cell suicide' (the most rapid and important mechanism); (2) apoptosis can also be triggered via a surface molecule called Fas (the 'death receptor') with which CTLs can interact via a complementary molecule induced on their surface called Fas ligand. CTLs are 'serial killers'; binding and release of cytotoxic mediators and delivery of a lethal hit to the target occurs in minutes (with death occurring a few hours later), allowing the CTLs to disengage and search out another victim. Interestingly, the same mechanisms are used by NK cells, although these employ a completely different recognition system (see Fig. 20.5 and Chapter 12). This is fortunate because one of the numerous ways in which viruses attempt to escape CTLs is by inhibiting

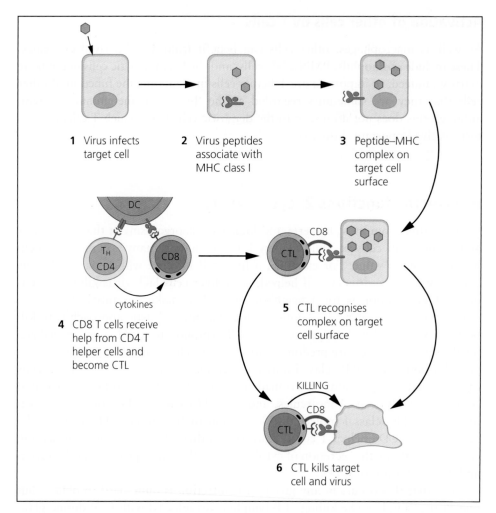

Fig. 20.4 Killing of virus-infected cells by cytotoxic T lymphocytes (CTLs). Note the involvement of different MHC molecules (class I) and T-cell surface molecules (CD8) from those used in the other T-cell-mediated responses (compare with Fig. 20.2). Generation of effector CTL from naïve CD8 cells requires involvement of antigen-presenting cells and CD4 T-helper cells which release cytokines and activate dendritic cells via expression of CD40L (not shown).

MHC class I expression, which would render CTLs ineffective but NK cells more effective! Other viral escape strategies include inhibition of caspases, Fas, and other parts of the apoptotic pathway (see Chapter 22).

Although CTLs are chiefly important in virus infections, they also act against other intracellular infections such as tuberculosis and malaria (liver stage). In the case of leprosy bacilli that infect the Schwann cells lining peripheral nerves, killing these could be counter-productive if it resulted in the liberation of still-living bacilli, which would then have to be dealt with by macrophages. CTLs are also involved in the rejection of transplants and possibly some tumours. Note that in addition to killing, CTLs can also secrete useful cytokines such as IFNγ, TNF, and

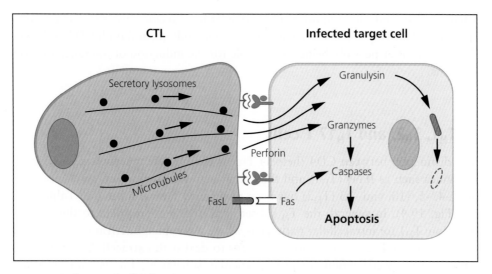

Fig. 20.5 Pathways of cell killing by CTLs. Target recognition causes secretory lysosomes to traffic to the contact site along microtubules within the CTL/NK cell. Transfer of granzymes (or cell-surface ligation of Fas–FasL) induces target cell apoptosis while the antimicrobial peptide granulysin kills intracellular pathogens such as *M. tuberculosis*.

lymphotoxin and it is not always possible to establish which function is the most important in a given infection.

■ T-cell memory

The immunity that follows viral infections such as mumps, measles, rubella, or smallpox is thought to involve both B and T cells. Experiments suggest that memory T cells can persist for many years through low level proliferation under the influence of IL-7 and IL-15. In mice this can occur without the need for stimulation via the T cell receptor but whether this really occurs in the complete absence of antigen in humans is very hard to prove. Certainly the generally longer-lasting protection from live than from killed vaccines, and the reported waning of protection against TB as BCG gradually disappears, suggest a role for antigen persistence. This point is discussed further in Chapters 21 and 28.

■ T-cell responses at mucosal surfaces

Just as with antibody, T cells may be required to act against pathogens that attempt to enter via the intestinal or respiratory routes. The lamina propria (see Chapter 19) contains CD4, NK, and memory CD8 T cells, which have been shown experimentally to contribute to protection against intestinal viruses, e.g. rotavirus. Moreover, oral vaccines prime this population while systemically injected ones do not, illustrating the specific homing pattern of gut-derived lymphocytes (see

Chapter 28) and the importance of delivering vaccines by the right route. Intraepithelial lymphocytes (see Fig. 19.5) also include γδ, and both CD4 and CD8 T cells, the latter possibly being responsible for the induction of tolerance to food antigens.

■ T$_H$1, T$_H$2, and T$_H$17 T cells

The distinction between CD4 (helper) T cells that secrete macrophage-activating cytokines such as IFNγ (T$_H$1) and those that activate B cells with cytokines such as IL-4, -5, -10, and -13 (T$_H$2) has been mentioned several times (see Table 19.1 and Fig. 19.4). In general, the T$_H$ subset activated is appropriate to the type of infection: T$_H$1 for intracellular pathogens where macrophage activation is required (Fig. 20.6) and T$_H$2 for antibody responses to deal with extracellular pathogens, with further specialization towards particular subclasses, for example IgA for intestinal infections and IgE for helminths (Fig 19.4).

Recently a third CD4 T-cell population has been described, preferentially secreting IL-17, a cytokine involved in neutrophil recruitment, and IL-22, which helps maintain the barrier function of epithelial cells. These T$_H$17 cells are mostly responsible for protection against extracellular bacteria and fungi, particularly at mucosal surfaces, but may also mediate pathology in allergic and autoimmune conditions. T$_H$1, T$_H$2, and T$_H$17 cells develop from a common precursor (T$_H$0) and the stimulus to their differentiation comes mainly from cytokines of the innate immune system. IL-12 (from dendritic cells, macrophages, and PMNs) favours the T$_H$1, IL-4 the T$_H$2, and a complicated mix of IL-1, IL-6, IL-23, and TGF-β the T$_H$17 pathway. As cells differentiate under the influence of these signals and polarize their functions they engage different transcription factors

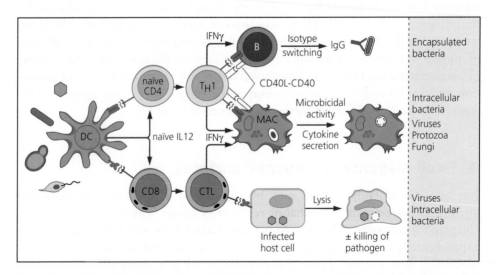

Fig. 20.6 Antimicrobial activities of type 1 CD4 T-cell responses and CTLs. Compare to Fig. 19.4.

(T-bet, GATA-3, and RORγt for T_H1, T_H2, and T_H17 respectively) and modify their chromatin to silence some genes and preferentially activate others, allowing for example T_H1 cells to make IFNγ but not IL-4. Since these populations secrete cytokines that tend to self-perpetuate their own population and suppress the others (e.g. the opposing effects of IFNγ and IL-4), responses usually remain predominantly of one or the other type, even when occasionally this is not the most appropriate (see Chapter 22 for examples of this from leprosy and EBV infection). Finally, polyfunctional CD4 T_H1 cells, which secrete a combination of IFNγ, IL-2, and TNF are of great interest as they produce large amounts of IFNγ per cell (compared to cells which secrete IFNγ alone), and may be the most protective T cell populations in some infections and vaccines.

SUMMARY

- T-cell-mediated responses not resulting in antibody production are referred to as 'cell-mediated'.

- The most important responses are the activation of macrophages, mainly by CD4 T_H1 T cells, the recruitment of neutrophils by CD4 T_H17 cells, and cytotoxicity, mainly of virus-infected tissue cells, by CD8 T cells.

- Activation of macrophages by T cells that recognize peptides+MHC class II molecules can improve their killing ability, and also promote their accumulation into granulomas. Eosinophils, neutrophils, and NK cells can also benefit from T-cell help via release of the appropriate cytokines.

- Cytotoxic T cells act by recognizing peptides+MHC class I molecules, binding to the infected cell, and releasing or activating molecules that give a suicide signal.

- Cell-mediated responses display long-lasting memory, primarily via the proliferative effects of cytokines, but the role of antigen cannot be ruled out.

Chapter 21

Regulation of immune responses and memory

Like most physiological processes, immune responses have the potential to damage their host unless properly regulated. In the case of innate immunity (complement, phagocytes, etc.; see Chapter 12) this is mainly a question of avoiding excessive responses and of focusing them as accurately as possible on the right (that is, the *foreign*) target. Often, however, some 'overspill' is unavoidable, as is shown, for example, by the inflammation and tissue damage that frequently accompany the elimination of a pathogen.

With adaptive responses there is the whole new problem of *lymphocyte proliferation*. The Persian legend of the grains of rice on the chessboard—one grain on the first square, two on the second, four on the next, and so on, culminating in a pile of rice weighing about 100 000 000 000 tons—gives a chilling idea of what could happen if clonal expansion of a B or T lymphocyte carried on unchecked. Several obvious factors would prevent this calamity, lack of available space and nutrients, for example. But Nature has seen to it that more subtle processes act to regulate the size of lymphocyte responses to somewhere near the optimum; that is, large enough to eliminate the pathogen if that is possible, but small enough to allow responses to other pathogens at the same time, with the added bonus of retaining *memory* to each one and mounting a stronger response if it reappears. In this chapter we review these regulatory processes, and we also consider some aspects of memory that have not already been discussed in Chapters 19 and 20.

We can distinguish four levels of control, as follows.

1. *Elimination* of antigen: since antigen is a requirement for the initiation of lymphocyte proliferation, the latter will tend to diminish as antigen disappears.
2. Once a population of lymphocytes has responded, the majority of them (more than 90%) will die by *apoptosis*. Those that survive will become memory cells.
3. Lymphocytes carry surface *receptors* which when ligated can induce inhibition of proliferation and/or function, particularly of B cells.
4. Lymphocytes can inhibit each other: the concept of *regulatory cells* (mainly T cells).

■ Elimination of antigen

Since the end result of a successful response, whether by B cells, T cells, or both, is the elimination of the inducing pathogen and therefore of its antigens, and since antigen is an essential part of the triggering process, a completely successful response does not really need to be turned off; it will simply die away as antigen disappears. Thus the rise and fall of an antibody response can be seen partly as an expression of antigen availability. However, as will be described in the following chapter, many successful pathogens have evolved strategies for avoiding complete elimination, while others recur so frequently that their antigens are present for months or years at a time. In such cases alternative means are required to avoid the chessboard scenario described above.

■ Apoptosis

The elimination of antigen-specific lymphocytes occurs by *apoptosis* (also known as 'programmed cell death' or 'cell suicide'). Unlike *necrosis*, this induces very little inflammation and is a normal part of all immune responses. Previously activated effector cells are particularly susceptible to apoptosis once their antigen, growth factors, and co-stimulatory signals are removed: so-called death by neglect. The mitochondria of these cells become leaky, allowing molecules such as cytochrome *c* to enter the cytoplasm, activate caspases, and induce apoptosis. Apoptotic cells shrink in size, with a characteristic 'laddering' of DNA, and break into small fragments that are removed by phagocytes.

■ Inhibitory receptors

The most striking example of receptor-mediated inhibition is the interaction between antigen–antibody complexes and the receptor on B cells known as FcγR II or CD32. When the IgG of an antigen–antibody complex binds to this molecule and at the same time the antigen binds to the B-cell immunoglobulin, an inhibitory signal is generated. This mechanism is referred to as *antibody feedback*. Clearly such a mechanism will not come into play until substantial amounts of IgG have been made and have bound to the antigen. Antibody feedback has important consequences, including: (1) the tendency of maternally derived IgG to inhibit antibody responses by the newborn—which is why vaccination against some common infections is usually delayed (see Chapter 28)—and (2) the prevention of Rhesus sensitization in RhD$^-$ mothers by RhD$^+$ infants; anti-RhD antibody being given immediately after birth to inhibit further anti-RhD antibody formation.

Other examples of receptor-mediated inhibition include some killer cell immunoglobulin-like receptors (KIRs) found on NK and T cells (see Chapter 12 and Fig. 12.9), and the molecules induced on T cells after activation, such as CTLA-4, which binds to B7 on antigen-presenting cells and gives the T cell an inhibitory signal to dampen down the response. The cytotoxic apparatus of CD8 T cells (see Chapter 20) may also have a regulatory role, since defects of perforins and lysosomal movement lead to overactive antiviral T-cell responses.

■ Regulation by T cells

This term covers two distinct kinds of cell: (1) T cells that are stimulatory for one type of immune response but inhibitory for another, and (2) T cells that are purely inhibitory.

Type 1, type 2, and type 17 T cells

Type 1 and type 2 helper cells have already been mentioned in Chapters 18 and 20, and Fig. 21.1 emphasizes their principal differences, namely that T_H1 cells secrete cytokines such as IFNγ, whose main stimulatory effects are on macrophages, T_H2 cells secrete cytokines such as IL-4 and IL-5, which stimulate eosinophils, mast cells, and basophils, and IgE production by B cells and T_H17 cells indirectly promote neutrophil recruitment via IL-17. Thus T_H1 cells are primarily active in responses to intracellular viruses and bacteria, T_H2 in antihelminth responses and T_H17 in resistance to extracellular bacteria and fungi. In addition, type 1 cytokines inhibit the generation and activity of type 2 cells and vice versa; for example IFNγ inhibits the proliferation of T_H2 cells, whereas IL-4 and IL-13 generate 'alternatively activated' macrophages (see Chapter 20 for more about these). Both IFNγ and IL-4 inhibit the generation of T_H17 cells. Finally, it is worth noting that these subsets are not entirely fixed and some cells which produce interesting mixtures of cytokines can occasionally be found during immune responses; CD4 T cells producing both IFNγ and IL-10 are found in leishmania infection, while IFNγ and IL-17 positive cells can be observed in experimental autoimmune disease.

Regulatory T cells

The separate existence of *suppressor T cells* was debated for many years (see Chapter 24) and they are now referred to as *regulatory T cells* (T_{reg} cells).

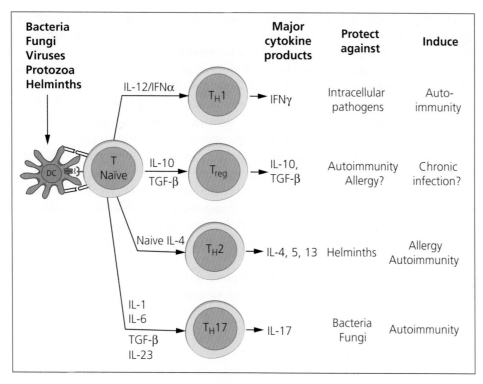

Fig. 21.1 Differentiation decisions of CD4 T cells. Naïve CD4 T cells can differentiate into T_H1, T_H2, T_H17, or inducible T_{reg} T cells according to the conditions present during antigen presentation which differ with the type of infection encountered. The recently discovered T_H17 subset promotes neutrophil-dependent protection against extracellular pathogens but has also been implicated in the generation of inflammatory diseases such as colitis, arthritis, and psoriasis.

Naturally occurring T_{reg} cells are present in all healthy individuals, express the transcription factor Foxp3, and are primarily reactive against self-antigens to prevent autoimmunity. In contrast, uncommitted peripheral T cells can be 'induced' towards a T_{reg} function in the presence of antigen and IL-10 and/or TGF-β. Induced T_{reg} cells specific for microbial antigens are often seen in chronic infections such as leishmaniasis, tuberculosis, and schistosomiasis, at least in experimental mice, and may have some role in pathogen evasion and survival strategy. T_{reg} cells are also suspected of helping to prevent overwhelming immune responses to the masses of commensal bacteria present in the gut. Regulatory T cells can act via either cell contact or inhibitory cytokines such as IL-10 and TGF-β (Fig. 21.1).

■ Therapeutic regulation

There are occasions when it may be necessary to deliberately down-regulate an immune response, most commonly by the use of *immunosuppressive* drugs. Reasons for immunosuppression include the hypersensitivity conditions to be described in Chapter 23 (allergies, granulomas, etc.), autoimmunity (Chapter 24), and, of course, the special situation of organ transplantation. As far as infectious disease is concerned, the major indication for inhibiting immunity is the excessive cell-mediated immune responses found in chronic diseases such as schistosomiasis, which in their efforts to kill and/or wall off the pathogen may end up destroying whole organs. In the case of allergies, it is usually more practical to inhibit the innate mechanisms actually causing the damage—mast cells, histamine, etc.— although preventing the initial IgE response would be the ideal strategy.

When pathology can be shown to be due to excessive cytokine activity, it might be possible to block or neutralize this; an example is the use of drugs or antibodies against TNF in conditions associated with bacterial endotoxins (with little success so far) or, more successfully, in chronic inflammatory conditions such as rheumatoid arthritis and psoriasis. But, in general, immunosuppression is likely to lay the patient open to *more* rather than *less* danger from infection. Table 21.1 lists the most commonly used therapies.

On the other hand, an inadequate immune response may benefit from being *enhanced*. Cytokines have been tried—for example, IFN and IL-2 for chronic

Table 21.1 Some commonly used immunosuppressive therapies

Drug/method	Target of action	Main applications
Corticosteroids	Cytokines (IL-1, -6; TNF), cell migration, inflammation	Hypersensitivities, autoimmunity
Cyclophosphamide	B cells	Autoimmunity
Azathioprine	Cell division	Organ grafting
Cyclosporin, Tacrolimus,	T-cell activation (IL-2)	Organ grafting
Rapamycin	T cell proliferation	Autoimmunity
Anti-lymphocyte antibodies (e.g. -CD3, -CD20)	Lymphocytes	Organ grafting, Non Hodgkins lymphoma, autoimmunity
Anti-cytokine antibodies (e.g. TNFα, IL–6)	Cytokines	Rheumatoid arthritis, Crohn's disease
Cytokine receptor antagonists (e.g. IL-1)	Cytokines	Systemic juvenile onset idiopathic arthritis
Anti-adhesion molecule	Integrins	Crohn's disease
Antibodies	e.g. VLA-4	Multiple sclerosis
Antihistamines	Histamine	Allergies
Sodium cromoglycate	Mast cells	Allergies

intracellular infections, multiple sclerosis (IFNβ)—and some tumours (again with limited success), and IFNγ and G-CSF for management of some primary immuno-deficiencies. Antibody-mediated blockade of CTLA-4, an inhibitor of T cell activation, has achieved recent success in the treatment of malignant melanoma and possibly also prostate cancer where many other attempts have failed. Various regimes, such as diet supplements, physical, and even mental disciplines, etc., may be beneficial too, although hard evidence is usually lacking. For enhancing antigen-specific responses, *vaccination* has proved so effective that it is a standard procedure and is given its own chapter (Chapter 28).

■ Memory

The generation of specific memory is one of the major virtues of adaptive immunity, ensuring that an individual responds progressively faster and more effectively with repeated exposure to a particular pathogen. It explains why one only gets diseases like measles once, and also why the measles vaccine works. Memory is a property of lymphocytes, both B and T, and is based on the development of *memory cells*, which differ in a number of ways from the B and T cells they are derived from (Table 21.2).

Table 21.2 Naïve, effector, and memory lymphocytes compared

	Naïve	Effector	Memory
B cells			
Location	Secondary lymphoid organs	Germinal centre, bone marrow	Secondary lymphoid organs
Surface markers	IgM, IgD	Low Ig, MHC class II	IgG, IgA, IgE
Activity	Minimal	Ig secretion, proliferation	Minimal, but rapid response on re-exposure
T cells			
Location	Secondary lymphoid organs (recirculating)	Sites of infection	Recirculating, gut, lung
Surface markers	CD44 low, CD45RA	CD44 high, CD45RO	CD44 high, CD45RO
	CD62L high	CD62L low	CD62L high or low
	CCR7 high	CCR7 low	CCR7 high or low
Activity	Minimal	Proliferation, cytotoxicity, cytokine secretion	Minimal, but rapid response on re-exposure

■ Generation of memory cells

We have already stressed what the results would be if all the possible progeny of a proliferating lymphocyte clone survived (the chessboard scenario) and described how in fact most of them eventually die. However, the opposite extreme would be equally disastrous, because if *all* of them died, the individual would then be left with no lymphocytes of the relevant specificity and would thus be specifically unresponsive, or *tolerant*, to that particular pathogen, and worse off than before. Memory cells exist to prevent this outcome. It is still not clear exactly how memory cells are generated: from a small population of 'rescued' effector cells otherwise destined to die, or separately from naïve cells stimulated by antigen. Nevertheless, they are adapted to survive for prolonged periods of time, at least in part by increasing expression of molecules which reduce cell death by apoptosis.

B cells

As already mentioned in earlier chapters, immunoglobulin molecules and plasma cells generated in the absence of T-cell help often survive for only a matter of weeks. However, long-lived plasma cells in the *bone marrow* can produce antibody for many months whereas memory cells in secondary lymphoid organs, though not making antibody, are maintained for decades. Thus some antibody is immediately available to deal with a second infection, and more can be made within a few days. It is still controversial whether or not the survival of memory cells requires the continued presence of small amounts of antigen, for example in the form of immune complexes on follicular dendritic cells. Experiments in mice suggest that memory cells can indeed survive in the complete absence of antigen (but mice do not last for 75 years as human memory does!; see Chapter 19). In favour of the idea of antigen persistence is that many pathogens are known to survive virtually indefinitely even in immune hosts, and that living viral vaccines often induce longer-lasting memory than killed ones, but another possible mechanism would be 'boosting' by cross-reaction between the antigens in question and other molecules in the environment.

T cells

Memory T cells appear to be a heterogeneous population with slightly different histories. Two main types are recognized: (1) effector memory T cells retain the adhesive properties of the original effector cells and preferentially migrate to epithelia in the skin and lungs, ready to respond immediately to re-exposure to the pathogen but with restricted proliferative capacity; (2) central memory T cells migrate like naïve T cells, expressing the homing receptors that allow them to recirculate through the blood and lymph nodes. On exposure to antigen, they proliferate strongly and then differentiate, providing a potent reserve, capable of generating large numbers of effectors. Both memory T cell types respond faster than naïve

T cells because of their increased numbers and susceptibility to activation. However, T cell responses do not appear to be prolonged in the manner described above for long-lived plasma cells, presumably because continuous production of the necessary cytokines would be too dangerous for the host.

■ Activation and response of memory cells

B cells

The superiority of secondary antibody responses is due to four properties of memory as compared to naïve B cells: (1) there are more of them specific for the antigen in question; (2) they differentiate into plasma cells more rapidly; (3) during the primary response, most of them switch from making the IgM isotype to IgG (or IgA); once switched, they remain as IgG or IgA producers from the start of the secondary response; (4) because of the high frequency of somatic mutation in the immunoglobulin genes during B-cell proliferation (mainly in germinal centres), a few cells emerge whose antibody has higher affinity for the inducing antigen. As antigen levels decline, these cells are preferentially selected for stimulation, so that the average affinity of the total antibody population rises ('matures'), sometimes by up to 100-fold. Both isotype switching and proliferation are greatly helped by T cells, so that high-affinity IgG tends to be made predominantly against protein antigens.

T cells

Memory T cells can be activated in three different ways, as follows. (1) By the same pathogen as that encountered before; note, however, that T cells do not show class switching or somatic mutation. (2) By a different pathogen which shares one or more antigens with the original inducing one, resulting in a secondary-type response to what should theoretically be a primary infection. This is known as *cross-reactive* or *heterologous* immunity, and could have important consequences as one ages and accumulates T-memory populations, enhancing one's response to a new pathogen in a way that might be beneficial (more rapid elimination) or harmful (more immunopathology; see Chapter 23). An example may be the curious fact that responses to one strain of influenza virus often consist mainly of activity against the strain first encountered, perhaps many years ago ('original antigenic sin'). (3) Unlike naïve T cells, memory cells can be activated by high local levels of cytokines induced by completely unrelated pathogens; this is called *bystander* activation and is particularly a feature of memory CD8 T cells, which can be driven by IL-12 and IL-18 to secrete large amounts of IFNγ. This differs from (1) and (2) above, in being independent of the T-cell receptor (TCR).

■ Maintenance of memory cells

Here, as already mentioned, the key question is whether long-lived *antigen* is needed to maintain long-lived *memory*. Only by being able to detect every single molecule of an antigen in the body (an impossible task) could this question be settled definitely, but cell-transfer experiments in mice suggest that while antigen certainly helps to keep memory up to optimal levels, it may not be strictly required; certainly cytokines (e.g. IL-7 for CD4 and IL-7 plus IL-15 for CD8 T cells) are important and may be sufficient, as in (3) above. Whatever the exact mechanism, multiple pools of memory cells to dozens or hundreds of different antigens are maintained. Presumably as new memory cells are generated others die, perhaps through competition for critical growth factors or other survival signals, but one can only marvel at the precision of the homeostatic mechanisms involved. However, over a lifetime, the relative frequency of T cells to different pathogens can become somewhat skewed—for example, persistent virus infections, in particular human cytomegalovirus, promotes the expansion of large numbers of virus-specific CD8 and CD4 T cells in healthy older people. The extent to which this contributes to the increased risk of infection and reduced response to vaccination in the elderly is the subject of much research.

SUMMARY

- Normally, immune responses die down as the stimulating antigen is eliminated.

- The death of effector B and T cells which are no longer active is mainly by apoptosis or 'cell suicide'.

- Other regulatory factors include binding of antigen–antibody complexes to B cells, and the interplay between various T-cell subpopulations releasing inhibitory cytokines.

- When responses are a danger to the host, they can be inhibited by suitable drugs ('immunosuppression').

- Memory ('secondary') responses are usually larger and faster than primary. This is due partly to increased numbers of B and T cells, but also to different properties of memory cells.

- Cells which mediate B and T cell memory are heterogeneous, with some providing immediate protection (long-lived plasma cells and effector memory T cells) and others in reserve (memory B cells and central memory T cells).

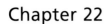

Chapter 22

How pathogens escape adaptive immunity

As the last five chapters have stressed, the key to adaptive immunity is the very high *specificity of recognition*. As compared with the relatively few pattern-recognizing receptors of innate immunity, B- and T-lymphocyte receptors can be generated to recognize a virtually infinite range of foreign molecules; it is certainly impossible to imagine a pathogen *none* of whose antigens would be recognized. Would-be successful parasites must therefore evolve ways of avoiding this recognition, in addition to those ways, already discussed in Chapter 13, of avoiding the disposal mechanisms of the innate immune system.

Every pathogen has its own approach to the problem of being recognized by B and T cells, but they can be grouped into three main categories:

1. attempts to *conceal* their presence from lymphocytes;

2. *variation* of surface antigens;

3. *suppression* or *modulation* of lymphocytes or lymphocyte function.

■ Concealment

Anything that intervenes between a microbial antigen and a B or T cell capable of recognizing it will obviously reduce the chances of inducing an immune response, or of restimulating already existing memory cells. Three fairly common things that can do this are:

1. cell membranes (the pathogen resides inside host cells);
2. cysts, usually of host origin, induced by the pathogen;
3. host-derived molecules taken up by the pathogen (and mimicry of host antigens by the pathogen).

Intracellular residence

Microbes that survive inside host cells are effectively protected against recognition by B lymphocytes, but as explained in Chapters 18 and 20, the MHC system betrays their presence to T lymphocytes and especially to the CD8 killers (Fig. 22.1). Viruses, in particular, have evolved a number of ways around this. They may interfere with the generation of MHC molecules in the endoplasmic reticulum, their transport to the cell surface, or their maintenance there (e.g. CMV, EBV, adenovirus, herpesvirus); alternatively they may prevent the host cell being killed by CTLs by inhibiting the caspase enzymes and other mechanisms leading to apoptosis (e.g. myxoma). Not only viruses but also larger pathogens such as *Chlamydia*, *Yersinia*, *Coxiella*, *Leishmania*, and *M. tuberculosis* can inhibit MHC and CD1 expression, co-stimulation, cytokine release, apoptosis, and indeed virtually anything that could lead to their demise. It is remarkable that in almost every case, successful pathogens rely on more than one single escape mechanism (see Table 22.1).

One vulnerable point in the life of an intracellular pathogen occurs when it attempts to spread to other cells or to infect another individual and is exposed to immune elements in blood or tissue fluid. The bacterium *Listeria monocytogenes* avoids this by the simple strategy of: (1) lysing the membrane of the phagosome in which it resides to enter the cytoplasm, and (2) causing a protrusion of the cell membrane to push into a neighbouring cell, which then buds off to leave the organism in a new phagosome, having never been exposed to the outside of any cell. Some viruses can pass directly into the outside world by shedding into structures that 'face outwards', for example the gut or the skin and its glands. Others

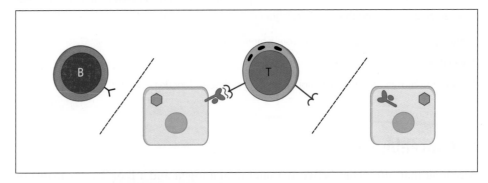

Fig. 22.1 An intracellular habitat protects against recognition by B cells (left). To avoid recognition by T cells, an intracellular pathogen must inhibit the function of MHC molecules (right).

Table 22.1 Mechanisms of pathogen interference with antigen-presenting cell function

Effect on APC	Examples of organism
Reduced endocytosis	CMV
Inhibition of phago-lysosome fusion or phagosome maturation	*M. tuberculosis*, *Chlamydia*, *Legionella*, *Salmonella*
Reduced MHC class II synthesis	*M. tuberculosis*, *Chlamydia*, *Toxoplasma*
Impaired MHC trafficking/expression	CMV, adenovirus
Reduced antigen processing	*Salmonella*
Reduced MHC class I synthesis/expression	*Salmonella*, *Yersinia*, HIV
Inhibition of proteasomes	*Yersinia*, EBV, CMV
Inhibition of TAP	HSV1, HSV2
Expression of non-functional MHC I-like decoys	CMV
Apoptosis of APCs	*Yersinia*
Inhibition of DC maturation	CMV
Over-expression of inhibitory molecules (e.g. IL-10, TGF-β, NO)	*M. tuberculosis*, *B. pertussis*, *Yersinia*
Impaired IL-12 production	Measles, *Leishmania*, *M. tuberculosis*, HIV
Destruction of lymphoid architecture	*Leishmania*
Reduced expression of CD1	*M. tuberculosis*
Impaired expression of co-stimulatory molecules	*L. donovani*

TAP, transporters associated with antigen processing.

do not spread at all but are content to reside, after a brief infection, in long-lived cells, e.g. varicella zoster virus (VZV; chickenpox) in the central nervous system, from which it can emerge decades later to cause a new skin infection (shingles). One could perhaps regard the DNA of the host cell as the safest hiding place of all; this is where retroviruses such as HIV persist so disastrously. Worse, one of the major sites of HIV growth is in the T cells and macrophages of the immune system itself (see *immunosuppression*, below).

Cysts

Cysts are a feature of some worm infections. Initially the cyst is of worm origin, but induces inflammation in surrounding tissue, with fibrosis and even calcification, so that the main bulk of it is host-derived. A striking example is the 'hydatid' cyst of the tapeworm *Echinococcus*, which can grow to enormous size: several litres of fluid containing millions of immature worms. Escaping worm antigens induce vigorous antibody responses, especially of the IgE class, but these antibodies cannot reach the worms inside the cysts. Instead, if antigen is released—for example during surgical operation—IgE bound to mast cells can precipitate severe allergic reactions (see Chapter 23). The tapeworm *Taenia* and the lung-fluke *Paragonimus* are two other worms that give rise to cysts.

Uptake of host antigens

Uptake of host antigens is another worm strategy, best illustrated by the blood fluke *Schistosoma*. The surface of these worms, which live free in the venous circulation and are therefore exposed to the entire range of immune components, becomes coated with host-derived molecules, including blood-group glycolipids, MHC molecules, and immunoglobulins of all kinds. The result is that, as far as the host recognition molecules are concerned, the worm is completely camouflaged and appears as 'self'. This strategy probably works better with slow-growing worms than it would with a rapidly dividing bacterium or protozoan whose surface area doubles every few hours.

Rather different in purpose are the viral genes increasingly being identified that appear to have been acquired from their hosts; these include a remarkable selection of cytokine-like and cytokine receptor-like molecules, presumably of use to the virus in manipulating the immune system for its own purposes (see also *immunosuppression*, below, and Table 22.2).

Antigen mimicry

There are several well-established cases where closely similar molecules are found on host cells and on a pathogen, which might be considered an attempt at disguise. A famous example is the myocardium-like antigen on the wall of Group A β-haemolytic streptococci, although this is probably more important as a cause of *autoimmunity* than as an escape mechanism for the pathogen, and is dealt with in Chapter 24.

■ Antigenic variation

This is one of the most cunning of all pathogen strategies, highly effective at confusing the recognition systems of adaptive immunity, and is found in all classes of pathogen from viruses to protozoa. The principle is that by continuously changing the shape of important surface antigens, or the sequence of critical peptides, the pathogen ensures that it induces a series of primary immune responses, rather than increasingly effective secondary responses, by B and T cells.

The classic example is the influenza virus. This RNA virus is covered with protein antigens of two kinds, haemagglutinin and neuraminidase, each of which

Table 22.2 Some examples of virus-coded cytokine and cytokine-receptor homologues

Virus	Cytokine/receptor	Function
Vaccinia	Epidermal growth factor	Cell growth
	IL-1β receptor	Blocks fever
	IFNα, β, γ receptors	Block IFN
EBV	IL-10	Anti-inflammatory
CMV	IL-10	Immunosuppressive
	Viral chemokine receptor	?
	TNF receptor	Inhibits secreted TNF
HHV6	IL-6, viral chemokine	Angiogenic
	Viral chemokine receptor	?
HHV8	IL-6, viral chemokine	B-cell growth, chemotactic antagonist
	Viral chemokine receptor	?
HIV*	IL-6, viral chemokine	Entry into cells
RSV*	IL-6, viral chemokine	Entry into cells

*RNA viruses; with these exceptions, viral homologues are characteristic of large DNA viruses.

exists in many different forms, known to virologists by number. Thus an attack of H1N1 ('Spanish') influenza would not protect you against the H2N2 ('Asian') or H3N2 ('Hong Kong') viruses (these are the major endemic human strains). A given strain of virus can change these antigens by mutation, producing minor alterations known as *antigenic drift*. Every few years, however, a more drastic change can occur by exchange of RNA between quite different influenza viruses, usually of human and bird origin, the recombination occurring in pigs, which are susceptible to both human and bird strains. This happens mainly in the Far East and is called *antigenic shift*. By spreading round the world, these new recombinant viruses ('escape mutants') are responsible for the major pandemics of influenza (Fig. 22.2 and see also Box 37.1).

A third type of variation is one that occurs during infection within a single individual, no doubt driven by the urgent need to escape the immune response. This is a particular feature of the AIDS virus, HIV. Not only does antigenic variation make the development of secondary responses impossible, but it also interferes with the design of vaccines. An ideal flu or HIV vaccine would have to contain all possible variants—a daunting task!

Also occurring during the individual infection is the slightly different type of antigenic variation displayed by the blood-dwelling protozoa that cause sleeping sickness, *Trypanosoma gambiense* and *Trypanosoma rhodesiense*. Like schistosome worms, these are at the mercy of all the immune components found

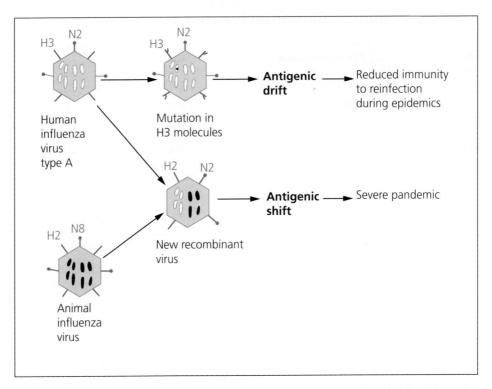

Fig. 22.2 The human influenza A virus is subject to antigenic variation of two kinds: drift (top) and shift (bottom).

in blood. However, the DNA of these parasites contains about 1000 quite different genes, each of which codes for a glycoprotein molecule with which the surface of the parasite can be completely coated. By a process of gene copying and translocation, any of these 1000 glycoproteins can be used as a coat protein. When the rapidly dividing trypanosome comes under attack from antibody, its progeny simply switch genes. Thus the host is obliged to make a series of primary responses (Fig. 22.3). Without drug treatment the disease is fatal, and with so many variants the prospects for a vaccine look fairly slim at present.

Antigenic variation is also a feature of malaria and of several bacterial diseases (e.g. relapsing fever due to *Borrelia recurrentis* and undulant fever due to *Brucella*, as well as infections with *N. gonorrhoeae* and *E. coli*). The antigenic diversity (or polymorphism) seen in so many pathogens, from adenoviruses and salmonellae to malaria, is simply the end result of antigenic variation over a time scale of years, leading to the coexistence of many different variants. For completeness, we should also mention that some pathogens display different antigens at different stages of their life cycle, so that the host may be immune to one stage and not another; a striking example is seen in schistosomiasis, where immunity to new infections by the larval stage allows the adult worms to lead a peaceful and uncrowded existence.

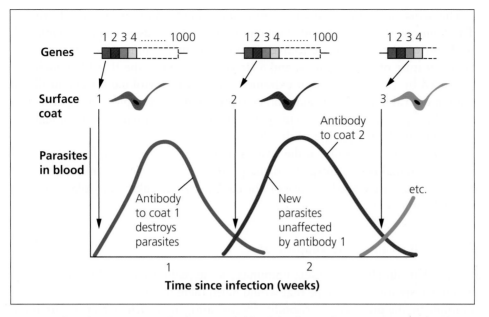

Fig. 22.3 The relapsing pattern of infection with blood-dwelling (African) trypanosomes is due to the repeated appearance and destruction of waves of parasites with completely different surface coat glycoproteins, each requiring a different specificity of antibody for its elimination. The host is thus prevented from developing memory, switching to IgG, etc.

■ Immunosuppression

During many infectious diseases, patients are found to be immunodeficient to some degree. There may be a reduction of T cells in the blood, or a failure to produce a good antibody response or switch from IgM to IgG (see Chapters 25 and 26). Immunosuppression is seen in measles, mumps, chickenpox, glandular fever, tuberculosis, leprosy, and many protozoal diseases. During measles, skin tests for tuberculosis become negative and susceptibility to a flare-up increases. Quite mild malaria has been shown to severely impair the ability of otherwise normal people to respond to some bacterial vaccines: a very important consideration in terms of public health programmes. Whether it actually helps the malaria parasite to survive is debatable, but there are examples in experimental animals where deletion of an immunosuppressive molecule undoubtedly helps the host to eliminate other infections. The wildly excessive T-cell responses induced by staphylococcal and streptococcal superantigens (see Chapter 18) could also be considered as an interference with normal immunity.

The above examples of immunosuppression are normally temporary and probably do no long-term harm. However, some pathogens cause severe and progressive immunosuppression; the classic example is HIV. Here the steady loss of CD4 (helper) T cells leads to a total inability to cope with intracellular parasites including viruses, mycobacteria, fungi, and protozoa. This terrible disease, the most common infectious cause of immunodeficiency, is discussed in more detail in Chapter 26.

The actual mechanisms involved in immunosuppression are extremely varied. The mimicry of cytokines and cytokine receptors by viruses, already mentioned, probably constitutes a very effective way of avoiding immune attack. It is particularly a feature of herpesviruses, and a striking example is the IL-10-like molecule produced by EBV. IL-10 is an extremely suppressive cytokine for cell-mediated immunity. Table 22.2 lists some other representative examples. In experimental mice, over-production of regulatory T cells (e.g. in leishmaniasis) is thought to contribute to the persistence of the chronic infection.

Suppression may operate at the level of tissues rather than cells, for instance the loss of germinal centre integrity in the protozoal disease leishmaniasis. Another rather special case is the blockage of normal lymph recirculation by filarial worms in elephantiasis.

Diversion of immune responses

Rather than simply suppressing immunity, some pathogens are able to *divert* the immune response from a type that would harm them to another, harmless type for example by the production of soluble 'decoy' antigens which attract the attention of the immune system away from the pathogen itself (see Table 22.2). Sometimes pathogens survive because the host mounts an ineffective response. Here the classic example is leprosy. This is caused by a mycobacterium similar to the tubercle bacillus, which is susceptible to T-cell-mediated but not antibody-mediated immunity. Many patients appear to achieve protective immunity without serious disease, but for reasons not fully understood, the infection sometimes induces excessive cell-mediated immunity, resulting in destruction of the bacilli and damage to host tissues, and sometimes strong but ineffective antibody responses. These two patterns of response, referred to as *tuberculoid* and *lepromatous*, respectively, represent the extremes of a 'spectrum' (Fig. 22.4), and a somewhat similar pattern is seen in cutaneous leishmaniasis. It has been proposed that the decisive event is the switching of the helper T cells towards the T_H1 or T_H2 type (see Table 18.1).

Polyclonal activation

Yet another variation on the theme of immunosuppression is the ability of some pathogens to activate large numbers of lymphocytes, most of which will not have the appropriate specificity to attack them. The staphylococcal superantigens that do this to T cells have already been mentioned, and also those T-independent antigens that activate B cells polyclonally such as LPS from Gram-negative bacteria (see Chapter 19). Many infections, particularly by protozoa such as those causing malaria and trypanosomiasis, are accompanied by high levels of antibody, much of which is not detectably specific for the pathogen. Likewise much of the high levels of IgE in worm infections are not specific for the infecting worm. It is reasonable to suspect (although hard to prove) that these useless lymphocyte responses restrict the host's ability to mount useful responses. Moreover, there is evidence that, because they may include anti-self responses, they may actually

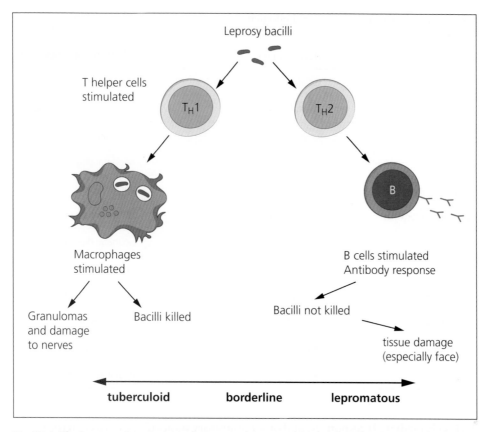

Leprosy bacilli

T helper cells
stimulated

T_H1

T_H2

B

Macrophages
stimulated

B cells stimulated
Antibody response

Granulomas
and damage
to nerves

Bacilli killed

Bacilli not killed

tissue damage
(especially face)

tuberculoid   borderline   lepromatous

Fig. 22.4 The 'spectrum' seen among leprosy patients may be related to the activities of subsets of T-helper cells. By releasing different cytokines, T_H1 and T_H2 cells induce different patterns of immune response, with different clinical consequences. What determines the choice of T_H1 or T_H2 pathway in different individuals is still unknown.

induce damage to host tissues. In fact polyclonal lymphocyte activation is believed to be the cause of some *autoimmune diseases* (see Chapter 24).

■ Pregnancy, transplants, and tumours

Although not directly related to infection, these special situations represent a challenge similar to that posed by pathogens to the immune system, namely how to survive in the face of immune attack. In the case of *pregnancy*, the problem has been solved by nature; despite the presence in the fetus of large amounts of foreign (paternal) HLA, *tolerance* is the rule. This is achieved by a number of separate strategies: Class I HLA antigens are lacking in the trophoblast, and the 'classical' NK cells that might be expected to react are inhibited by a special embryo-derived antigen, HLA-G. In addition the maternal immune system, at least in the local environment, appears to be set at a level favouring T_H2 (antibody) rather than

Table 22.3 Some congenitally acquired infections

Pathogen	How acquired	Effect on fetus/newborn
Toxoplasma	via placenta	eye, ear, brain damage
Rubella virus	via placenta	eye, ear, brain damage
Cytomegalovirus	via placenta	eye, ear, brain damage
Syphilis	via placenta	neonatal disease
Herpes simplex virus	via placenta	encephalitis
Varicella zoster virus	via placenta	childhood zoster
Malaria (rare)	via placenta	neonatal disease
HIV	via placenta and during birth	neonatal disease
Hepatitis B	during birth	neonatal disease
Gonorrhoea	during birth	conjunctivitis
Chlamydia	during birth	conjunctivitis
Candida	during birth	neonatal thrush

T_H1 (cell-mediated) responses, and other inhibitory molecules such as α-fetoprotein are also involved. Excessive T_H1-type responses are thought to contribute to repeated miscarriage which is, rather surprisingly, commoner when maternal and paternal HLA are closely matched. The placenta has an important role in infection due to the ability of certain pathogens to cross it and infect the fetus (Table 22.3).

Tumours represent the opposite situation, an unwanted mass of 'self' tissue that manages to avoid elimination. The best evidence that the immune system can to a certain extent restrict tumour growth comes from the increased tumour incidence in immunodeficient or immunosuppressed individuals, and from 'knock-out' mice: NK, T cells, both CD4 and CD8, and several cytokines, notably TGFβ and IFNγ, all play a role. Recently cytokine therapy and tumour 'vaccines' have had some success in particular tumours. Finally, a *transplant* (e.g. a kidney) constitutes a challenge for which nature is not prepared; how to make a completely foreign organ survive and function in a new host. Here, despite decades of immunologically-inspired approaches, the most successful regime is still carefully controlled immunosuppression by drugs such as cyclosporin, a fungal product that inhibits the synthesis of the cytokine IL-2 in T cells.

SUMMARY

- Successful pathogens need mechanisms for escaping innate and adaptive immunity if they are to survive more than a short time.

- Concealment, for example inside cells, is effective, but makes spread to another host more difficult.

- Antigen variation is highly effective against adaptive immunity and is a serious impediment to vaccine development.

- Suppression and/or diversion of immune responses may not only permit pathogen survival but increase susceptibility to unrelated infections.

Chapter 23

Disease due to adaptive immunity I: hypersensitivity

The way in which lymphocytes respond, amplifying a tiny minority of specific cells into large clones with powerful potential to damage their target, makes it all the more important for the responses to take place against the right target and in the right place. Unfortunately this does not always happen precisely, with the result that host tissues can also be damaged, the actual damage being inflicted frequently by elements of the innate immune system (refer back to Chapter 14 for a reminder of how innate immunity itself can also overreact). Tissue damage caused in this way is called *immunopathology*, or sometimes *hypersensitivity*. If lymphocytes actually start to respond to the host's own (i.e. self) antigens, this is called *autoimmunity*. Autoimmunity is an abnormal response and will be discussed in the following chapter; here we consider the unwelcome side effects of 'normal' responses against perfectly ordinary non-self antigens.

All over the world, one system of nomenclature is used to classify these effects: it is the one introduced in 1958 by Gell and Coombs, who divided up the causes of hypersensitivity as shown in Table 23.1.

■ Type I (allergic) hypersensitivity

This is by far the most common type of immunopathology, since about one person in six suffers from some kind of allergy. The fundamental problem is that IgE antibody can do harm as well as good, triggering off acute inflammatory reactions where they are not needed. Hay fever is an example. Most people can inhale the pollen grains, dust particles, etc. that the air is full of without ill effect, either coughing them up or phagocytosing them. However, some people have the tendency

Table 23.1 Mechanisms of hypersensitivity: the Gell and Coombs classification

Type, name	Mediated by	Example
I, *allergic*	IgE antibody and mast cells	Hay fever
II, *cytotoxic*	IgG antibody, complement, phagocytes	Rejection of blood transfusion
III, *complex-mediated*	Soluble antigen–antibody complexes, polymorphs, complement	Glomerulonephritis
IV, *cell-mediated*	T cells, cytokines	TB granuloma
V, *stimulatory* (added later)	Antibody to hormone receptors	Thyrotoxicosis

to make large amounts of IgE against a particular animal or plant antigen; their mast cells and basophils pick this up via their Fcε receptors, and when the antigen comes along again, activating the mast cell by cross-linking two or more receptors, the cells degranulate, release a number of preformed mediators (Fig. 23.1 and Table 23.2), and initiate a local inflammatory reaction. Such reactions are called *allergic* and people with this tendency are called *atopic*. As hinted in Chapter 12, inflammation can be most useful in getting blood and blood components to the site of an infection, but if it occurs in the nose and eyes every time a pollen grain settles there it is just a nuisance. Likewise in the skin (urticaria). If it occurs in the bronchi it can be dangerous, causing attacks of asthma. And if it occurs all over the body it can even be fatal, as very occasionally happens with the *anaphylaxis* following a bee-sting or a penicillin injection.

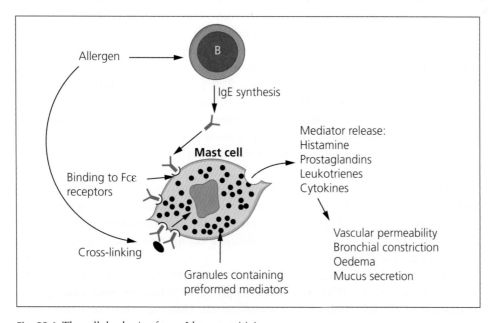

Fig. 23.1 The cellular basis of type I hypersensitivity.

Table 23.2 Mast-cell-derived mediators of hypersensitivity

Mediator	Biological effects
Preformed in granules	
Histamine	Vascular permeability increase, bronchoconstriction
Chemotactic factors	Attract PMNs and other cells
Platelet-activating factor	Release of factors causing vascular permeability
Heparin	Anticoagulant
Newly formed after activation	
Prostaglandins	Pain, fever
Leukotrienes	Attract cells

Despite intensive study, the reasons why one person makes a large amount of IgE to one molecule and a second to another, while a third is not allergic to anything, are not understood, but it has been thought, like the leprosy spectrum (see Fig. 22.4), to be related to the pattern of cytokine production by T-helper cells, T_H2 cells favouring allergy by releasing IL-4, IL-5, and IL-13, and T_H1, and T_{reg} cells tending to inhibit this. It is worth mentioning that for IgE 'a large amount' is a relative term, since even a 1000-fold increase in serum IgE level leaves it as the minority immunoglobulin class (look back to Table 17.1).

To test for allergy, a small amount of the suspected allergen is injected into the skin, and if there is IgE on the local mast cells, a red, swollen 'immediate hypersensitivity' reaction comes up within 10 min. This is mediated by the granule contents of triggered mast cells, including histamine and lipid mediators such as prostaglandins, leukotrienes, and platelet-activating factor. It is followed a few hours later by a 'late phase reaction' involving recruited eosinophils, basophils, T_H2 T cells, and neutrophils, but not the T_H1 cells and macrophages typical of delayed (type IV) responses. The skin test subsides by the following day, but in asthma the response is prolonged and contributes to the pathology. The incidence of allergy in the Western world, but not in the tropics, has increased dramatically in the last decades, and the reason for this has been the subject of much debate (see below).

Although most antigens causing allergy (allergens) are non-microbial, allergy and infection are linked in a number of ways. Most striking are the worm infections. As mentioned in the previous chapter, escape of antigen from a hydatid cyst can precipitate massive anaphylaxis, a dreaded complication of surgical removal of large cysts (Fig. 23.2).

Roundworms like *Ascaris*, which sometimes visit the lung, can precipitate violent asthmatic attacks. Why worms are so prone to induce so much non-specific as well as specific IgE antibody is not understood. However, there is evidence that

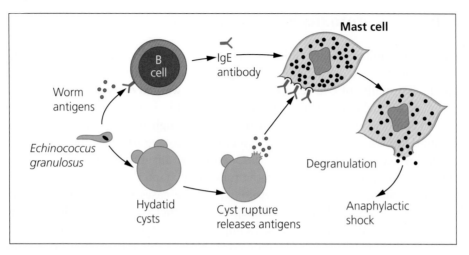

Fig. 23.2 Anaphylaxis, with vascular collapse, following rupture of a hydatid cyst, illustrates the mechanism of type I hypersensitivity. Less severe symptoms, often localized to one organ (e.g. the lung), may occur in other worm infections.

specific IgE and eosinophils constitute a killing mechanism against some worms, and that mast-cell degranulation in the gut helps remove parasites by increasing peristalsis and mucus production, so there may be some protective advantage. Some of the symptoms of respiratory virus infections may also be due to type I hypersensitivity, although it can be difficult to distinguish these from the effects of the virus itself (sneezing, mucus secretion, etc.). In addition, a viral infection of the upper respiratory tract may trigger allergy or asthma in an already atopic individual (e.g. to pollen).

Most interesting of all is the proposed link between childhood exposure to infectious disease and the later development of allergy: the *hygiene* hypothesis. According to this idea the increased level of allergic disease in developed countries is due to the later and lesser exposure to various pathogens, perhaps especially enteric organisms. The mechanism was thought to operate via changes in the T_H2/T_H1 balance, but since the incidence of T_H1-mediated autoimmune diseases is also on the increase, a more likely explanation is that infections in early life stimulate the development of regulatory mechanisms. These might include, for example, the secretion of IL-10 by T_{reg} or other cells in response to a range of microorganisms. IL-10 has a 'damping down' effect on almost all immune responses, both innate and adaptive, and has been referred to as the 'homeostatic' cytokine. Another indirect link between infection and allergy is the unfortunate tendency of many *antibiotics* to induce allergic reactions, with penicillin being the most obvious example (see Chapter 29 for further details). The clinical importance of these responses is clearly shown in young boys with a rare X-linked mutation in Foxp3, a key transcription factor in a subset of T_{regs}, who suffer from allergy and autoimmunity and can die by two years of age if not treated.

■ Type II (cytotoxic) hypersensitivity

Here it is the ability of IgG antibody to destroy cells by causing them to be either phagocytosed or lysed by complement (IgM will do the latter too) that causes the trouble. Normally, of course, IgG is just what is wanted to get rid of pathogens, but in two special circumstances phagocytosis and lysis are not wanted. One case is when removal of the cells is not desired, although they are foreign, obvious examples being a blood transfusion or a bone-marrow graft. The other is when the IgG is directed against self; this is *autoimmunity*, an important complication of some infections, to be discussed in the following chapter. Sometimes included in this group, though not actually cytotoxic, are the cases where antibody against *hormone receptors* can bind to the receptor and either stimulate or inhibit it; thyroid diseases are the best-validated examples of this but there is no clear link to infection. However, some authorities prefer to call this type V hypersensitivity. The killing of liver cells infected with hepatitis B virus by CTLs is an essential part of recovery, but may go too far, leading to chronic, or in rare cases fatal, hepatitis. On the other hand, too weak a CTL response may allow persistent infection, the *carrier* state.

■ Type III (immune complex-mediated) hypersensitivity

Here, too, IgG antibody is involved, but the damage is actually initiated by soluble complexes of antigen and antibody. The antigen may be self (autoantibodies to DNA are particularly important in some chronic diseases) or of microbial origin. The damage is due to the fact that, though of course complexing with antigen for subsequent removal is the whole point of making antibody, large amounts of antigen–antibody complexes cannot always be removed from the blood rapidly enough, and tend to end up in the tissues or, more seriously, in the walls of small blood vessels. Here they can be attacked by the combination of PMNs and complement (both of which are involved in the protective effects of antibody, see Chapter 12 and Table 17.1). Under these conditions, PMNs may release their toxic contents and damage the blood vessel. Platelets also contribute to the damage. The skin and the renal glomerulus are two particularly vulnerable sites, but any small vessel can be affected. Prolonged immune-complex deposition in the kidney is one of the commonest causes of *glomerulonephritis*, which in turn is the commonest cause of renal failure. Several infectious diseases are among the causes of glomerulonephritis (Table 23.3) and quite often an infectious organism is suspected but cannot be identified.

In the pre-penicillin days when injection of horse antibodies was the only treatment for bacterial pneumonia, etc., immune complexes formed between the horse immunoglobulins and human antibodies against them, deposited at several sites in the body, gave rise to the syndrome of *serum sickness*, with damage to

Table 23.3 Glomerulonephritis and other forms of vasculitis can be caused by immune complexes formed during the course of various infectious diseases; these would all be regarded as examples of type III hypersensitivity

Organ(s) affected	Infectious organism	Condition
Renal glomerulus	Hepatitis B virus	Chronic hepatitis
	Staphylococcus	Endocarditis
	Streptococcus	Post-streptococcal infection
	Treponema pallidum	Secondary syphilis
	Plasmodium	Malaria
	P. falciparum	malignant tertian
	P. malariae	quartan
	Schistosomes	Schistosomiasis
Other blood vessels	Hepatitis B	Acute hepatitis
(in skin, joints, etc.)	*Mycobacterium leprae*	Leprosy
	Hepatitis B?, TB?	Polyarteritis nodosa
	Dengue virus	Haemorrhagic fever

skin, kidney, and joints; generally this got better when the injections were stopped. The modern use of 'humanized' monoclonal antibodies has eliminated this complication.

■ Type IV (cell-mediated) hypersensitivity

This term refers to the harmful aspects of cell-mediated immune responses, the principal one being excessive *granuloma* formation. As explained in Chapter 20, the formation of a granuloma may sometimes be the best way to control an intracellular infection that even activated macrophages cannot totally eliminate; the solid mass of macrophages, fibrous tissue, etc., being an effective 'walling-off' device as well as providing enhanced killing potential. However, very numerous confluent granulomas can displace so much normal tissue that they interfere with normal function. Moreover, some of them tend to become necrotic at the centre. This combination of *fibrosis* and *cavitation* is a frequent end-result of pulmonary tuberculosis (Fig. 23.3). In some diseases (e.g. sarcoidosis) granulomas form but no microbial cause can be identified. In others, the organism is known, but not the mechanism. An example is *farmer's lung*, a serious hypersensitivity reaction to fungal spores (and some animal products) whose pathogenesis seems to include features of both type III and type IV.

Just as allergic status can be measured by an immediate skin test (see above), the level of cell-mediated hypersensitivity can be detected by a *delayed* skin test. For

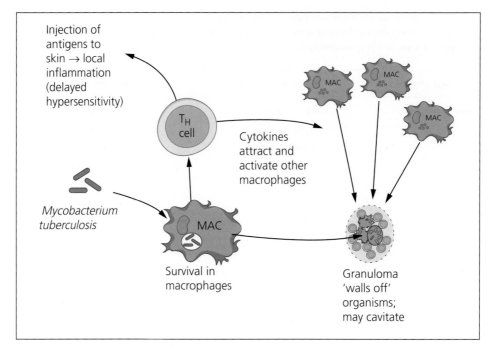

Fig. 23.3 Granuloma formation in tuberculosis, and the elicitation of a positive delayed (Mantoux) skin test, are both dependent on the existence of mycobacterial antigen-specific T cells (CD4, T_H1 type). Both phenomena are covered by the term type IV hypersensitivity. For further details see Fig. 20.3.

example, if an intradermal injection of purified protein antigens from the tubercle bacillus (purified protein derivative, PPD) encounters specific T-helper cells, a local inflammatory reaction, with oedema and cellular infiltration (mainly monocytes and T_H1 cells), develops over the next 2–3 days: a positive *delayed-type hypersensitivity* (DTH) test. DTH tests are often named in relation to the substance injected for the disease in question; thus tuberculin (for TB), lepromin (for leprosy), and leishmanin (for leishmaniasis). Note, however, that a positive Mantoux (tuberculin) test does not guarantee that the patient is 'immune' to TB, merely that there has been previous exposure, so that one cannot automatically equate delayed hypersensitivity with protection. During infections where the pathogen is not eradicated (e.g. tuberculosis, schistosomiasis) chronic DTH may lead to fibrosis due to an increase in collagen synthesis by fibroblasts at the site under the influence of macrophage-derived TGF-β. Another situation where cell-mediated reactions harm tissues is the killing of virus-infected cells by CTLs (see Fig. 20.4). On balance this is beneficial in disposing of the virus, but nevertheless there is damage to the host which can reach serious levels, as in the case of hepatitis and some respiratory viral infections. The damage to the liver in hepatitis B, which may occasionally be life-threatening, is mainly due to CTLs, since the virus itself is not cytopathic.

SUMMARY

- Adaptive immune responses can damage host tissues in several ways.

- IgE antibody attached to mast cells and cross-linked by pathogen-derived antigen can trigger inflammatory (allergic) reactions. These are particularly common in worm infections.

- Cytotoxic killing of intracellular viruses and their host cell can damage vital organs, such as the liver.

- Antigen–antibody complexes that become attached to blood vessel walls, e.g. the renal glomerulus, can induce local inflammation and organ damage.

- T cells over-stimulated by persistent intracellular pathogens can attract and activate macrophages into a granuloma.

Chapter 24

Disease due to adaptive immunity II: autoimmunity

CHAPTER CONTENTS

- Self-tolerance
- Polyclonal lymphocyte activation
- Antigen mimicry
- Release of sequestered antigens

- Anomalous antigen presentation
- Anomalous cytokine production
- Autoimmunity, autoimmune disease, and genetics

In the previous chapter, several examples were given where damage to host tissues is due to an adaptive response against 'self' antigens. This is called *autoimmunity*, and represents a failure of normal tolerance to 'self' by T and B lymphocytes. Of the large number of possible underlying causes, two stand out: *infection* and *genetic predisposition*. However it must be admitted that there are considerable areas of ignorance as to precisely what goes wrong in individual diseases, but five mechanisms can be identified as fairly well established.

1. polyclonal activation of anti-self B or T lymphocytes;

2. activation of anti-self B or T lymphocytes by antigens closely similar to self: *molecular mimicry*;

3. release of sequestered antigens;

4. anomalous antigen presentation;

5. anomalous cytokine production.

■ Self-tolerance

Before discussing these further, we need to understand how autoimmunity is normally avoided (Fig. 24.1). Why do some B and T lymphocytes not recognize and respond to 'self' antigens, considering that their receptors are produced by a random recombination of genes and should be able to recognize virtually everything, instead of being unresponsive, or *tolerant*, to self?

Tolerance develops at two levels, firstly in primary lymphoid organs where lymphocytes are first generated (central tolerance) and secondly, since this process is never perfect, by additional mechanisms in the periphery (peripheral tolerance). In the case of B cells, engagement of the B-cell antigen receptor in the bone marrow by self antigens blocks maturation and if continued leads to death of cells with the highest affinity for self (although many self-reactive cells with low affinity still escape). T cells are 'vetted' by means of a two-stage selection process in the thymus, and the great majority of those that recognize *self MHC plus a self peptide* are eliminated. This means that in the periphery few or no T cells will respond to *unaltered* self, and therefore a B cell, even if it does recognize a self antigen, will generally not get help from a T cell and will instead become 'anergic'. This ensures that only low-affinity IgM antibody is normally made against self antigens, and only those of the 'repeating epitope' kind (see Fig. 19.2). There are also mechanisms for rendering T cells anergic in the periphery, under the influence of special 'tolerogenic' dendritic cells which do not express the cytokines and co-stimulatory molecules that drive productive T-cell responses to microbial antigens. Repeated antigenic stimulation can also lead to ligation and activation of 'death receptors' (e.g. of Fas by FasL) resulting in apoptosis and deletion of self-reactive T cells.

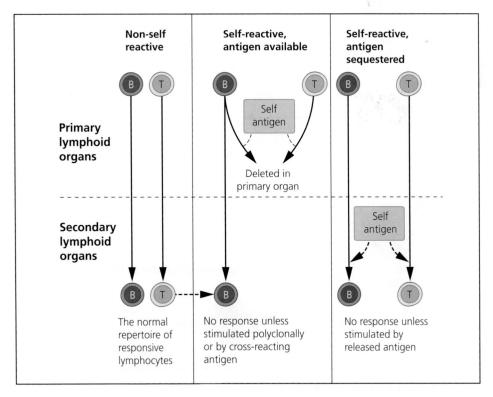

Fig. 24.1 Self-tolerance in B and T cells is maintained in several ways. For further details, see text.

Defects in this death pathway predispose to autoimmunity. In addition, regulatory T cells generated in the thymus of normal individuals can react against self antigens and inhibit autoimmune T-cell responses.

■ Polyclonal lymphocyte activation

This embargo on responses by self-reactive B cells, however, can be broken by molecules with the property of triggering responses by all, or a high proportion of, lymphocytes. In the case of B cells, such molecules include some from bacteria such as LPS, from protozoa—notably malaria and trypanosomes—and viruses such as EBV and hepatitis C. Infections of all these kinds are accompanied by high levels of IgM antibody, most of which is not directed at the microbial antigens, but some of which may be directed against self. Usually this is not serious, and the autoantibodies disappear when (and if) the infection is cleared. But it has been suggested that in some diseases associated with IgG autoantibodies (for example

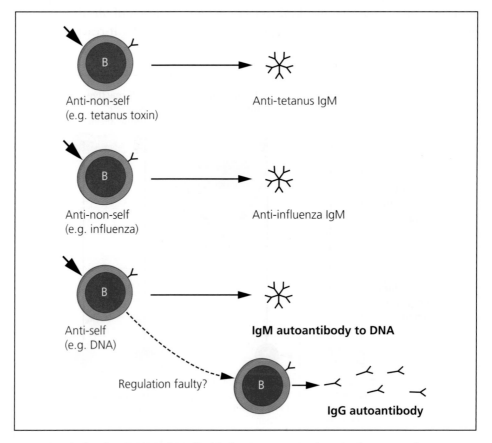

Fig. 24.2 Polyclonal activation of B cells (black arrows) may induce the formation of autoantibody by any self-reactive cells that have escaped elimination in the bone marrow.

systemic lupus erythematosus and rheumatoid arthritis), the above process has got out of control (Fig. 24.2). Possibly in these cases the T cells are being activated by *superantigens* from bacteria or viruses (see Chapter 18), although at present it is thought that these are more important in exacerbating already activated autoimmunity than in initiating it.

■ Antigen mimicry

Another way round the absence of self-reactive T cells is for an antigen to carry both 'self' and 'non-self' determinants, thus partially *mimicking* its host and bypassing the lack of self-reactive T cells. Provided a B cell can recognize the self portion and a T cell the non-self portion, the T cell will supply help, resulting in a full-blown antibody response to the self portion. An example is the group A *Streptococcus*, which happens to carry an antigen (the M protein) very similar to one on mammalian heart muscle, kidney, and joints. Antibodies to this antigen can therefore damage these organs, and this explains the myocarditis seen in rheumatic

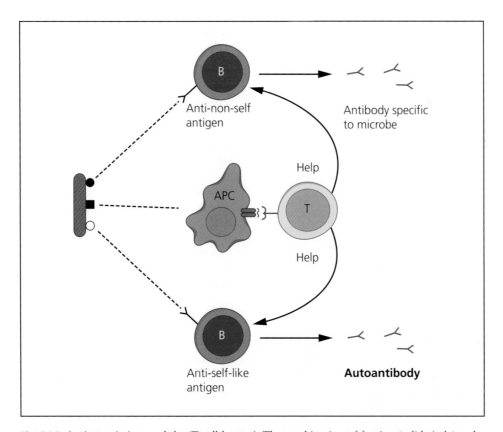

Fig. 24.3 Antigen mimicry and the 'T-cell bypass'. The combination of foreign (solid circle) and self (open circle) antigens on a microbe (left) allows a T-dependent autoantibody response, bypassing the lack of self-reactive T-helper cells.

Table 24.1 Some examples of molecular mimicry between pathogens and their hosts

Pathogen	Mimicked molecule
Viruses	
Vaccinia	IL-1 receptor
EBV	IL-10
CMV	β2 Microglobulin, chemokine receptor
Herpes simplex	Complement receptor 1
Polio	Acetylcholine receptor
Hepatitis B	Myelin basic protein
Rabies	Insulin receptor
Adenovirus	α Gliadin* (a wheat component)
Herpes (monkey)	IL-8 receptor
HIV	Astrocyte antigen
	Platelet antigen
Sarcoma viruses (cat, mouse, etc.)	Host oncogenes
Bacteria	
Group A streptococci	Human myocardial myosin*
Klebsiella	HLA B 27*
Meningococcus	Fetal brain (NCAM)
Treponema (syphilis)	Cardiolipin* (a phospholipid)
Mycoplasma	Blood group I antigen*
Campylobacter jejuni	Peripheral nerve gangliosides*
Fungi	
Candida	Complement receptor 3
Protozoa	
Plasmodium (malaria)	Thymus hormone
Trypanosoma cruzi	Human heart and nerve antigens
Worms	
Schistosoma	Glutathione transferase

*For asterisked items there is reasonable evidence that they are involved in the induction of autoimmunity.

fever. Figure 24.3 illustrates this mechanism and Table 24.1 lists some other examples of molecular mimicry by microbes. Another way of arriving at the same result is for a foreign molecule to bind to a host cell and supply a 'carrier' antigen for normal T cells to recognize; this is thought to be what happens when penicillin, which binds to red blood cells, causes an autoimmune haemolytic anaemia.

Molecular mimicry can also operate at the T-cell level, because MHC–peptide binding (see above) is *degenerate*; that is, one MHC molecule can bind more than one peptide, provided certain critical amino acid residues are present. Thus a microbial peptide could be similar enough to a self-peptide to trigger T cells which can go on to respond to unaltered self (one can imagine that if *all* T cells were deleted that recognized 'near-self', very few would be left to cope with non-self!). Once one self peptide has been recognized, others on the same molecule may be drawn in, the concept of *epitope spreading*. Many examples have been found in animal experiments. One group of antigens that display great similarity between microbe and host are the *heat-shock proteins* released during tissue damage and able to activate CD8 T cells as well as many innate immune mechanisms.

Mimicry of the streptococcal kind is sometimes cited as an example of pathogens trying to escape the immune system, but whether it actually contributes to this is debatable. There are many much more effective escape mechanisms open to the pathogen. On the other hand, the mimicry of cytokines and signalling molecules by viruses may be a major element in pathogen survival (see Chapter 22).

■ Release of sequestered antigens

Whatever the mechanism of tolerance, if B and T lymphocytes do not meet a self antigen, they cannot develop tolerance to it. This is particularly the case with lens and sperm proteins. Thus if the corresponding organ is damaged, the lymphocytes will see the antigens as foreign and mount an immune response. This can happen in the testis during mumps, and accounts for a small proportion of male sterility (see Fig. 24.1).

■ Anomalous antigen presentation

One of the striking findings in organs affected by autoimmunity—for example the thyroid and the pancreatic islets—is the appearance of MHC class II antigens on cells where they are normally absent. It is thought that this may be due to local production of cytokines, especially IFNγ, perhaps in response to viral infection. One result might be that thyroid or islet cells can now present antigens to T cells, including their own surface or secreted molecules, which in turn would allow B cells to make antibodies against them (Fig. 24.4). Another possibility would be that the pathogen increases co-stimulatory activity; the experimental use of mycobacteria as *adjuvants* for autoimmunity may be an example of this. This whole concept still requires firm proof, but it illustrates another way in which infection might lead indirectly to autoimmunity.

■ Anomalous cytokine production

Infection or other sources of tissue damage may provoke inflammation, with the resulting production of cytokines with effects on antigen presentation sufficient to

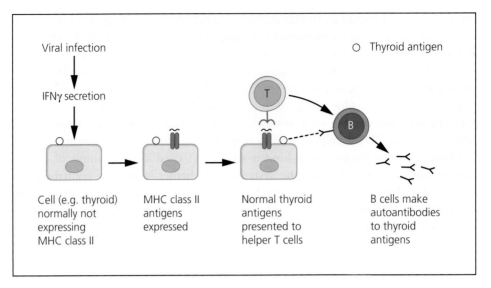

Fig. 24.4 The 'anomalous' MHC expression hypothesis for autoimmunity. Note that the abnormal MHC expression could also be secondary; that is, due to cytokines produced during an already established autoimmune thyroiditis.

attract and trigger T lymphocytes in the vicinity with specificities unrelated to the pathogen. This is known as the 'bystander effect' and might be a risk of using powerful adjuvants with vaccines. Indeed vaccines have frequently been blamed for the onset of autoimmune disease, though the evidence is still not compelling.

■ Autoimmunity, autoimmune disease, and genetics

Finally, it should be stressed that the presence of *autoantibodies* does not automatically lead to disease, and in fact it has only been proved for a few diseases that they are actually caused by the autoantibodies rather than vice versa; these include thyrotoxicosis, myasthenia gravis, and the skin disease pemphigus. Others, such as diabetes, may be largely T-cell-mediated, whereas others, such as haemolytic anaemia, can be due to normal immune responses against foreign antigens that happen to bind to self cells, in this case red blood cells (see above).

Studies in twins and large families leave no doubt that there is a strong genetic element in almost all autoimmune diseases, but that many genes are involved. However a striking feature is the predominance of particular HLA types, presumably reflecting the importance of T cells in these responses. In one group of rheumatological diseases, headed by ankylosing spondylitis, the association is with B27, possibly because of mimicry of this molecule by bacterial antigens. A range of other autoimmune diseases is more weakly associated with the combination B8 DR3, and here the suspicion is that the control of cytokine responses is defective. There may also be defects in genes such as Fas, required for T-cell deletion. Interestingly, autoimmune diseases in general are less common in tropical countries, perhaps due to a protective effect by protozoal or worm infections.

SUMMARY

- Autoimmunity (anti-self reactivity) is normally held in check by screening T and B cells before release from the thymus or bone marrow, together with regulatory mechanisms in peripheral organs.

- These safeguards may break down during infection for several reasons, including polyclonal lymphocyte activation, antigenic mimicry of host antigens by pathogen, and inflammatory effects on bystander lymphocytes.

- The tendency to generate autoimmune reactions is under complex genetic control, notably by genes at the HLA locus.

Chapter 25

Immunodeficiency II: primary defects of adaptive immunity

First, look back at Chapter 15 to be reminded about the difference between primary (genetic) and secondary (acquired) immunodeficiency. As you will see from Fig. 15.1, primary immunodeficiencies affecting the adaptive immune system—that is, *lymphocyte* function—are about five times more common than those affecting innate immunity (complement, phagocytes, etc.), which were discussed in Chapter 15. Note, however, that in terms of total incidence, secondary immunodeficiencies (see Chapter 26) outnumber them both considerably.

Just as with the innate defects, primary adaptive immunodeficiencies are inherited, so that they are either X-linked or autosomal. Depending on the nature of the defect, it may show up at an early or a late stage of lymphocyte differentiation, affecting T cells, B cells (i.e. antibody), or both (Fig. 25.1). Of course, since much antibody formation depends on healthy T cells, a pure T-cell defect may present with an antibody problem too. Generally the defect becomes evident because of repeated or unusual infections or a failure to respond to vaccination. Diagnosis, formerly based on the clinical condition, can now usually be made with great precision by identifying the abnormal or missing gene.

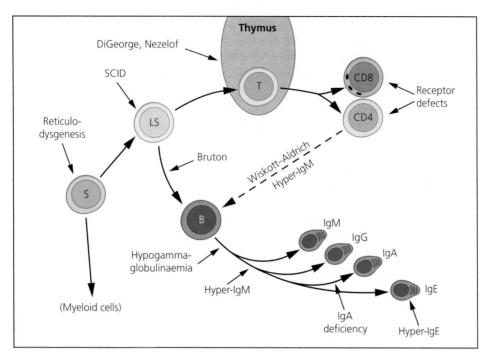

Fig. 25.1 A simplified scheme of haemopoiesis, showing the site of the defect in the major lymphoid immunodeficiencies. LS, lymphoid stem cell; S, bone marrow stem cell; SCID, severe combined immunodeficiency.

■ Defects affecting T and B cells

Defects that act at the earliest precursor stages in the bone marrow, or on some function vital to both types of cell, will show up as a combination of T and B cell deficiency.

1. *Reticular dysgenesis*. A bone-marrow stem-cell failure, incompatible with survival.

2. *Ataxia telangiectasia*. A defect in the normal mechanism by which damaged DNA is repaired, with multiple consequences, both to the immune system (hypoplastic thymus, IgA deficiency) and elsewhere (brain, liver, skin).

3. *Wiskott–Aldrich syndrome*. An X-linked combination of defects at the level of platelets (bleeding), skin (eczema), and antibody formation to polysaccharides (infection with capsulated bacteria). The defect is in the WASP protein responsible for cytoskeletal function, required for normal cell morphology, movement, and adhesion, including T–B cell interaction.

4. *Severe combined immune deficiency (SCID)*. A heterogeneous group of defects at the level of lymphocyte precursors. The common feature is a severe reduction or absence of T cells, with variable reductions in B (and NK) cells. There are several types: (1) the most common is an X-linked defect in the cytokine receptor chain

γ_c, shared by many cytokine receptors including those for IL-2, -7, and -15, required for the maturation of lymphoid stem cells; (2) a lesion in enzymes of the purine pathway, either adenosine deaminase (ADA) or less frequently, purine nucleoside phosphorylase (PNP), allowing a build-up of dATP or dGTP, which are toxic to lymphoid stem cells; (3) mutations can occur in the recombinase genes (e.g. RAG-1/2) needed for the proper rearrangement of germ-line V, D, and J segments into functional TCR or immunoglobulin genes.

■ Defects affecting T cells

1. *DiGeorge syndrome*. A failure of embryonic development of the third and fourth pharyngeal pouches, resulting in absence of the thymus and parathyroids, with facial and cardiac abnormalities. Cases usually present rapidly with tetany due to the lack of parathyroid hormone; the immunological defect was originally noticed when affected babies developed massive vaccinia infections following the smallpox vaccine and on X-ray the thymus shadow was seen to be missing. Treatment with fetal thymus grafting has shown some success, but spontaneous improvement may occur due to compensatory non-thymic development of T cells.

2. *Nezelof syndrome*. Somewhat similar to the above, but with normal parathyroids.

3. *PNP deficiency* (see above). This may affect only T-cell development.

4. *T-cell receptor (TCR)*. Defects in TCR-associated signalling molecules such as ZAP-70 and CD3 will also affect T-cell development.

5. *MHC and antigen-presentation defects*. There may be absence or low levels of MHC molecules, or defects in the processes by which they pick up and transport antigen within the antigen-presenting cells. In *bare lymphocyte syndrome* there is a reduction or absence of HLA class II (BLS-II) or class I (BLS-I).

■ Defects affecting B cells and antibody

1. *Agammaglobulinaemia* (Bruton's disease). An X-linked absence of B cells and thus of immunoglobulin, caused by a number of different mutations in the tyrosine kinase gene. There may also be intermittent reductions in neutrophils. Patients typically present with pyogenic infections. The disease was first spotted in 1952 in a boy with recurrent pneumonia, thanks to the newly invented immunoelectrophoresis technique for demonstrating immunoglobulins in the serum (Fig. 25.2).

2. *Hypogammaglobulinaemia*. More commonly, low levels of IgG or IgA are found, often with normal numbers of B cells in the bone marrow, but a failure

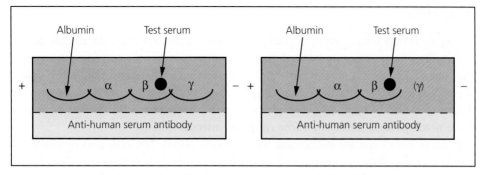

Fig. 25.2 Immunoelectrophoresis of (left) normal and (right) agammaglobulinaemic serum. Note the absence of the precipitation arc corresponding to the gammaglobulins.

to develop properly into plasma cells. The heterogeneous nature of this group of defects is reflected in the name *common variable immunodeficiency.*

3. *Selective IgA deficiency* is remarkable in being quite common (about 1 in 500 white people) and often symptomless. In some, this is associated with loss of a receptor for cytokines involved in B cell activation (TACI).

4. *X-linked hyper-IgM syndromes.* These are mutations which have their effect on the B-cell IgM–IgG switch. The best known are caused by a mutation in the gene for the CD40 ligand on T cells, which is involved in the switch from IgM to IgG, etc., and also T-cell–macrophage interaction. As a result there are raised levels of IgM and reduced levels of IgG and IgA, an absence of germinal centres and somatic hypermutation, and sometimes defects in cell-mediated immunity. A second type is caused by a mutation in an enzyme, AID (which stands for activation-induced cytidine deaminase), leading to giant germinal centres.

5. *Hyper-IgE syndrome (Job syndrome).* Characterized by raised serum IgE and repeated skin and lung infections, particularly with *Staph. aureus.* These patients have mutations in STAT3, an important transcription factor involved in cytokine receptor signal transduction and have impaired production of IL-17.

■ Clinical aspects of primary immune deficiencies

Although they are rare, primary immune deficiencies represent one of the best opportunities for immunological principles to be applied to human disease (another, *vaccination*, was established long before anything was known about immunology). Infant lives which would certainly have been lost until a few decades ago are now being saved regularly, chiefly in specialist centres where diagnosis and treatment can be carried out.

Diagnosis

Severe recurrent infections in a young child should always alert the doctor to the possibility of a primary immune deficiency, particularly if the infection is an unusual one. To some extent the nature of the infection will suggest where the defect is (see Table 26.7 in the following chapter for a summary). Note that, because of the cooperation of antibody, complement, and phagocytic cells, defects of any of these predispose to much the same range of infections.

Routine tests exist for measuring blood T-cell, B-cell, NK-cell, and myeloid-cell numbers, using flow cytometry and monoclonal antibodies against specific cell surface markers (e.g. CD3, CD4, and CD8 for T cells, T_H cells, and CTLs, respectively). Serum antibody levels are easily measured using enzyme-linked immunosorbent assay (ELISA). T- and B-cell function can be assessed broadly by their proliferative and cytokine response on culture with various mitogens, e.g. phytohaemagglutinin (PHA) for T cells, or specific 'recall' antigens. The oxygen burst in neutrophils (e.g. for chronic granulomatous disease) can be checked with the NBT test: a simple rapid colour change. Where a particular gene defect is suspected, Northern blotting/PCR (for mRNA) or gene sequencing (for DNA) can be applied. Although there will undoubtedly be further refinements, these kinds of test can usually indicate whether there is a significant immune defect or not. Unfortunately there remain patients with clearly increased susceptibility to, for example, upper-respiratory viruses or skin infections, in whom no obvious defect can be traced. In fact the extent to which *minor ill-health* has an immunological basis remains a field that has hardly been explored.

Treatment

Treatment of an immunodeficient patient can be directed (1) at reducing their infection(s), and/or (2) replacing the defect.

Reducing infection

Obviously avoiding likely sources of infection makes sense; for example a patient with a T-cell deficiency should not come in contact with cases of TB or be given live vaccines such as BCG, MMR, and oral polio vaccine. Very severe immunodeficiency may require complete isolation: a very distressing and expensive process. For infections with identified organisms, chemotherapy is the mainstay—antibacterial, antifungal, etc. as appropriate (see Chapter 29) as well as antibiotic prophylaxis. Some conditions respond to cytokines, the best example being the effect of repeated injections of IFNγ in some cases of CGD and of G-CSF for severe congenital neutropenia.

Replacement therapy

Most patients with hypogammaglobulinaemia can be kept healthy by monthly injections of pooled normal human immunoglobulin. This is a vivid demonstration that normal people have protective levels of antibody against common pathogens.

Another, perhaps surprising, form of replacement therapy is the transfusion of normal red blood cells for ADA deficiency, but of course neither of these nonself-renewing treatments constitutes a cure. For this it is necessary to permanently replace the defective *cell* or *gene*.

Haemopoietic stem cell transplantation

All the cellular components of the immune system are derived ultimately from haemopoietic stem cells in the bone marrow, so a successful graft of normal marrow (or even in some cases peripheral blood) should theoretically be able to replace any of them. In practice, because of its dangers (see below) this is reserved for severe cases, notably SCID (over 400 successful treatments of this condition have been carried out worldwide to date) but also other severe deficiencies. A good HLA match between host and donor is desirable (giving more than 80% success rates), not so much to avoid rejection (the patients are already immunodeficient!) but to prevent *graft-versus-host* (GVH) disease. This is the situation where the injected marrow attempts to reject the host, causing severe damage to epithelial cells in the gut, liver, and skin, which is frequently fatal. It is minimized by (1) ensuring the best possible HLA match; (2) depletion of T cells with potential reactivity against host HLA from the marrow before grafting; (3) prior administration of the cytokine granulocyte colony-stimulating factor (G-CSF) to the donor in order to increase the number of stem cells in the blood or marrow; and (4) in some cases, the use of purified stem cells.

Gene therapy

Gene therapy is the most logical approach, since most primary defects are of a single gene, and even a partial restoration of levels of the missing protein may be quite beneficial. However, being still experimental, this technique is reserved for life-threatening conditions, particularly SCID. A normal version of the defective gene can be inserted into the patient's own T cells or, better, stem cells, using a suitable retrovirus, modified so as not to be pathogenic (Fig. 25.3). The major problems so far are (1) the rather low efficiency of gene insertion, and (2) the inability to control where the new gene is inserted. In a γ_c-SCID gene-therapy trial, long-term (>10 years) reconstitution of T cell but not NK cell function led to most children leading normal lives, albeit in some cases with some still needing infusions of immunoglobulins. However, four of these nine children developed leukaemia due to insertion into a site on the chromosome involved in the control of haemopoiesis (the *LMO2* gene) of which one died, the others being in remission following successful anti-cancer treatment. Similar trials are continuing, often in patients in whom bone-marrow transplantation has already failed, with no adverse effects so far. However, new approaches are also being tried for targeting the corrective gene into a 'safe' site in the genome, and selecting only those cells with the correct insertion, which could then be cloned and injected.

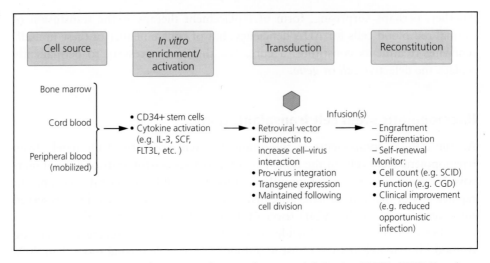

Fig. 25.3 The major approaches to gene therapy of immune deficiencies. FLT3L, FLT3 ligand; SCF, stem-cell factor.

SUMMARY

- Lymphocyte development and function can be deficient for genetic reasons at many levels.

- Very rarely, T cells are absent because of a failure of the thymus to develop (DiGeorge syndrome).

- More commonly, B cells are completely or relatively deficient (agamma/hypogammaglobulinaemia).

- There are also defects that show up in both T and B cells (severe combined immunodeficiency).

- Therapy consists of replacing the missing factor (e.g. antibody) or, more experimentally, the defective gene.

Chapter 26

Immunodeficiency III: secondary immunodeficiency and AIDS

In contrast to the inborn primary immunodeficiencies already described, secondary immunodeficiency results from some influence *external* to the immune system—infection, malnutrition, etc. (see below)—ranging from the slightly increased risk of infection following surgery to the severe and progressive immune failure of HIV/AIDS. Most adult immunodeficiency falls into this category, and since both innate and adaptive immunity can be affected, they will be discussed together here. In fact the defects in secondary immunodeficiencies are usually multiple and complex, so that the only effective treatment is to remove the external cause, if possible. The principal causes are listed in Table 26.1. Note that several forms of medical treatment can themselves cause *iatrogenic* immunodeficiency.

Table 26.1 The commonest causes of secondary immunodeficiency

Condition	Main causes	Major elements affected
Malnutrition	Protein-energy, iron, zinc deficiency	Antibody
Infection	HIV, CMV, EBV, measles, TB, leprosy, *Brucella*, syphilis, malaria, sleeping sickness	T cells
Tumours	Lymphoid: myeloma, CLL, Hodgkin's, NHL, other	Multiple
Trauma	Burns, wounds, surgery	Cytokines, monocytes
	Splenectomy	Clearance from blood
Medical treatment	Drugs: steroids, azathioprine, cyclophosphamide; X-irradiation	Neutrophils
Protein loss	Diarrhoea, nephrotic syndrome, burns	Multiple
Other	Diabetes, renal failure, haemochromatosis	Multiple

CLL, chronic lymphoid leukaemia; NHL, non-Hodgkin's lymphoma.

■ Malnutrition

When either total calorie or protein intake falls below a certain level, antibody production is severely affected and, to a lesser extent, complement levels and phagocytes. There may also be atrophy of lymphoid tissues, especially the thymus, and loss of T-cell function. This is probably the main reason why infections normally regarded as minor, such as measles, can be so severe in the tropics, the complications including pneumonia, otitis, diarrhoea, and massive haemorrhagic rashes. It is estimated that a million children die each year from measles worldwide. A normal intake of iron (see below) and zinc is also necessary for healthy immunity, and the effects of these and other food supplements including vitamins on chronic infection and in the elderly are currently being tested. Vitamin D, derived from food (such as cod liver oil) and from exposure to sunshine has been suspected for years to improve resistance against infection. It is now believed to have pleiotropic effects on antigen presenting cells, T cells, and B cells and to induce the synthesis of antimicrobial peptides which can kill *M. tuberculosis*. Vitamin A (retinoic acid) has important effects on T lymphocyte differentiation, promotes the migration of lymphocytes to the gut and increases production of regulatory T cells while reducing T_H17 responses. Interestingly, a few diseases (e.g. typhus) appear to be *less* severe in malnourished patients, and here one would suspect that the symptoms may themselves be immunological in nature (see Chapter 23). Note that malnutrition may itself be secondary to renal failure, drug therapy, etc.

Iron

Iron metabolism is strictly controlled and either deficiency or excess can increase susceptibility to infection (see Table 26.2). On the one hand iron is a key co-factor of many host enzymes involved in immune function, particularly the ROI responsible for killing pathogens in neutrophils. On the other hand many bacteria, fungi, and protozoa require adequate concentrations of iron for their own growth, and some have multiple siderophores which scavenge iron from the environment. There is thus a competitive battle for iron between host and pathogen. In malaria, iron deficiency may actually reduce the severity of infection because of the parasite's need for healthy red cells to grow in, and there is also the special case of sickle-cell anaemia, in which heterozygotes for the abnormal haemoglobin HbS are relatively resistant to *Plasmodium falciparum*. Some cytokines (e.g. IFNγ, TNF) can decrease the available iron pool by raising the level of the iron-binding protein ferritin. Neutrophil-derived lactoferrin has the same effect.

Iron overload is seen in several situations (see Table 26.2) and can have deleterious effects on the function of macrophages, neutrophils, NK cells, and lymphocytes.

■ Infection

The ability of some infections to cause immunodeficiency, thus predisposing the patient to other infections, is of great interest and importance, and the AIDS epidemic has brought home to the developed world the way in which infectious organisms can interact with one another in the same host. A successful treatment for AIDS (e.g. highly active anti-retroviral therapy, or HAART; see page 242), if globally available, would relegate such organisms as *Pneumocystis carinii*, still a cause of death in AIDS patients (and the clue that led, in 1981, to the first description of the disease), to the small print of microbiology textbooks where it previously languished.

HIV and AIDS

The human immunodeficiency viruses HIV-1 and -2 are unique in that their primary target of attack is the cells of the immune system, to which they cause

Table 26.2 The balance between iron deficiency and overload

Iron deficiency	Iron overload
Dietary	Haemochromatosis (see text)
Blood loss	Dietary
	Chronic hepatitis C
	Blood transfusion
	Thalassaemia

progressive damage to the point where the patient succumbs, usually to another infection. The reason the immune system is singled out is that HIV uses as its cell receptor the CD4 molecule (see Chapter 18), which is found mainly on T-helper cells, dendritic cells, and macrophages, but also on some other cells including parts of the brain. Entry also requires a second host molecule, usually a chemokine receptor whose normal function is the control of cell migration (see Chapter 12). The two best known are CCR5, the receptor used by so-called 'macrophage trophic' viruses which appear early in infection, and CXCR4, used by 'T cell tropic' strains which arise later. Following an initial interaction with CD4, one of the viral surface antigens, known as gp120 (where gp stands for glycoprotein), binds to these receptors and allows the virus to enter and multiply, predominantly in mucosal and peripheral lymphoid tissues (such as lymph nodes), spreading from cell to cell by budding. The requirement for the CD4 molecule means that T cells and antigen-presenting cells are mostly affected. There are also variable effects on antibody responses, the mechanisms of which are unclear. Vaccination with pneumococcal polysaccharides is not recommended in HIV-positive people in Africa, since it is only effective in the early stages of HIV infection, whereas the polysaccharide-protein conjugate vaccine does provide significant protection against the increased risk of pneumococcal pneumonia in these individuals. Some immunopathological consequences of infection may actually be reduced; for example, the systemic spread of *Candida* and the formation of cavities in TB.

Spread to a new host can occur by sexual contact, contaminated blood, or from mother to newborn. It was assumed originally that infection with HIV simply destroyed helper T cells, but it is almost certainly not as simple as this, and a number of other possible mechanisms have been proposed (Table 26.3). Even in advanced disease, not more than about 1% of CD4 T cells in the blood actually contain the virus, although the numbers are much higher in lymph nodes where the virus replicates.

HIV-1 and -2 are retroviruses (see Fig. 2.2), and contain a number of unusual genes that help to control their replication and integration into host DNA (Table 26.4). They are closely related to two African animal immunodeficiency viruses; HIV-1 is thought to have reached humans from chimpanzees and the less frequent HIV-2 from the simian immunodeficiency virus (SIV) of sooty Mangabey monkeys. Both monkeys and chimpanzees appear to be able to maintain their T-cell levels despite persistent infection, and do not develop AIDS, perhaps because of *less* vigorous general immune activation.

An important feature is that HIV, and especially gp120, contains five *hypervariable regions*, V1–V5, remarkably subject to antigenic variation, especially V3 (at least 20 times more than influenza), both between patients and within a single individual. In addition, the variable rather than conserved regions of the molecule tend to be immunodominant, the molecule tends to be unstable and few are expressed on the surface of infected cells, and binding of antibodies to neutralizing epitopes is masked by sugars. Both antibody and cytotoxic T cells are therefore only transiently effective. This is unfortunate because gp120 would otherwise be an ideal molecule on which to base a vaccine since it is essential for infection. Thus

Table 26.3 Numerous theories have been advanced to explain why HIV, without infecting all T-helper cells, causes a progressive loss of their numbers and function

---

Direct effects on T cells

    *Lysis by HIV (infected cells only)

    *Suppressed production, thymic failure

    *Persistent immune overactivation, clonal expansion, death (*apoptosis)

    Fusion (syncytium formation) and death

Immune mediated destruction

    Killing by CD8 cytotoxic cells (infected cells, and cells binding HIV antigens)

    Killing by antibody dependent cell mediated cytotoxicity

    Selective loss of memory cells

Immunosuppression

    By free gp120 molecules blocking CD4 function

    By T_H2 cytokines (IL-4, IL-10) inhibiting protective T_H1 responses

    *Of antigen-presenting cell function by loss of follicular dendritic cells

---

Autoimmunity

    To CD4 or other T-cell antigens

    To uninfected cells binding HIV antigen

    To self-MHC due to cross-reaction with HIV

---

*Currently most favoured.

HIV poses the same problem as influenza but much worse and despite intensive research no effective vaccine has been developed (see Table 27.2 for details of the clinical trials performed to-date). Vaccine approaches started by inducing antibody responses to gp120, went on to generate cytotoxic T cells against the virus and now involve simultaneous induction of both these responses from the same vaccine using prime-boost strategies.

Initially, single antiviral drugs were not as successful as originally hoped (see Chapter 29) due to rapid acquisition of resistance, and treatments aimed at stimulating immune function, for example administration of cytokines such as IL-2 or IFNγ, have been disappointing. However, a combination of three or more drugs, aimed at different targets—so-called HAART—is effective (Table 26.5). Paradoxically, patients treated in this way may undergo severe tissue reactions caused by their recovering T cells responding to their opportunists such as Mycobacteria spp., CMV, and Pneumocystis: 'immune reconstitution disease'. However, HAART does not eradicate reservoirs of latent HIV and viral loads can rebound rapidly upon cessation of treatment. Many other strategies to completely eradicate the virus are under consideration, including the use of small interfering RNA sequences to silence or degrade viral mRNA (see also Chapter 31).

Table 26.4 HIV genes and their function

Gene	Function encoded
5'-LTR	LTR promoter, enhancer, DNA integrating
gag	Core proteins p24, p17, p7
pol	Reverse transcriptase, protease, integrase, RNAse
vif	Viral infectivity factor
vpr	Weak transcriptional factor, etc.
tat	Transactivator, replication protein
rev	Regulator virion proteins
vpu	Virion budding, reduced CD4 expression
env	gp160 (cleaved to gp120, gp41) envelope proteins
nef	Negative regulatory factor, reduced CD4 and MHC expression
3'-LTR	Links to 5'-LTR

LTR, long terminal repeat; pol, polymerase.

Table 26.5 Some drugs used in the treatment of HIV infection

Class	Examples
Nucleoside analogue RT inhibitors	AZT, ddl, abacavir, *emtricitabine
Nucleotide analogue RT inhibitors	*tenofovir
Non-nucleotide RT inhibitors	efavirenz, etravine, rilpivirine
Protease inhibitors	*ritonavir, saquinavir, atazanavir

*Often used in combination (triple therapy). Many other similar combinations are also effective . RT: reverse transcriptase.

The classic course of HIV infection includes four distinguishable stages (Table 26.6). Following infection there is usually an acute, symptomatic illness, when there is a burst of viral replication and temporary depletion of CD4 T cells. This is brought under control (but not eliminated) by a robust cytotoxic CD8 T cell response. Virus specific antibodies are also generated, which are useful for diagnosis but their role in immunity seems limited. A prolonged period of clinical latency then follows, such that the average time between infection and fully developed AIDS is approximately 10 years. However, it is now evident that not all

Table 26.6 Infection with HIV normally leads to a steady progression of symptoms as the number of CD4 T cells falls, but some features (*) are not always seen

Stage	Main symptoms	Blood tests		
		HIV antigen	Antibodies to HIV	CD4 T cells/µl
Acute	Glandular fever-like illness*	+ ↓ −	− ↓ +	1000
Persistent generalized lymphadenopathy*	Enlarged lymph nodes	−	+	
Symptomatic (pre-AIDS)	Weight loss, fever, diarrhoea, opportunist infections	−	+	c.500
AIDS	Kaposi's sarcoma, lymphomas, major opportunist infections, encephalopathy*, neuropathy, dementia*	+	+	200 or less

For a list of the common opportunist infections, see Table 26.7.

infected individuals progress at the same rate (the disease was only recognized in 1981) and it is widely believed that other factors contribute to the final outcome. These may include other viruses and microorganisms, MHC type, age, nutrition, and possibly the precise strain of HIV contracted. Individuals with a 32 base pair mutation in their CCR5 co-receptor are more resistant to infection and if infected also have a modest delay in the onset of AIDS. In a few others, so called 'long-term non-progressors' or 'elite controllers', virus loads are either low or very low and there is no obvious disease despite being infected for some 15 years; these people are subject to intense study in order to identify exactly how they are preventing the otherwise inevitable destruction of their immune systems. Nevertheless, the steady increase in numbers—perhaps 50–60 million people infected and over 20 million deaths—and the impact of HIV on a disease like TB, which was hitherto thought to be coming under control but is now ravaging tropical countries, make HIV the most feared of all infectious organisms and a huge challenge to everyone concerned with infectious disease at any level. The theory that AIDS is not caused by HIV at all is not taken seriously now.

Other infections

No other infection has such a disastrous effect on the immune system as HIV, but the immunosuppression caused by the other infections listed in Table 26.1 can be quite serious. For example, quite mild malaria can impair the response to pneumococcal and meningococcal vaccines, as was demonstrated in Nigeria by giving a course of antimalarial therapy before vaccination. Furthermore, severe non-typhoidal *Salmonella* infection is a common complication of *P. falciparum* malaria in Africa. Polyclonal activation of lymphocytes (e.g. of B cells by EBV, malaria, and leprosy, and of T cells by staphylococcal superantigens) no doubt contributes to the immunosuppression seen in these diseases, although whether this benefits the pathogen is hard to establish. Measles, by infecting T lymphocytes and antigen-presenting cells, suppresses cell-mediated immunity and can cause TB to flare up. Similarly, many deaths attributed to influenza are actually the result of an increased risk of secondary bacterial pneumonia. The way in which herpesviruses interfere with the cytokine network has been mentioned in Chapters 13 and 22, and in this case it seems likely that the immunosuppression does have a survival advantage to these very persistent pathogens.

■ Other causes of immunodeficiency

Tumours

Space-occupying tumours growing in the bone marrow (e.g. leukaemia, myeloma, metastases) can directly inhibit leucocyte production. Others (e.g. Hodgkin's lymphoma) can do the same by secreting inhibitory cytokines. Remember also that anticancer therapy, whether irradiation or chemotherapy, will inhibit the production of all actively dividing cells, including immunological ones, the effect being most rapid and severe on short-lived cells such as polymorphs.

Trauma and sepsis

The systemic inflammatory (shock) reaction following massive endotoxin release in Gram-negative sepsis has been mentioned in Chapter 14. In survivors, this may be followed by a stage of over-compensation during which inflammatory and immune responses are damped down and susceptibility to other infections increased. A similar phenomenon can occur after major trauma, blood loss, burning, and even post-operatively (Fig. 26.1). The exact mechanisms are unclear but may include the production of inhibitory cytokines such as IL-10 and TGF-β, and treatments such as plasmapheresis (to remove inhibitory molecules) or the administration of stimulatory cytokines are being considered.

Splenectomy carries the special risk of infection with capsulated bacteria (and the otherwise harmless protozoal parasite *Babesia*), which are normally cleared by this organ. Splenectomized patients are generally vaccinated against *S. pneumoniae* as a precautionary measure.

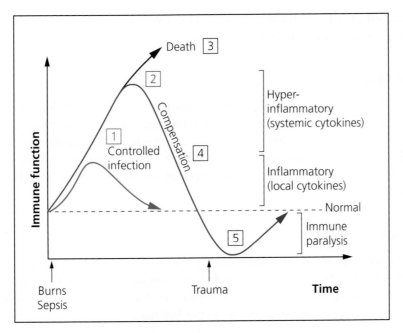

Fig. 26.1 The possible effects on the immune system of septic or post-traumatic shock. (1) Control of infection, with local cytokine production and transient inflammation; (2) hyper-inflammatory reaction with systemic cytokine levels, which may lead to either (3) death, or (4) compensatory anti-inflammatory control mechanisms; (5) immune paralysis.

Medical treatment

In addition to chemotherapy for cancer, a number of deliberately immunosuppressive drugs are used to reduce inflammation and various immunopathological conditions. A list of these is given in Table 21.1. Inevitably they carry with them the risk of infection.

Protein loss

In conditions of increased glomerular permeability (the nephrotic syndrome), in addition to albumin, immunoglobulins and complement components may be lost into the urine, resulting in an increased susceptibility to bacterial infection.

Diabetes

Skin, soft tissue, and bone infections are well-known complications of diabetes. The main lesion is a failure of neutrophils and monocytes to increase their background level of antimicrobial activity (motility, phagocytosis, intracellular killing), and may be partly related to the raised blood sugar itself and the metabolic stress this causes. Infections of the extremities are particularly common and, combined with the effects of the disease on small blood vessels, may lead to necrosis and gangrene, sometimes requiring amputation.

Renal failure

Most cellular elements, but especially neutrophils, may be impaired in chronic renal failure, resulting in an increased risk of bacterial sepsis and poor responses to vaccination, which is particularly important in renal dialysis patients who have a higher risk of exposure to hepatitis viruses. Renal transplantation, with its associated immunosuppressive regime, will of course exacerbate the danger of infection.

Haemochromatosis

In this condition of iron overload, which may be primary (due to a mutation in the HLA-related *Hfe* gene) or secondary to overconsumption of iron, repeated blood transfusion, and haemolytic anaemias, bacterial and fungal infections are common (see above for a discussion of iron balance).

Immunity in the elderly

As the production of new T cells declines and existing cells approach the end of their proliferative lifespan, the population is increasingly composed of memory cells. B cells, and cell–cell interaction, are also progressively impaired. TB, pneumonia, urinary infection, and reactivation of herpesviruses (e.g. VZV) are more common with age, and so is autoimmunity. In some cases, elderly individuals respond less well to vaccination. However, studies on centenarians have shown remarkably normal levels of general immune competence.

■ Infections in the immunodeficient patient

Whatever the cause of the immunodeficiency, the resulting pattern of infection depends on the component affected; indeed, with a knowledge of immunology one can more or less predict it. Broadly speaking, defects of phagocytes, complement, or antibody predispose to infections with extracellular organisms, especially bacteria and fungi, and T-cell defects to intracellular infections, including most viruses but also several important bacteria, fungi, and protozoa (see Table 26.7 and refer back to Chapters 15 and 25 for more details).

Treatment of secondary immunodeficiency

The mainstay of treatment is to treat the infection, and if possible the original cause. On a worldwide scale, *malnutrition* is by far the most common cause of

Table 26.7 The major infections encountered in immunodeficient patients fall into two main sets: (top) those depending on antibody, complement, and phagocytes for their control and (bottom) those depending mainly on T-cell-mediated responses

Deficiency	Major infections expected			
	Viruses	Bacteria	Fungi	Protozoa and worms
Phagocytes		*Staphylococcus, Streptococcus, Pseudomonas*	*Candida Aspergillus*	
CGD Splenectomy		*Staph.*, etc. Pneumococcus, Meningococcus	*Aspergillus*	*Babesia*
Complement		*Staphylococcus, Streptococcus, Pseudomonas*		
Lytic pathway		*Neisseria*		
Antibody	Enteroviruses	*Staphylococcus, Streptococcus, Haemophilus,* Pneumococcus	*Pneumocystis*	*Giardia*
T cells	CMV, HSV, EBV	*Listeria, M. tuberculosis, M. leprae, Mycoplasma*	*Candida, Aspergillus, Histoplasma, Pneumocystis, Cryptococcus*	*Strongyloides*
AIDS	CMV, HSV, EBV, HHV8	*Mycobacteria* (including *M. avium*)	*Cryptococcus, Candida, Pneumocystis*	*Cryptosporidium, Toxoplasma, Leishmania*

Note the importance of fungal infections in both groups.

such infections, which is particularly disastrous for tropical countries since they are also exposed to a much wider range of infectious organisms, many of which (e.g. most protozoa and worms) are restricted to these areas. The effect of adequate nutrition (and clean water) on the incidence of infection in the tropical world would probably outweigh the effects of all the vaccines and antibiotics in existence.

SUMMARY

- Most immunodeficiency is due to external (i.e. non-genetic) causes, and is referred to as 'secondary'.

- The two major factors worldwide are malnutrition and AIDS.

- Infections in immunodeficient patients depend on the immune element that is defective, for example in AIDS (T cell), intracellular pathogens such as the tubercle bacillus predominate, whereas in malnutrition (antibody), lung, ear, and intestinal infections are most common.

Tutorial 3

For many people this will be the most difficult part of the book, the activities of lymphocytes being so unlike those of any other type of cell. By attempting the following essays, you will discover where your weak spots (if any) lie, and which chapters may need going over again, supplemented by some further reading from the list at the end of the book. Some suggestions for your answers are given in the section at the back of the book (p. 372).

1.   *I assume . . . that all antibody molecules contain the same polypeptide chains . . . the antigen causes the polypeptide chains to assume a configuration complementary to the antigen.*   (Pauling 1940)

   . . . in the animal there exist clones of (lymphocytes) each carrying immunologically reactive sites corresponding . . . to one potential antigenic determinant. . . . When an antigen is introduced it will make contact with a cell of the corresponding clone . . . and stimulate it to produce more globulin molecules of the cell's characteristic type.   (Burnet 1959)

   How do we know Burnet was right and Pauling wrong?

2. Why does an individual B cell retain only one out of hundreds of heavy-chain V genes but a full set of C genes?

3. Without T cells, there would be no need for MHC molecules. Discuss.

4. Any successful parasite must be able to vary its antigens. Discuss.

5. The development of *memory* is the hallmark of the lymphocyte. Is it?

6. If a pathogen is to be eliminated, some damage to host tissues is inevitable. Is it?

7. An 8-year-old boy who had recovered normally from chickenpox 4 years earlier, but who suffered repeated attacks of pneumonia, failed to respond to several injections of a standard pneumococcal polysaccharide vaccine. What was wrong with him and what did his physician do?

Further reading and information

Textbooks

Abbas, A. K., Lichtman, A. H., Pillai, S. *Cellular and Molecular Immunology.* Saunders, 7th edn., 2011.

Delves, P.J., Martin, S.J., Burton, D.R., Roitt, I.M. *Roitt's Essential Immunology.* Wiley Blackwell, 12th edn., 2011.

Kindt, T. J., Goldsby, R. A., and Osborne, B. A. *Immunology.* W. H. Freeman, 6th edn., 2007.

Murphy, K.M. *Janeway's Immunobiology.* Garland Science, 8th edn., 2011.

Websites

http://image.bloodline.net/ (colour images of blood cell morphology.)

www.cellsalive.com/clips.htm (commercial website offering video images of events in microbiology and immunology such as phagocyte chemotaxis, cytotoxic T cell killing, etc.)

www.immunology.org/ (website of the British Society for Immunology.)

http://www.aai.org/ (website of the American Association of Immunologists.)

http://www3.niaid.nih.gov/ (website for the National Institute of Allergy and Infectious Diseases (National Institutes of Health, USA).)

http://www.rndsystems.com/research_topic.aspx?r=4 (RD systems site offering succinct reviews with colour figures on cytokine biology and other topics in immunology and inflammation such as wound healing, etc.)

http://www.emmanet.org/ (extensive list and details of knockout mice.)

Recent reviews and articles

Innate immunity

Berzins, S. P., Smyth, M. J., Baxter, A. G. 'Presumed guilty: natural killer T cell defects and human disease'. *Nat Rev Immunol.* 2011, Feb; 11 (2):131–42.

Bianchi, M. E. 'DAMPs, PAMPs and alarmins: all we need to know about danger'. *Leukoc Biol.*, 2007, Jan.; 81 (1): 1–5.

Chow, A., Brown, B. D., Merad, M. 'Studying the mononuclear phagocyte system in the molecular age'. *Nature Reviews Immunology.* 2011, 11, 788–98.

Elinav, E., Strowig, T., Henao-Mejia, J., Flavell, R. A. 'Regulation of the antimicrobial response by NLR proteins'. *Immunity.* 2011, May 27; 34 (5):665–79.

Finlay, B. B., McFadden, G. 'Anti-immunology: evasion of the host immune system by bacterial and viral pathogens'. *Cell*, 2006, Feb. 24; 124 (4): 767–82.

Flannagan, R. S., Cosío, G., Grinstein, S. 'Antimicrobial mechanisms of phagocytes and bacterial evasion strategies'. *Nat Rev Microbiol.* 2009, May; 7 (5): 355–66.

Ham, H., Sreelatha, A., Orth, K. 'Manipulation of host membranes by bacterial effectors'. *Nat Rev Microbiol.* 2011, Jul. 18; 9 (9): 635–46.

Ip, W. K., Takahashi, K., Ezekowitz, R. A., Stuart, L. M. Mannose-binding lectin and innate immunity. *Immunol Rev.* 2009, Jul; 230 (1): 9–21.

Iwasaki, A., Medzhitov, R. 'Regulation of adaptive immunity by the innate immune system'. *Science.* 2010, Jan. 15; 327 (5963): 291–5.

Kawai, T., Akira, S. 'Toll-like receptors and their crosstalk with other innate receptors in infection and immunity'. *Immunity.* 2011, May 27: 34 (5): 637–50.

Krysko, D. V., Agostinis, P., Krysko, O., Garg, A. D., Bachert, C., Lambrecht, B. N., Vandenabeele, P. 'Emerging role of damage-associated molecular patterns derived from mitochondria in inflammation'. *Trends Immunol.* 2011, Apr; 32 (4): 157–64.

Lambris, J. D. 'Complement evasion by human pathogens'. *Nat Review Microbiol,* 2008, 6: 132–42.

Levine, B., Mizushima, N., Virgin, H. W. 'Autophagy in immunity and inflammation'. *Nature.* 2011, Jan. 20; 469 (7330): 323–35.

Mallevaey, T., Selvanantham, T. 'Strategy of lipid recognition by invariant natural killer T cells: "one for all and all for one"'. *Immunology.* 2012, Jul.; 136 (3): 273–82.

Mantovani, A., Cassatella, M. A., Costantini, C., Jaillon, S. 'Neutrophils in the activation and regulation of innate and adaptive immunity'. *Nat Rev Immunol.* 2011 Jul.; 25; 11 (8): 519–31.

Murray, P. J., Wynn, T. A. 'Protective and pathogenic functions of macrophage subsets'. *Nature Reviews Immunology.* 2011, 11: 723–37.

Netea, M. G., Wijmenga, C., O'Neill, L. A. 'Genetic variation in Toll-like receptors and disease susceptibility'. *Nat Immunol.* 2012, May 18; 13 (6): 535–42.

Pedra, J. H., Cassel, S. L., Sutterwala, F. S. 'Sensing pathogens and danger signals by the inflammasome'. *Curr Opin Immunol.* 2009, Feb; 21 (1): 10–6.

Ribet, D., Cossart, P. 'Pathogen-mediated posttranslational modifications: A re-emerging field'. *Cell.* 2010, Nov. 24; 143 (5): 694–702.

Sacks, D., Sher, A. 'Evasion of innate immunity by parasitic protozoa'. *Nat. Immunol.*, 2002, Nov. 3 (11): 1041–7.

Schaible, U. E., Kaufmann, S. H. 'Iron and microbial infection'. *Nat Rev Microbiol.* 2004, Dec.; 2 (12): 946–53.

Schroder, K., Tschopp, J. 'The inflammasomes'. *Cell.* 2010, 140, 821–32.

Shelburne, C. P., Abraham, S. N. 'The mast cell in innate and adaptive immunity'. *Adv. Exp Med Biol.* 2011; 716: 162–85.

Skattum, L., van Deuren, M., van der Poll, T., Truedsson, L. 'Complement deficiency states and associated infections'. *Mol Immunol.* 2011, Aug; 48 (14): 1643–55.

Sun, J. C., Beilke, J. N., Lanier, L. L. 'Adaptive immune features of natural killer cells'. *Nature.* 2009, Jan. 29; 457 (7229): 557–61.

Sun, J. C., Lanier, L. L. 'NK cell development, homeostasis and function: parallels with CD8 T cells'. *Nat Rev Immunol.* 2011, Aug. 26;11 (10): 645–57.

van der Poll, T., de Boer, J. D., Levi, M. 'The effect of inflammation on coagulation and vice versa'. *Curr Opin Infect Dis.* 2011, Jun; 24 (3): 273–8.

van der Poll, T., Meijers, J. C. 'Systemic inflammatory response syndrome and compensatory anti-inflammatory response syndrome in sepsis'. *J Innate Immun.* 2010, 2 (5): 379–80.

Whitsett, J. A. 'Review: The intersection of surfactant homeostasis and innate host defense of the lung: lessons from newborn infants'. *Innate Immun.* 2010, Jun.; 16 (3): 138–42.

Wilkins, C., Gale, M. Jr. 'Recognition of viruses by cytoplasmic sensors'. *Current Opinion in Immunology.* 2010, Feb.; 22 (1): 41–7.

Williams, A., Flavell, R. A., Eisenbarth, S. C. 'The role of NOD-like Receptors in shaping adaptive immunity'. *Current Opinion in Immunology.* 2010, Feb.; (1): 34–40.

Adaptive immunity

Belosevic, M. 'Immune evasion strategies of trypanosomes: a review'. 2012, *J Parasitol.* 98(2): 284–92.

Cohen, M. S., Shaw, G. M., McMichael, A. J., Haynes, B. F. Acute HIV-1 Infection. *N Engl J Med.* 2011, May.; 19; 364 (20): 1943–54.

Collette, J. R., Lorenz, M. C. 'Mechanisms of immune evasion in fungal pathogens'. *Curr Opin Microbiol.* 2011, Sep.; 26. 14(6): 668–75.

Daniel, L., Barber, B. B., Andrade, I. S., Sher, A. 'Immune reconstitution inflammatory syndrome: the trouble with immunity when you had none'. *Nature Reviews Microbiology.* 2012, Feb.10: 150–6.

Deenick, E. K., Ma, C. S. 'The regulation and role of T follicular helper cells in Immunity'. *Immunology.* 2011 Dec.; 134 (4): 361–7.

Fishbein, A. B., Fuleihan, R. L. 'The hygiene hypothesis revisited: does exposure to infectious agents protect us from allergy?' *Curr Opin Pediatr.* 2012, Feb; 24 (1): 98–102.

Goodnow, C. C., Vinvesa, C. G., Randall, K. L., Mackay, F., Brink, R. 'Control systems and decision making for antibody production'. 2010, *Nature Immunol.* 11: 681–8.

Hacein-Bey-Abina, S., von Kalle, C., Schmidt, M., Deist Wulffraat, N., McIntyre, E., Radford, I., Villeval, J. L., Fraser, C. C., Cavazzana-Calvo, M., Fischer, A. 'A serious adverse event after successful gene therapy for X-linked severe combined immunodeficiency'. *N. Engl. J. Med.*, 2003, Jan. 16: 348 (3): 255–6.

Harding, C. V., Boom, W. H. Regulation of antigen presentation by Mycobacterium tuberculosis: a role for Toll-like receptors. *Nat Rev Microbiol.* 2010 Apr; 8(4): 296–307.

Hewitson, J. P., Grainger, J. R., Maizels, R. M. 'Helminth immunoregulation: the role of parasite secreted proteins in modulating host immunity'. *Mol Biochem Parasitol.* 2009, Sep; 167 (1): 1–11.

Horst, D., Verweij, M. C., Davison, A. J., Ressing, M. E., Wiertz, E. J. 'Viral evasion of T cell immunity: ancient mechanisms offering new applications'. *Curr Opin Immunol.* 2011, Feb; 23 (1): 96–103.

Jiang, X., Chen, Z. J. 'The role of ubiquitylation in immune defence and pathogen evasion'. *Nat Rev Immunol.* 2011, Dec 9; 12 (1): 35–48.

Kita, H. 'Eosinophils: multifaceted biological properties and roles in health and disease'. *Immunol Rev.* 2011 Jul., 242 (1): 161–77.

Locksley, R. M. 'Nine lives: plasticity among T helper cell subsets'. *J Exp Med.* 2009 Aug. 3; 206 (8): 1643–6.

Maizels, R. M., Pearce, E. J., Artis, D., Yazdanbakhsh, M., Wynn, T. A. 'Regulation of pathogenesis and immunity in helminth infections'. *J Exp Med.* 2009 Sep.; 28; 206 (10): 2059–66.

Maizels, R. M., Smith, K. A. 'Regulatory T cells in infection'. *Adv Immunol.* 2011; 112: 73–136.

Masopust, D., Picker, L. J. 'Hidden memories: frontline memory T cells and early pathogen interception'. *J Immunol.* 2012, Jun. 15; 188 (12): 5811–7.

McHeyzer-Williams, M., Okitsu, S., Wang, N., McHeyzer-Williams, L. 'Molecular programming of B cell memory'. *Nat Rev Immunol.* 2011, Dec. 9; 12 (1): 24–34.

Min, B., Brown, M. A., Legros, G. 'Understanding the roles of basophils: breaking dawn'. *Immunology*, 2012, Mar., 135 (3): 192–7.

Neefjes, J., Marlieke, L. M., Jongsma, P. P., Bakke, O. 'Towards a systems understanding of MHC class I and MHC class II antigen presentation'. *Nature Rev Immunol.*, 2011, 11: 823–36.

Nimmerjahn, F., Ravetch, J. V. 'Fcγ Receptors as regulators of immune responses'. *Nature Rev Immunol.*, 2008, 8: 34–47.

Noriega, V., Redmann, V., Gardner, T., Tortorella, D. 'Diverse immune evasion strategies by human cytomegalovirus'. *Immunol Res.* 2012, Mar. 28.

Oladiran, A., Paige, C., Bishai, W. R. 'Penitentiary or penthouse condo: the tuberculous granuloma from the microbe's point of view'. *Cell Microbiol.* 2010, Mar; 12 (3): 301–9.

Pepper, M., Jenkins, M. K. 'Origins of CD4(+) effector and central memory T cells'. *Nat Immunol.* 2011 Jun.; 12 (6): 467–71.

Picard, C., Casanova, J. L., Puel, A. 'Infectious diseases in patients with IRAK-4, MyD88, NEMO, or IκBα deficiency'. *Clin Microbiol Rev.* 2011, Jul; 24 (3): 490–7.

Prentice, A. M., Gershwin, M. E., Schaible, U. E., Keusch, G. T., Victora, C. G., Gordon, J. I. 'New challenges in studying nutrition-disease interactions in the developing world'. *J Clin Invest.* 2008, Apr.; 118 (4): 1322–9.

Romani, L. 'Immunity to fungal infections'. *Nat Rev Immunol.* 2011, Apr; 11 (4): 275–88.

Schatz, D.G., Ji, Y. 'Recombination centres and the orchestration of V(D)J recombination'. *Nature Reviews Immunology,* 2011, 11: 251–63.

Schroeder, H. W., Cavacini, L. 'Structure and function of antibodies', *J Allergy Clin Immunol.,* 2010, 125, S41–52.

Sheridan, B. S., Lefrançois, L. 'Regional and mucosal memory T cells'. *Nat Immunol.* 2011 Jun; 12 (6): 485–91.

Shlomchik, M. J., Weisel, F. 'Germinal center selection and the development of memory B and plasma cells'. *Immunol Rev.* May 2012, 247 (1): 52–63.

Sprent, J., Surh, C. D. 'Normal T cell homeostasis: the conversion of naive cells into memory-phenotype cells'. *Nat Immunol.* 2011, Jun.; 12 (6): 478–84.

Strugnell, R. A., Wijburg, O. L. C. 'The role of secretory antibodies in infection immunity', 2010. *Nature Rev Microbiol.,* 8: 656–67.

Vyas, J. M., Van der Veen, A. G., Ploegh, H. L. 'The known unknowns of antigen processing and presentation'. *Nat Rev Immunol.* 2008, Aug., 8 (8): 607–18.

Weaver, C. T., Hatton, R. D. 'Interplay between the TH17 and TReg cell lineages: a (co-)evolutionary perspective'. *Nat Rev Immunol.* 2009, Dec.; 9 (12): 883–9.

Weng, N. P., Araki, Y., Subedi, K. 'The molecular basis of the memory T cell response: differential gene expression and its epigenetic regulation'. *Nat Rev Immunol.* 2012, Mar. 16; 12 (4): 306–15.

Wherry, E. J. 'T cell exhaustion'. *Nat Immunol.* 2011, Jun.; 12 (6): 492–9.

Wilke, C. M., Bishop, K, Fox, D., Zou, W. 'Deciphering the role of Th17 cells in human disease'. *Trends Immunol.* 2011, Dec.; 32 (12): 603–11.

Young, D., Hussell, T., Dougan, G. 'Chronic bacterial infections: living with unwanted guests'. *Nat. Immunol.,* 2002, Nov. 3 (11): 1026–32.

Zhang, N., Bevan, M. J. 'CD8(+) T cells: foot soldiers of the immune system'. *Immunity.* 2011 Aug. 26; 35 (2): 161–8.

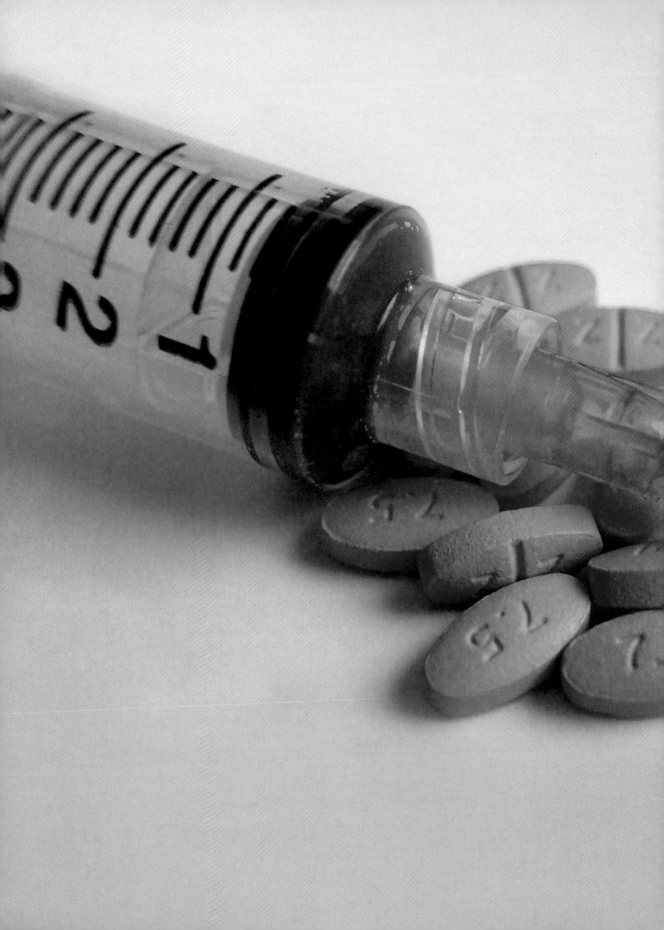

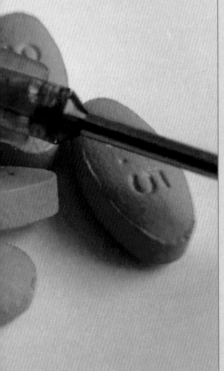

Part 3

The host–pathogen balance

Chapter 27
Epidemiology

In the previous sections of this book we have described the world of pathogens and that of the immune system, treating each element more or less in isolation. However, the real world does not consist of clean cages of highly inbred mice exposed under laboratory conditions to a single clone of identical pathogens, but of large groups of individuals, genetically different and living in different circumstances, irregularly exposed to a large array of pathogens, also genetically highly variable and frequently interacting among themselves. In this last section we consider this balance between human populations and their pathogens with two crucial aims in mind: (1) to *understand* the 'real world' situation, and (2) where necessary to try and *control* it. In the three following chapters we discuss the available control strategies; here we shall look at some of the factors that determine the incidence and distribution of infectious diseases; that is, their *epidemiology*. The science of epidemiology has developed a language of its own, and Table 27.1 lists some of the terms commonly used by workers in this field.

■ Diagnosing, monitoring, and predicting disease

In order to study the epidemiology of an infectious disease, one must first be confident of being able to diagnose it. Diagnosis can be clinical, microbiological, or immunological.

Table 27.1 The language of epidemiology

Term	Meaning
Prevalence	The proportion (percentage) of individuals with an attribute (e.g. disease, antibody) in a population
Incidence	The number of new events (e.g. disease, seroconversion) in a susceptible population
Seroprevalence	The proportion of antibody- or antigen-positive individuals
Seroconversion	The detection of antibody or antigen for the first time
Endemic	Constantly present in the population
Epidemic	Occurring in an unusually high incidence in a population
Pandemic	A worldwide epidemic
Sporadic	Apparently unrelated cases (i.e. not epidemic)
Outbreak	One or more new cases in a single area, possibly related
Incubation period	Time between exposure and symptoms
Reproduction rate	The average number of susceptible individuals infected by a single case (often referred to as R_0)
Subclinical infection	Disease with few or no symptoms
Carrier	An infected individual, who may be symptomless, able to infect others
Reservoir	A site from which infection may originate
Zoonosis	An infection with an animal reservoir
Vector	A living agent transmitting a pathogen
Nosocomial	Acquired in hospital
Mortality	The prevalence or incidence of death in a population
Morbidity	The prevalence of disease in a population
Herd immunity	Resistance in a population due to some, but not all, being immune
Quarantine	Restriction of movement to prevent spread
Retrospective study	Comparison of groups, measured retrospectively
Prospective study	Planned comparison of groups following exposure

1. *Clinical diagnosis* is often easy, particularly during epidemics (e.g. childhood virus infections), in endemic areas (e.g. malaria during the transmission season), or when the symptoms and signs are characteristic (e.g. elephantiasis). However,

clinical diagnosis is an art rather than a science; it is never absolutely precise and—especially in children—frequently wrong.

2. *Microbiological diagnosis* is usually precise, but it must be remembered that finding a pathogen does not prove that it is causing the disease in question. The methods used include simple microscopy with or without special stains (for bacteria, fungi, protozoa), culture in agar media (mainly for bacteria, particularly for assessing antibiotic sensitivity), or in animal cells (for viruses), electron microscopy (for viruses), and DNA/RNA sequencing (mainly for studying variation). The use of monoclonal antibodies, usually coupled to fluorescent dyes, allows extremely rapid and specific identification of pathogens and their antigens. Detection of antigen is particularly helpful as it denotes an ongoing infection.

3. *Immunological diagnosis* is valuable when the pathogen is hard to find or identify. It is essentially retrospective and does not prove the presence of an infection, merely that it has occurred. The principal responses measured are specific antibody, T-cell proliferation/cytokine release, and skin tests. Since B and T cells recognize *antigens* rather than whole pathogens, there is sometimes the problem of cross-reaction, but immunological screening can be very useful in monitoring the spread of epidemics and the success of vaccine campaigns. In addition, antibodies are most useful reagents for detecting microbial antigens in the laboratory (see above).

Theoretical epidemiology

It has become possible to create mathematical models of disease spread, given certain basic numerical values. These include the number of susceptible individuals in a population, the duration of the infectious state, the distance over which spread occurs, and in the case of vector-borne diseases, the duration of the infectious state for the vector. Models of this kind have been particularly valuable in predicting the periodicity of epidemics and the proportion of a population that would need to be immunized, or of animals that would need to be culled (see prion disease, Chapters 8 and 31) for a disease to die out, and in general their calculations have agreed closely with already known facts. For example, the elimination of measles would require a vaccination uptake of at least 95% whereas smallpox was eradicated with only about 80% of the world's population being vaccinated. Mathematical models are also useful in planning drug trials where drug resistance is expected.

Practical epidemiology

The epidemiology of any given disease depends on four main factors, all of which need to be understood by those working in the 'real world'.

1. the *host* and its variables, such as lifestyle, immune competence, genetics;
2. the *pathogen* and its variables, such as virulence factors, genetics;

3. the degree of *contact* between the two, which depends on the numbers of pathogens in the environment and the means by which they spread;

4. the effect, if any, of *treatment* or *preventive measures* (vaccines, drugs, public health strategy).

We shall illustrate these points in relation to three diseases, one viral (AIDS), one bacterial (TB), and one protozoal (malaria), which together make up a large percentage of the total world burden of morbidity and mortality caused by infection, and all of which are currently on the increase, and two even more numerically important conditions, infantile respiratory disease and diarrhoea, which are not due to a single pathogen (global mortality figures approximate).

■ HIV and AIDS (1.8 million deaths per year)

It is estimated that following a single exposure to HIV, there is up to a 10% chance of becoming infected, a much lower rate than that of the common childhood viruses, which is almost 100%. The rate of disease progression is then related to the total viral load, and is monitored mainly by following T-cell numbers in the blood. As far as can be judged (the virus was only identified some 30 years ago and the first contact between this animal virus and human populations probably occurred not more than about 50 years ago) the morbidity and mortality in those infected and not treated are very close to 100%, the exceptions being mainly individuals genetically lacking the 'second receptor' for the virus. One can imagine that if humans were exposed to HIV for long enough, this defective genotype, having a strong survival advantage, would spread quite rapidly through the populations at risk, as the sickle gene appears to have (see malaria, below). At present the very high morbidity and mortality are due to two main causes: the severe damage to the immune system, which limits effective immunity, both against HIV itself and against a whole range of *opportunists*, and the extremely high level of antigenic variation, which renders what immunity there is against HIV ineffective and vaccination difficult. The major vaccine trials that have been completed to date are listed in Table 27.2, with a small margin of success observed in the most recent trial (Rv144) which targeted production of both antibody and T cell responses in the same vaccine. Only two strategies of control are currently available: limitation of *contact* and *chemotherapy* (see Table 26.5). Monitoring is by peripheral T-cell counts and the detection of complications (see Table 26.6).

AIDS is one of the few diseases to have emerged within living memory (see Chapter 37 for a discussion of some others) and the observations that unravelled its pathogenesis are a good example of epidemiology in action. The alarm was given by a sharp rise in the incidence of pneumonia due to *Pneumocystis carinii*, previously considered a harmless parasite (1981). Other opportunistic infections were noted in the same individuals, along with skin tumours (Kaposi's sarcoma), low blood T-cell counts, and severe weight loss. Evidently a new form of immunodeficiency had suddenly appeared. Consideration of the type of patient affected

CASE STUDY 27.1 HIV/AIDS

Presentation

(1) A 25-year-old man went to his doctor with a fever and a mild rash. The doctor found some enlarged lymph glands and realized that HIV infection was a possibility. He suggested a blood test for the virus but did not insist when the patient refused. Three months later he felt worse and had lost some weight. He was married, but admitted to occasional homosexual encounters. After discussion with his family he agreed to be tested again and the result was positive for both antibody and HIV antigen. It was explained to him that he had HIV but not (yet) AIDS. (2) Other important means of spread include infected mother to child; shared needle use; blood transfusion; hospital accidents.

Diagnosis

The demonstration of HIV antigen and antibody on two separate tests is sufficient to prove infection. Progress is measured mainly by following the plasma viral load (e.g. by PCR), by the T-cell count (<350/µl instead of the normal 500–1000/µl is considered the threshold for drug treatment), and by the development of complications such as opportunist infection.

Therapy and prevention

Drugs have been increasingly effective against HIV, the present standard regime, known as Highly Active Antiretroviral Therapy or HAART, consisting of a protease inhibitor plus at least two others from a list of inhibitors of fusion, reverse transcriptase, integrase, or viral processing. Opportunist infections are treated as they arise with the appropriate antibiotic. As the case described above emphasizes, ethical considerations are important; the diagnosis of HIV infection is a severe blow, and a common policy on disclosure, informed consent, and compliance has not yet been universally adopted. The result of vaccine trials so far has been disappointing (see Table 27.2 below), and public health campaigns targeted at changing sexual attitudes, increasing use of condoms, promoting male circumcision, and controlling other sexually transmitted diseases which increase the risk of HIV transmission remain the best hope of preventing infection. The recent findings that HAART also reduces the risk of transmitting the virus to others has raised the question of whether global delivery of HAART to all infected individuals could stop the HIV epidemic. However, this is financially impossible, drug therapy needs to be for life, has significant side effects and long-term treated individuals still die earlier than healthy controls despite management of their viral burdens.

revealed that they were mostly (1) male homosexuals, (2) intravenous drug abusers, or (3) haemophiliacs requiring injections of human clotting factor VIII. Clearly the common element was the transfer of blood or body fluids, which immediately suggested an infectious agent, and by 1983 a French group had identified a virus, later baptized HIV (now HIV-1). Since this time the balance of infection has shifted so that heterosexual transmission is now the most common route. Sequencing of the HIV genome and comparison with other viruses strongly suggested an origin in African primates. It is a frustrating thought that, with the possible exception of mother–child transfer, all the means by which HIV spreads could *theoretically* be prevented by changes in human behaviour, such as promoting safe sex and the avoidance of needle sharing. By contrast, infections transmitted by the aerosol route (e.g. TB) are almost impossible to avoid.

Table 27.2 The major HIV vaccine clinical trials completed to-date.

Trial	Vaxgen	AIDSVAX	STEP	Rv144
Year	2003	2003	2007	2009
Number enrolled	5000	2500	3000	16,000
Target group	Men sex Men	IV drug users	at risk	at risk
Immune objective	Ab	Ab	T cells	Ab + T cells
Antigens	gp120	gp120	gag/pol/nef	gag/pol/env + gp120
Vaccine type	protein/alum	protein/alum	Adenovirus	Canarypox/protein
PROTECTION[1]	NO	NO	WORSE?[3]	31%
CONTROL[2]	NO	NO	NO	NO

[1] testing for protection against infection with HIV, [2] testing whether vaccinated individuals who still get infected will have lower viral loads, [3] an increased risk of HIV infection was observed in individuals with evidence of pre-existing antibody responses to the adenovirus component of the vaccine (Adenovirus serotype 5) prior to vaccination. See also Chapter 28 for an explanation of the vaccine strategies described here.

■ Tuberculosis (1.3 million deaths per year)

Unlike AIDS, TB is an ancient scourge of mankind. *M. tuberculosis* is fairly common in the air we breathe, and it is estimated that one-third of the world population is infected. However, fewer than 10% of these individuals show symptoms, whereas in many others the development of a positive skin (Mantoux) test indicates that they have responded immunologically and acquired a level of cell-mediated immunity to the bacterium, without having eliminated it completely, because a change of general health status can be sufficient to 'light up' the disease (see below). Disease activity is monitored clinically, radiologically, and microbiologically, a positive sputum test being a particular danger sign because of the risk of infecting others. This precarious balance between host and pathogen is mainly due to the ability of the bacteria to survive inside phagocytic cells and even inside granulomas composed of large numbers of phagocytes and other immunological cells; antigenic variation between pathogen strains does not seem to be a major factor.

On the other hand many variables influence the ability of the host to keep the infection down, of which the most important appear to be: (1) the general level of immune competence, which can be compromised by malnutrition, stress, other diseases, and particularly HIV infection (see Chapter 26 for a discussion of this and other secondary immunodeficiencies); (2) the widely used BCG vaccine, which undoubtedly gives some protection at the population level, although more effectively in children and to a very different extent in different countries; (3) the

---

CASE STUDY 27.2 Tuberculosis

Presentation

A 60-year-old retired paint factory worker complained to his doctor of chronic productive cough and fatigue. He was a non-smoker, but the doctor diagnosed a prolonged recovery from a cold 3 months earlier and prescribed across-the-counter remedies. A month later the cough was worse and the patient had lost half a stone (about 3 kg). On questioning he admitted to heavy night sweats. He was sent to hospital for a chest X-ray.

Diagnosis

On a chest X-ray active tuberculosis shows up as consolidation with loss of lung air spaces and/or cavitation. The most reliable proof is the finding of the organism *Mycobacterium tuberculosis* (or occasionally some related species) in the sputum. TB antigens can also be detected by PCR. A positive tuberculin (Mantoux) delayed hypersensitivity skin test shows that there has been exposure at some time, however it may become negative in acute cases.

Therapy and prevention

The mainstays of treatment are the drugs isoniazid and rifampicin, which may have to be prolonged for 6 months or more. However resistance to these and other drugs is becoming more widespread. At the same time family and other contacts should be screened for early symptomless disease. The standard vaccine is BCG, given in infancy in countries with high prevalence, but this is only partially effective in adults and new vaccines are under investigation and trial.

Risk factors that predispose to severe TB include HIV infection, diabetes, and inhalation of silicates (possibly significant in the case described above).

---

presence of other mycobacteria in the local environment, which may affect the response to both TB itself and to the BCG vaccine; and (4) genetic differences between individuals, affecting mainly intracellular pathogens. These include mutations in the IFNγ receptor and IL-12 genes, the transporter gene Slc11a1 (see Chapter 9) and, more weakly, the HLA class II allele DR2 and numerous other candidate genes. New vaccine candidates are listed in Table 27.3.

Before the days of antibiotics, treatment of active TB relied on the isolating and restful effect of sanatoria, usually at high altitude, but the present level of control has been largely achieved by BCG, together with chemotherapy, which both kills the organisms and reduces transmission. Drug treatment is typically a combination of, isoniazid, rifampicin, ethambutol, and pyrazinamide for 2 months followed by 4 months (or longer) of isoniazid and rifampicin. None of these drugs are infallible and all have side effects. The increasing extent of drug resistance of *M. tuberculosis* is a global problem, with multi-drug (MDR) strains resistant to these 'front-line' antibiotics and extremely-drug (XDR) strains resistant to first and some 'second line' antibiotics. There has been a recent report from India of a totally drug resistant form of *M. tuberculosis*—a 'nightmare scenario', the impact of which has still to be determined. The global HIV epidemic has also profoundly changed the epidemiology of tuberculosis, particularly in sub-Saharan Africa. The loss of CD4 T cells dramatically impairs resistance to infection, increasing the risk

---

CASE STUDY 27.3 Malaria

Presentation

(1) A 6-month-old child was brought to the doctor in an African village with convulsions and developing coma. Since one in three of all outpatients in the area turn out to have malaria, this was the obvious diagnosis. (2) A 28-year-old nurse was returning from holiday in Brazil when her flight was re-routed for a one-night stop in Dakar, Senegal. Two weeks later she reported that she was coming down with the flu. An astute house physician did a blood smear and recognized the characteristic intra-erythrocytic parasite: to her surprise she had malaria. (3) Malaria can also, exceptionally, be transmitted by a blood transfusion from an infected individual.

Diagnosis

When microscopy is available, a blood film is sufficient. In a thin film the species of *Plasmodium* can usually be identified, but with low parasite levels, a thick film needs to be done too. The latter can detect down to 10 parasites per microlitre of blood. In the field, a rapid dipstick test on a single drop of blood will pick up a parasite antigen, but the sensitivity is about 20 times less than a blood film.

Therapy and prevention

For acute cases, intravenous artesunate or quinine can be life-saving. Prophylaxis for travellers depends on the known sensitivity/resistance of the parasites in the area to be visited: common drugs are malarone, mefloquine, proguanil, chloroquine, doxycycline. For the population in endemic areas, bed nets impregnated with the insecticide permethrin have given the best results. Despite extensive research and numerous trials, there is still no really effective vaccine (but see p. 266).

---

of developing active disease after exposure from 10% in a lifetime to 10% per year. HIV-infected TB patients have high mortality rates and have a greater risk of recurrence after treatment. They are more likely to have extrapulmonary disease, a sign that their immune system cannot prevent dissemination from the lung, but paradoxically may also have lower amounts of bacteria in their sputum since the tissue damage which usually results in cavities and release of bacteria is immune-mediated. This may reduce their chances of spreading the infection to another person but since there are so many HIV–TB infected people, they still contribute substantially to the spread of tuberculosis in the community. Indeed, the coexistence of HIV and *M. tuberculosis* in a population represents pathogen–pathogen interaction at its worst.

■ Malaria (1.1 million deaths per year)

Caused by four species of the protozoon *Plasmodium*, this disease is normally restricted to tropical areas by the distribution of the *Anopheles* mosquito vector, which plays an essential role in the pathogen's complex life cycle. However, the huge increase in migration and travel (2 000 000 people are estimated to cross a

Table 27.3 Major candidate vaccines in development and evaluation against tuberculosis

Vaccine Type	Description	Stage
Modified BCG		
BCG30	rBCG overexpressing Ag85A	Phase I (on hold)
VPM1002	rBCG/urease deleted + listeriolysin	Phase II
AERAS 422	rBCG expressing Ag85A/Ag85B/Rv3407 + perfringolysin	Phase I halted due to safety concerns
Attenuated M. tuberculosis		
MTBVAC	M. tuberculosis (phoP/fad D26 deleted)	experimental
Killed or mixed components		
RUTI	detoxified, fragmented *M. tuberculosis* in liposomes	Phase II
Mw	killed *Mycobacteria indicus pranii* (non pathogenic saprophyte)	Phase III
Subunit (Viral vector)		
MVA85A/AERAS 485	Modified Vaccinia Ankara expressing Ag85A	Phase IIb
AdAg85A	rAdenovirus expressing Ag85A	Phase I
AERAS 402/CrucellAd35	rAdenovirus expressing Ag85A/Ag85B/ Mtb10.4	Phase I
Subunit (protein + adjuvant)		
M72	MTB32A-MTB39A fusion protein + AS01 or AS02 adjuvant	Phase II
Hybrid 1	Ag85B-ESAT 6 fusion protein in IC31 or CAF01 adjuvant	Phase I/II
HyVac 4/AERAS 404	Ag85B-TB10.4 fusion protein + IC31 adjuvant	Phase I
H56	Ag85B-ESAT6-Rv2660c fusion protein + IC31 adjuvant	Phase I

See also Chapter 28 for an explanation of the vaccine strategies described here.

national boundary every day) means that cases of malaria are increasingly seen in the non-tropical world. The only reliable diagnostic marker is the finding of parasites in a blood film.

In the endemic areas themselves, the pattern of disease is determined by numerous factors, as follows.

1. The distribution of the *vector*, at low altitudes and near swampy water.
2. The *age* of the infected individual; young children harbour more parasites and are more likely to die of complications such as anaemia and cerebral malaria, probably because of the slow development of immunity. Adults who have acquired a partial level of immunity sufficient to keep parasite numbers low

and symptoms absent can lose this after 6 months away from the endemic area, suggesting that repeated boosting is required to maintain protection.

3. Extensive surface antigenic variation by the blood-stage parasite, to the point where every member of a village may carry a different variant; this variability is enhanced by the possession of a clear sexual stage in the parasite life cycle, allowing rapid reassortment of parasite genes.

4. Genetic differences between individuals. This may operate at the level of the red blood cell: absence of the Duffy blood-group antigen prevents the entry of *P. vivax*, whereas heterozygotes for HbS (the sickle-cell trait) show partial resistance to *P. falciparum*. The latter has had the interesting effect of helping to maintain what is otherwise a deleterious gene in endemic areas, at the expense of those unfortunate enough to be homozygous, who suffer life-threatening sickle-cell anaemia: this is a good example of *balanced polymorphism*. There is also a link between severity and HLA type, probably mainly due to linkage between alleles of the HLA and TNF genes; TNF is thought to play a role in both protection and disease.

Malaria displays important interactions with other infections. It is immunosuppressive (though much less so than HIV) and even mild malaria has been shown to interfere with the effectiveness of vaccines against *S. pneumoniae* and *N. meningitidis*. It also appears to be a co-factor, along with EBV, for the development of Burkitt's lymphoma. Here the mechanism is not so clear, but suppression of the CTL response to virus-infected B cells may be one element. Since the realization that vector control (e.g. by DDT) is not as simple as was thought, numerous other strategies have been tried. Experimental vaccines have been devised against the liver stage, the infected red cell, the free (merozoite) blood parasite, and even the sexual stage (to block transmission by preventing the mosquito stage). Table 27.4 summarizes the leading candidate vaccines, with RTS,S showing the most promise and currently being evaluated in a multi-centre Phase 3 clinical trial of some 15 000 individuals in 7 different African countries. However, effective control still relies on minimizing contact (by mosquito nets, etc.) and the careful use of chemotherapy; unfortunately drug resistance has occurred to virtually every drug and the pharmaceutical industry is engaged in a literal race against the pathogen.

■ Acute infantile respiratory disease (3.5 million deaths per year)

One in five deaths in children under 5 are due to infections of the lower respiratory tract—bronchitis, bronchiolitis, and pneumonia. Social and nutritional deprivation is a common predisposing factor. Transmission is by droplet. Mortality from the major bacterial causes—*Streptococcus pneumoniae*, *Haemophilus influenzae*, *Bordetella pertussis*, and *Corynebacterium diphtheriae* has fallen dramatically where effective vaccines and antibiotics have been widely used, so that viral

---

CASE STUDY 27.4 Acute Respiratory Disease

Presentation

A 9-month-old boy was referred to hospital because of a 5-day constant 'barking' cough and, more recently, breathing difficulty with wheezing. He was one of a family of five in a small flat, and had been a month premature. He was only breast-fed for a few days. He had had the first round of vaccinations against diphtheria, pertussis, *Haemophilus B*, the pneumococcus, and measles. A provisional diagnosis of viral pneumonia was made, but he was given an injection of chloramphenicol to cover possible bacterial infection and admitted to the ward.

Diagnosis

A stained film of sputum followed by culture will rule out the commonest bacterial causes of pneumonia such a *S. pneumoniae* and *H. influenzae*, bearing in mind that these may be superimposed on the primary viral infection. If available, ELISA or PCR tests on a nasal or throat swab may confirm the diagnosis. In the case described here, the causative agent turned out to be respiratory syncytial virus (RSV).

Treatment and prevention

The majority of patients recover with supportive treatment – fluids, oxygen if required, and a bronchodilator. Secondary bacterial infections are treated with the appropriate antibiotics. A monoclonal antibody, given by inhalation, can be used in susceptible infants (immunodeficiency, congenital heart or lung defects). RSV infection, which is virtually universal and mild in older children, does not induce lasting immunity, but a vaccine would be highly desirable since it is the earliest infection(s) that are most likely to be fatal.

---

infections, notably RSV, are now more common causes of pneumonia in these countries. Vaccines against RSV are still experimental, but a monoclonal antibody, palivizumab, is quite effective in prophylaxis and the antiviral drug ribavirin, given by inhalation, has been successful in severe cases. Other viral causes of pneumonia include, influenza, parainfluenza, and measles; secondary bacterial infection is a common complication. In the case of influenza, the role of animals has to be taken into account (see Box 37.1).

■ Infantile diarrhoea (2.5 million deaths per year)

When all deaths from diarrhoea are considered together—and they are not always easy to tell apart—they are the second commonest cause of death under the age of 5. Viruses and bacteria play a roughly equal role in this mortality. The symptoms range from a mild 'stomach flu' to extreme dehydration, as in Case Study 27.5. The key symptoms, not all of which are found with every pathogen are: frequent watery stools, abdominal pain, vomiting, and fever. With some bacteria, the stools may be bloody ('dysentery'). Spread is predominantly by the faecal-oral route, though animal vectors are sometimes involved.

Table 27.4 Some major candidate vaccines in development and evaluation against *Plasmodium falciparum*

Vaccine Type	Description	Stage
Pre-erythrocytic:		
RTS,S	Circumsporozoite (CS) 9 central tandem repeat + C-terminal region fused to Hepatitis B S antigen adjuvanted with AS01E	Phase 3 (completion 2015)
Adenovirus-RTS,S	CS in Adenovirus 35 and RTS,S in AS01 as heterologous prime-boost	Phase 1
ChAd63/MVA ME TRAP	liver stage antigen ME TRAP expressed in simian Adenovirus and MVA vectors for heterologous prime-boost	Phase 2
Adenovirus CS	CS antigen expressed in Adenovirus 35	Phase 1
PfSPZ	radiation attenuated sporozoites	Phase 2
Pf GAP p52⁻/p32⁻	genetically attenuated sporozoites with double gene deletion	Phase 1
Blood stage:		
ChAd63/MVA MSP1	merozoite surface protein 1 expressed in simian adenovirus and MVA for heterologous prime-boost	Phase 2
FMP2.1/AS02A	recombinant *E.coli* expressed apical membrane antigen 1 (AMA 1) in AS02A adjuvant	Phase 2
MSP 3 [181–276]	MSP3 long synthetic peptide in alum adjuvant	Phase 1
GMZ2	fusion protein of MSP 3 and GLURP in alum adjuvant	Phase 2
AMA 1/C1	AMA 1 in alhydrogel adjuvant plus CPG 7909	Phase 2
NMRC-M3V-Ad-PfCA	adenovirus expressing CS plus adenovirus expressing AMA 1	Phase 1

See also Table 34.1 and Chapter 28 for an explanation of the vaccine strategies described here.

The two most important viruses are *rotavirus* and *norovirus*, each responsible for about half a million deaths per year. Mild infections are virtually universal in infants, becoming rarer as a degree of immunity develops. This is shorter-lived with norovirus than rotavirus, thus the latter is rare in adults and two vaccines are currently in use with the backing of the WHO.

Common bacterial causes include, in roughly descending order of frequency, *E. coli* (particularly ETEC), *Campylobacter jejuni*, *Shigella*, *Salmonella*, and cholera. These all secrete toxins, which may act by directly damaging the gut epithelium (e.g. *Shigella*, *Salmonella*) or by interfering with salt and water transport (e.g. cholera, ETEC). One protozoan organism, *Cryptosporidium parvum*, has come to the fore, mainly in adults, thanks to the HIV epidemic. As an opportunist

---

CASE STUDY 27.5 Infantile Diarrhoea

Presentation

An 18-month-old boy was brought to the clinic in a North African town. The mother complained that he had been crying all night and now was not responding and looked lifeless. On questioning she said his stools were 'loose'. On examination he was severely dehydrated and his garments were soaked in watery faeces. Oral rehydration was started and preparations made for intravenous hydration, but the child died 20 minutes later.

Diagnosis

The most likely cause of this child's illness is infection with rotavirus or one or other species of enteropathic bacteria, of which enterotoxic *Escherichia coli* (ETEC) is the commonest. Diagnosis can usually be made by light or electron microscopy and culture of the faeces and, if available, PCR for particular antigens.

Treatment and prevention

In acute cases such as this one, rehydration is vital. 500 million sachets per year of an 'oral rehydration therapy' (ORT) combination containing sodium and potassium chloride, citrate, and glucose have been supplied by UNICEF. If a bacterial cause is identified, appropriate antibiotics will also be needed. Vaccines are available for rotavirus, cholera, and—still experimental—*E. coli*. However the principal factors contributing to the high incidence and mortality from infantile diarrhoea are: (1) contaminated water supplies and (2) parental ignorance—well exemplified by this case.

(see Chapter 26) it can disseminate and cause life-threatening disease in AIDS patients rather than the usual self-limiting diarrhoea.

■ The value of epidemiology

We have looked at only five diseases and there are dozens of others, each with its special and interesting epidemiological features (see Chapters 31–35). What is the use of all this knowledge? The answer is that without it, the chances of controlling any infectious disease would be practically nil. A classic example is the detective work carried out in 1855 by the London doctor John Snow, who used detailed maps of disease incidence and the London water supplies to pinpoint the source of cholera, hitherto rampant in some parts of the city. This was a case where *public health* measures were clearly called for. On the other hand the massive incidence of soil-derived tetanus during the early months of trench warfare in the First World War—a disease already known to be due to a toxin that could be neutralized by antibody—was an indication for passive immunization with antibody, soon to be replaced by active immunization by a *vaccine*. Finally, the susceptibility of the ever-present *Staphylococcus* to penicillin and the non-availability of a vaccine was the impetus for the modern science of *chemotherapy*. In the next three chapters we shall look at these three contrasting ways of controlling infectious disease.

SUMMARY

- The science of epidemiology attempts to understand and manipulate disease at the population level.

- Epidemiologists have to take into account the methods and accuracy of diagnosis, knowledge of all relevant pathogen and host factors, means of spread, interaction with other diseases, and the likely success of control measures.

Chapter 28

Control of infectious disease: vaccination

Immunization makes use of the ability of the adaptive immune system to learn and improve. It may be *active*, inducing the immune system itself to acquire a permanently enhanced resistance to a particular pathogen, or *passive*, where preformed antibody is introduced into the individual to be protected (see below). Active immunization directed at a specific organism is known as *vaccination*, in commemoration of Edward Jenner's pioneering work (1797) on the prevention of smallpox by scarification with vaccinia (cowpox). Smallpox has now been eradicated (1980) but ever since Pasteur showed in the 1880s that it was possible to immunize against other infections, the general term 'vaccination' has been retained (Box 28.1).

The function of a vaccine is to induce *memory* without causing *disease*, so that the pathogen itself, on first contact with the patient, provokes a secondary rather than a primary response, and a response of the right kind to be effective; that is, antibody or T-cell-mediated, systemic or mucosal. Thus all our current vaccines are prophylactic, given before exposure to the organism (only the rabies vaccine being also effective after exposure, see later). In general, vaccines are more successful when mimicking a normally effective immune response (e.g. measles) than when

Box 28.1 Jenner and Pasteur, a study in contrasts

The first vaccine?

From fifteenth-century China, via eighteenth-century Turkey and the wife of the British Ambassador, the practice of sniffing dried smallpox crusts to protect against the disease reached the England of George I. A later modification was injection of tiny amounts of material from smallpox lesions. This risky procedure of *variolation* spread throughout Europe, inducing protection but also occasional mortality. In 1774 an English farmer, Benjamin Jesty, encouraged by the tradition that country girls who had had cowpox never got smallpox, tried cowpox on his own family, during a smallpox epidemic. His two sons were protected but his wife became quite ill and he did not publicize the result. Edward Jenner, a general practitioner, did the same 22 years later. He injected material from Sarah Nelmes' cowpox lesion into 8-year-old James Phipps, deliberately challenged him with live smallpox, and established the first scientifically tested vaccine. First published in 1798, by 1800 the procedure was world-famous, hailed as a major breakthrough by Napoleon, Jefferson, and the learned European societies, although resisted elsewhere on religious grounds, as in some quarters it remained until the final eradication of smallpox in 1980.

A long wait for the second

Since there was no understanding of viruses or of immunity, there was no intellectual framework into which the success of Jenner's vaccine could be fitted. Not until the germ theory of Koch and Pasteur took shape almost a century later, in the 1870s and 1880s, could the vaccine idea be tried rationally on other diseases. It was Louis Pasteur, already famous for his work on fermentation and the demolition of 'spontaneous generation', who took the plunge by showing that chickens could be protected against cholera and sheep against anthrax, using 'stale' bacilli. By carrying out his experiments in the full public gaze, Pasteur took enormous risks but acquired enormous fame, crowned by his immunization of young Joseph Meister against rabies in 1885. Emil Behring (later von Behring), Karl Fraenkel, and Shibasaburo Kitasato in Berlin had shown by 1890 that diphtheria toxin could also be made into a vaccine, and moreover that it was *antibody* that caused the protection, thus initiating the era of modern immunology. Pasteur's greatest rival, Robert Koch, joined the vaccine hunt with his tuberculosis extract *tuberculin*, which proved to be a disaster and he escaped to Egypt with his new young wife. Nevertheless, the principle of vaccination had been thoroughly established. No really convincing successor to Jenner's living cowpox virus emerged, and future vaccines were to be either killed organisms, inactivated toxins, or pathogens—mostly viruses—attenuated by repeated culture or, in modern times, by genetic manipulation.

trying to improve upon partial or absent immunity (e.g. TB, HIV). The aim of a vaccine is ideally to prevent *infection* occurring at all, but there are special situations, for example vector-borne diseases like malaria and leishmaniasis, where a vaccine that only prevents *transmission* has been contemplated.

■ Requirements for a vaccine

There are not vaccines for every disease; this is because a vaccine, to be worth bringing into use, must satisfy four criteria. It must be (1) effective, (2) safe, (3) stable, and (4) affordable.

Effectiveness

The best vaccines are very effective indeed. As mentioned in Box 28.1, smallpox was eventually eliminated by 1980, infection with one of the three strains of polio virus (type 2) has not occurred since 1999 and in 2011 the world was declared free of rinderpest, an important disease of cattle which destroyed precious livestock in tropical regions. Several other viral diseases have been targeted by the World Health Organization for eradication within the next generation; these include polio (the most realistic), measles, rubella, and mumps. Whether or not this is achieved, there is no doubt that in the developed world these four diseases have essentially disappeared as major public health threats and the same is true for the 'toxic' bacterial diseases tetanus and diphtheria (Fig. 28.1). It is estimated that vaccination currently saves some 3 million lives per year, a figure that could increase to 5 million if vaccines were available universally.

At the other end of the scale, there are vaccines that, although undoubtedly beneficial, stand no chance at present of eradicating the corresponding disease; examples are influenza, rabies, and BCG (the TB vaccine). Note that it may not always be necessary to vaccinate every single member of the population. When most individuals are protected and few are susceptible, transmission is reduced (so-called *herd immunity*) and the disease may eventually die out. A recent example is where adults who have not been vaccinated show a reduced incidence of pneumococcal disease in communities where only the young children have received the new generation of conjugate vaccines. Rarely, an attenuated strain may actually replace the pathogenic type in the environment, as is happening with live polio vaccine in water supplies, so that individuals may become immunized without knowing it.

The reasons for reduced effectiveness differ. In the case of influenza, antigenic variation (see Fig. 22.2) makes it hard to match the vaccine to the current virus strain, requiring manufacturers to make a new vaccine effectively every year. For the pneumococcus, there are over 90 different serotypes, requiring complicated mixtures of antigens to cover the dominant strains in each geographical region. With rabies, there is a vast animal reservoir beyond the reach of the vaccinator. With BCG, the problem is that it works much better in adults in some parts of the world than others, for reasons that are not fully understood but probably reflect the influence of other mycobacteria in the local environment as well as genetic differences between human populations. However, the use of BCG in the tropics is universal since it provides good protection against disseminated tuberculosis in children. Any new vaccine is likely to be based on a better version of BCG and/or boosting this response with some form of sub-unit vaccine.

Individual genetic differences, particularly in HLA antigens with their role in presenting peptides to T cells (see Chapter 18), can determine the success or failure of vaccines based on single, small peptides, making a 'universal' peptide vaccine—for example to tuberculosis—difficult to achieve. Instead, larger fragments or whole proteins are used, allowing each individual to respond to one or more peptides within this structure, and making it more likely to be immunogenic in a

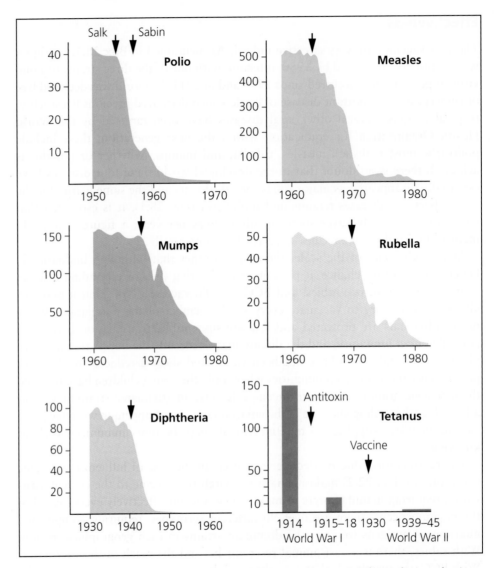

Fig. 28.1 The impact of vaccination on six major diseases. The arrows indicate the introduction of general immunization in each case. Polio, measles, mumps, and rubella show cases per 10 000 in the USA; diphtheria shows cases per million in the UK; tetanus shows cases per 10 000 in British Army troops (also showing the dramatic protective effect of passive antibody).

genetically diverse population. Polysaccharide vaccines are inefficient at inducing memory in young children, but this can be overcome by coupling them to a protein carrier—either one from the same organism (e.g. *H. influenzae*) or one to which most people would be primed (e.g. tetanus toxoid). Finally, there are diseases where no vaccine is currently available at all: leading examples are the common cold, staphylococcal infections, and virtually all fungal, protozoal, and worm infections. The reason is usually technical, but may also be economic. Opportunist

Table 28.1 The main vaccines in use, with some important diseases where vaccines are still lacking

	Virus	Bacteria	Fungi	Protozoa or worms
In general use	Polio, measles, mumps, rubella, hepatitis B	Diphtheria, tetanus, pertussis, BCG (in tropics), *Haemophilus*		
Mainly for those at risk	Influenza, yellow fever, hepatitis A, rabies, VZV, rotavirus, papilloma	BCG, cholera, typhoid, Pneumococcus, Meningococcus, plague, anthrax		
Vaccines not available	Adenovirus, rhinovirus, herpesviruses, respiratory syncytial virus, HIV*	*Staphylococcus*, Gp A *Streptococcus*, Gonococcus, syphilis, leprosy†, *Chlamydia*	*Candida*, *Pneumocystis*, *Cryptococcus* etc.	Malaria*, *Leishmania*, trypanosomiasis, schistosomiasis, filariasis hookworm*

Measles, mumps, and rubella vaccines are usually given simultaneously, as are diphtheria, tetanus, pertussis, *Haemophilus*, and killed polio vaccines.

*Trials have been carried out with experimental vaccines. In parasitic diseases, the anti-malaria vaccine RTS,S is the most advanced and currently in a large scale Phase III study. Trials of a promising new hookworm vaccine were recently stopped due to adverse reactions in individuals with prior exposure to the parasite, but an alternative antigen with less evidence of pre-existing immunity in endemic populations is now progressing with considerable hope of success.

†BCG gives some protection against leprosy.

infections, against which healthy individuals do not need to be vaccinated (e.g. CMV, *Pneumocystis*) are a special case; it will be interesting to see whether vaccination in the early stages of immunodeficiency will delay the onset of the opportunistic infection. Table 28.1 summarizes the major diseases for which effective vaccines currently do and do not exist.

Safety

Safety is an increasingly critical consideration. One must remember that vaccines are the only medical treatment administered to perfectly healthy people, and 'vaccine accidents'—real or imaginary—can lead to public alarm and enormously expensive litigation. Live attenuated vaccines are the most vulnerable because of the real possibility of reversion to the pathogenic 'wild' type. Here established vaccines differ enormously: BCG is estimated to have lost some 100 genes from the wild-type *M. bovis*, whereas some polio vaccine strains have mutations in 10 genes or fewer (see below). Other important safety problems are listed in Table 28.2.

Table 28.2 The main safety problems with vaccines

The vaccine

   Attenuated organisms revert to wild type (e.g. polio types 2, 3)*

   'Killed' organisms not properly killed (has happened with polio)

   Inclusion of toxic material (e.g. typhoid, pertussis)

   Contamination by animal viruses

   Contamination by egg proteins (hypersensitivity)

   Cross-reaction with 'self' (autoimmunity)

The patient

   Immunodeficiency (attenuated organisms may cause serious/fatal disease)*

   Local inflammatory reactions, often to the adjuvant

   Worsening of disease by increasing immunopathology

   Hypersensitivity to vaccine (e.g. tetanus)

   Interference between vaccines given together (fortunately rare)

   Induction of inappropriate response (e.g. respiratory syncytial virus, dengue)

   Patient already exposed (therapeutic vaccination, e.g. HIV)

---

*Those asterisked are the most important. In general, living attenuated vaccines are not given to immunodeficient patients.

Partly for these reasons, and partly because of the low profitability of vaccines compared to chemotherapy (see Chapter 29), some pharmaceutical companies nowadays are still cautious of embarking on vaccine development.

Stability

Stability becomes particularly important where vaccines are used far from their site of manufacture, and is again chiefly a problem for living vaccines, where maintenance of the 'cold chain' between producer and consumer requires conscientious monitoring at all stages of the journey (see below).

Affordability

Most vaccines are remarkably cheap; indeed, vaccination has been called the most cost-effective form of preventive medicine ever invented. For example, the cost of vaccinating a child against measles, pertussis, diphtheria, tetanus, polio, and TB is less than US$20. However, it must be borne in mind that for some tropical countries, even a few pence per person per year may exceed the available health budget. Moreover, some vaccines are definitely not cheap; the hepatitis B vaccine still costs around $60 per individual, having fallen from $125! The technology exists to make each vaccine more and more complicated—containing increasing number of antigens in a single dose—however this can also increase the price dramatically and, as in the case of a new pneumococcal conjugate vaccine, can require up to a year per batch to manufacture. To develop a *new* vaccine is extremely expensive (see below) but delivering existing vaccines is also costly and requires both the healthcare infrastructure and the political will to make it happen. Each year almost 2 million children die from vaccine preventable diseases and 23 million remain unvaccinated. Part of the problem is the time taken for successful vaccines which are already in use in developed countries to then be adopted in low-income settings. It is estimated that in the more than 10 years it took for the *H. influenzae B* vaccine to come into use in less well-developed countries some 6 million children died of this disease. One of the biggest advances in vaccine financing was the launch in 2000 of the Global Alliance for Vaccines and Immunization (GAVI). This brings together donor governments, pharmaceutical companies, international aid agencies, and other groups such as the Bill and Melinda Gates Foundation to provide a concerted effort for vaccine funding in the poorest countries in the world. In some cases, pharmaceutical companies provide their vaccines at reduced cost (while charging regular prices in the developed world) and can be offered guaranteed pricing for their products for up to 10 years to encourage them to find the huge investment required to develop new vaccines.

■ Established vaccines

To induce memory requires exposure of the immune system to an antigen or set of antigens identical or closely similar to those on the infectious organism. This can be achieved in a number of ways, some established and some still experimental (Table 28.3). For practical purposes, the essential distinction is between *living* and *non-living* vaccines.

Living vaccines

Living vaccines have been outstandingly successful with viral diseases, from smallpox onwards. In fact, smallpox was unusual in that an animal virus existed with sufficient antigenic similarity to immunize (mainly via T cells) against the human disease, but which was unable to survive more than a few weeks in the human host. The same principle has been tried with some other viruses (e.g. rotavirus), with success; a similar concept underlies the once-favoured use of the vole bacillus to immunize against human TB, and of the practice of leishmanization, in which

Table 28.3 The antigens used in vaccination are of various kinds: some examples are given of each type

Type of antigen	Examples
1. Whole organisms	
Living (e.g. from animals)	Vaccinia (for smallpox)
Killed	Rabies, influenza, polio (Salk), hepatitis A, pertussis, typhoid, cholera
2. Attenuated (i.e. mutant) organisms	
Randomly mutated	Measles, mumps, rubella, polio (Sabin), yellow fever, VZV, BCG, typhoid
Site-directed*	Cholera, typhoid
3. Antigenic fragments	
Inactivated toxins (toxoids)	Tetanus, diphtheria
Capsular polysaccharides	Meningococcus, Pneumococcus, _Haemophilus influenzae_
Surface antigen	Hepatitis B
Bacterial pili	Gonococcus*, _E. coli_*
4. Peptides/proteins	
Gene-cloned	Hepatitis B, malaria*
Synthetic	Foot-and-mouth disease (cattle)
5. Genes cloned into living vectors*	e.g., TB antigens in vaccinia*
6. DNA*	Influenza*, malaria*, TB*

*Still experimental; that is, used in trials or animal models only.

a deliberately induced cutaneous infection gave some protection against the more serious visceral leishmaniasis.

Living vaccines are in general more immunogenic because they are still capable of some growth and they tend to locate to the site where protection is required; for example the oral (Sabin) polio vaccine induces better intestinal IgA levels than the killed (Salk) vaccine, which is injected intramuscularly. However, live vaccines suffer from three drawbacks: (1) instability if a complete _cold chain_ is not maintained from factory to clinic; (2) the danger of _reversion_ to the non-mutant (wild) type; and (3) their ability to cause serious disease in _immunodeficient_ individuals (Table 28.2). In the days of smallpox vaccination, the first sign of severe T-cell deficiency (see Fig. 25.1) in children was sometimes the development of spreading and eventually fatal infections with the supposedly non-virulent vaccinia virus, and these babies, if given BCG, risked dying of 'disseminated BCG-osis', effectively a new, man-made disease. A reminder of the danger was the death from vaccinia of three patients in Zaire, immunized with the virus containing a cloned antigen from HIV as part of an attempt to protect against AIDS. The WHO has recently changed its policy and no longer recommends giving BCG vaccine to children known to be HIV positive due to the risk of severe infection, although in practice this is not easy to implement in low-income countries where HIV testing is not adequate. Reversion was seen in some early polio vaccine campaigns, which was subsequently explained by the discovery that some of the original 'attenuated' strains (Types 2 and 3) contained only two new mutations; in contrast, Type 1 contained 57 mutations and has not reverted. On the other hand, *over*-attenuation would be self-defeating, since the vaccine might not behave like the live infection in which case it would, in effect, be 'dead'.

Attenuation

Most live vaccines are produced by *attenuating* a normal human pathogen. Originally this was a lengthy process of inducing random mutation by imposing unusual growth conditions (low temperature, abnormal host cell, etc.) and selecting the mutants that have lost virulence but retained antigenicity. A better way to do this nowadays is through recombinant DNA technology and sequencing of the full genome, allowing the deliberate deletion of, for example, known virulence factors or undesired antigens as well as reducing the risk of reversion. However, the existing attenuated viral vaccines were all produced by the original approach (aptly termed 'genetic roulette'). Only one bacterial vaccine has been produced by attenuation—the *bacille Calmette–Guérin* (BCG) for TB, which took over 10 years and 200 passages of *M. bovis* to develop.

Non-living vaccines

Compared to living ones, non-living vaccines are relatively safe. They range from whole organisms killed by heat, formalin, β-propiolactone, etc., to so-called subunit vaccines—purified, chemically defined components of the organism; for example, the polysaccharide capsules of *Streptococcus pneumoniae*, the surface coat protein of the hepatitis B virus, or the inactivated toxins ('toxoids') of the tetanus and diphtheria bacilli (Table 28.3). Since the injected antigen does not proliferate or localize in the way a living vaccine can, killed and sub-unit vaccines are generally less immunogenic and need to be given more than once, usually by intramuscular injection and often with an *adjuvant* (see below). The safety problems are restricted to (1) failure to kill the organisms properly, and (2) the inclusion of toxic material; the increased risks of adverse reactions seen with the original whole cell whooping-cough vaccine, probably mediated at least in part by the presence of endotoxin, led to a change to a safer (but less immunogenic) acellular sub-unit vaccine (Fig. 28.2). There is the further problem that a more purified antigen, lacking the 'pathogen-associated molecular patterns' of the whole organism (see Chapter 12), may not trigger an optimal response through failure to activate innate immunity- placing great emphasis on inclusion of adjuvants in the preparation (see below).

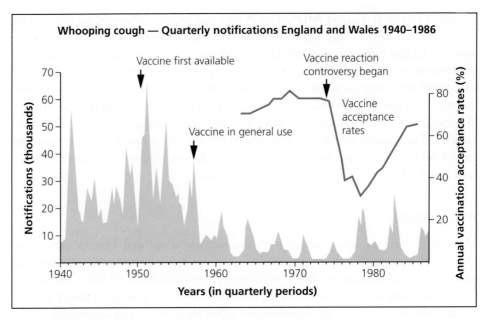

Fig. 28.2 The introduction of a vaccine against *Bordetella pertussis* infection (whooping cough), which reached about 90% of the population by 1956, reduced the incidence of the disease dramatically, although periodic epidemics still occurred. Anxiety that the vaccine could cause serious neurological reactions led to a fall in the numbers vaccinated and a prompt increase in cases (1978, 1982), some fatal. This illustrates both the medical and the social aspect of vaccination. With acknowledgement to Dr N.S. Galbraith and the PHLS Communicable Disease Surveillance Centre, London, UK.

Adjuvants

Often an immune response and/or the development of memory can be enhanced if another substance is injected together with the antigen. It was discovered 70 years ago that aluminium salts had this property and many vaccines, such as the tetanus and diphtheria toxoids, are still given in an emulsion with aluminium hydroxide as an *adjuvant* (and found only in 2008 to act via the NOD-like receptor Nlrp3). Their main effect is to induce local inflammation as well as retain the antigen for a longer period. However, this is a fine balance as excessive inflammation, leading to local tissue reactions and fever, as was seen in animals given complete Freund's adjuvant, is not clinically acceptable. After a long wait, a new generation of adjuvants is now available, based on improved understanding of pattern recognition, antigen presentation, and the role of dendritic cells and cytokines. Currently, the leading adjuvants are based on activation of TLR molecules through detoxified LPS, such the monophosphoryl lipid A (MPL) used in the AS01/2 adjuvant series, or mimics of viral double-stranded RNA such as polyICLC which activate both TLR3 and MDA-5, one of the RIG-like viral sensors. It seems that simultaneous triggering of innate immune responses through more than one signalling pathway may provide the best response. The artificial lipid vesicles known as *liposomes*, used for drug delivery and also in the cosmetics industry, and the somewhat similar immunostimulating complexes (ISCOMs), have also had considerable success as vehicles to transport antigens into antigen-presenting cells. Some enterotoxins (*E. coli*, cholera) have shown promise as adjuvants for mucosal vaccines whereas plasmid DNA has its own adjuvanticity via the activation of TLR9. Indeed, some cytokines themselves have considerable adjuvant activity (IL-1, IL-2, IL-12, IFNγ) but most strategies now employ adjuvants that induce the simultaneous production of multiple cytokines rather than injecting the cytokine itself. Choosing the right adjuvant can determine the success or failure of sub-unit vaccines—for example, the leading malaria vaccine candidate RTS,S was ineffective in humans until the same antigen was reformulated some years after its original discovery with MPL containing adjuvants. In achieving the best activation of the innate immune system, good adjuvants not only activate robust protective immunity but also reduce the amount of antigen needed per vaccine dose and even the number of doses, important advantages in reducing the cost and time taken to confer protection in a population.

Long- and short-term vaccines

One exception to the rule that a vaccine must induce memory occurs when the requirement for protection is only temporary (the 'tourist vaccine'). For example the induction of a strong primary antibody response, even without any memory, would be enough to protect against many infections for 3–6 months, although another course would be needed for a subsequent visit. Ideally, of course, manufacturers aim at a single-dose vaccine that evokes long-term immunity. However, the apparent lifelong duration of protection by some infections (e.g. mumps, measles) may be slightly misleading, since recovered individuals will be regularly 'boosted' by exposure to infected contacts; the same process would also make the duration of protection by a vaccine appear longer than it really was. Here the danger is that as the disease is progressively eliminated from the population, as measles, etc. may soon be, this boosting will disappear and vaccination may need to be repeated more often. Boosting is already recommended for vaccines where there is no regular exposure, for example every 10 years for tetanus.

Route of vaccination

Until recently, most vaccines were given intramuscularly, with the exception of the attenuated polio vaccine which is given orally. In fact the oral route should be ideal for all pathogens that enter via the intestine (as polio does), so that immunity is generated where it is most needed. Several other successful live attenuated vaccines are given via this route such as those against rotavirus and typhoid. It is even possible to express viral antigens in plants, which might lead to the attractive prospect of an edible vaccine. However, overcoming the natural tendency for sub-unit vaccines presented in the gut to induce tolerance rather than immunity is a major problem and the focus of new efforts in adjuvant design. There is also some evidence that live oral vaccines do not work as well in poor tropical countries, perhaps due to particular enteric infections, impaired gut maturation, and even maternal antibodies from milk at the time of vaccination. Intranasal and inhaled vaccines have also been tried experimentally for appropriate pathogens, again, their advantage being the generation of immunity at the site of first contact with many organisms including *M. tuberculosis* and the influenza virus; a new, more broadly cross-protective flu vaccine now given intranasally is the most successful example of this approach to date.

When and whom to vaccinate

In general, vaccines are given as early as possible, with certain qualifications. BCG, given at birth in tropical countries, is delayed until school entry where the risk of exposure to TB is less. The measles, mumps, rubella vaccine is delayed for at least a year to allow maternally transmitted antibody to disappear, because this would otherwise reduce vaccine efficiency. Polysaccharide vaccines are usually delayed because children under 2 years respond poorly. Some vaccines are restricted to those 'at risk'; for example, *Streptococcus pneumoniae* for the very young or elderly, influenza when an epidemic is expected, and yellow fever for travellers to endemic areas.

■ Other vaccine strategies

Vaccine development is currently at a very interesting stage thanks to several promising new molecular biological techniques (see Table 28.3). First in the field was the production of protein antigens by *recombinant DNA* methods; the present hepatitis B vaccine, made by cloning the gene for the surface antigen in yeast, has replaced the original vaccine derived from the blood of carriers of the disease. Alternatively, small *peptides* can be produced synthetically, as has been shown in animals with a foot-and-mouth disease capsid protein, although here, as mentioned above, host genotypic variation may become an important factor. An advantage of this method is that epitopes aimed at B and T cells can be coupled together in appropriate proportions; for example, four epitopes for each cell type.

An alternative approach is to insert the desired gene into a living virus or bacterium (suitably attenuated) which, administered as a vaccine, will express and induce immunity to the inserted protein: so-called *vaccine vectors*. Modified Vaccinia Ankara (MVA), a further attenuated version of the smallpox vaccine, is the most common vector used, along with other pox viruses such as fowlpox or canarypox and even yellow fever vaccine. Human adenoviruses are also used but may be less immunogenic in the tropics where the majority of people already have pre-existing immune responses to this vector, prompting the search for adenovirus strains which are less common in the environment, and even the use of monkey adenoviruses such as those from chimpanzees. Some bacteria (*Salmonella*, BCG),

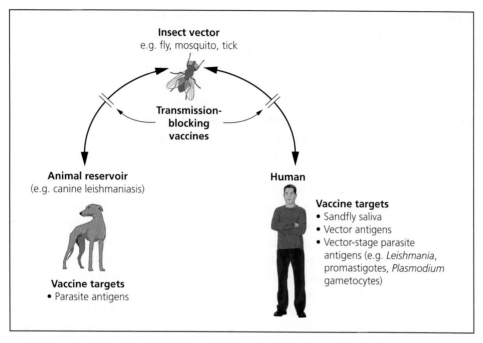

Fig. 28.3 Strategies for transmission-blocking vaccination for vector-borne diseases.

have also been proposed as vaccine vectors. Finally, it is possible to simply inject the gene for the vaccine antigen itself—the *DNA vaccine*—coupled to a suitable promoter, intramuscularly; surprisingly, muscle cells will express the corresponding protein and induce immunity. Unfortunately, DNA vaccines on their own have been somewhat disappointing, but combinations of DNA vaccination, protein in adjuvant or live vectors—the 'heterologous prime-boost' strategy—are increasingly used and are a good way to induce cytotoxic (CD8) T-cell immunity, which is important in the case of HIV, TB, etc. The recent advances in genomics (see Chapter 9) have greatly facilitated the search for genes and/or proteins with selected suitable qualities for vaccine candidates. This so-called 'reverse vaccinology' allows the rapid *in silico* reduction of thousands of potential antigens to a more manageable number (usually less than one hundred) which can then be tested for efficacy in preclinical models.

Another novel approach, for use with vector-borne diseases, is the 'transmission-blocking vaccine' (see Fig. 28.3).

■ Immunological correlates of protection

Virtually all the vaccines in routine use mediate protection by inducing antibodies which either neutralize toxins and viruses or opsonize bacteria for uptake and killing by neutrophils and macrophages. Of course, apart from the pure polysaccharide vaccines, which are T-cell independent, these also induce specific CD4 helper

T cells to achieve this high-affinity antibody response. For these vaccines, the antibodies produced are a correlate of protection broadly defined as a biological response that accurately predicts protection by the vaccine (you will also come across related terms such as *biomarkers* and *surrogates of protection*). Relatively simple assays which measure the quantity, quality (e.g. avidity, IgM versus IgG), and function of the antibody response are used to determine whether an individual has responded to a vaccine (i.e. seroconverted) and is predicted to be resistant to infection (sero-protected). These assays include ELISA, virus neutralization and opsonophagocytosis/killing assays, the latter used in assessment of vaccines against encapsulated bacteria.

However there is an urgent need in other diseases, such as malaria, tuberculosis, and HIV, for vaccines which act more directly via the induction of CD4 and CD8 T cells. Here, vaccine developers measure the amount of T-cell proliferation or cytokine production (most commonly IFNγ) from peripheral blood cells of a vaccinated person following re-stimulation with vaccine antigens *in vitro*. These assays are expensive and technically more difficult than measuring antibodies, particularly when applied to large-scale clinical trials, although simply using diluted whole blood rather than purified mononuclear cells (PBMC) has made such studies much easier. New techniques now allow measurement of multiple rather than single T cell functions: for example using flow cytometry to count the frequency of T cells that produce different combinations of three or more key cytokines (so-called polyfunctional T cells producing IFNγ/IL-2/TNF) and the use of bead array methods to measure the concentration of 20 or more different cytokines and chemokines in each sample. This 'measure everything' approach is taken to its extreme in the exciting use of whole genome transcriptional microarrays to measure vaccine responses, where a single drop of blood can give a 'signature' of expression of some 46 000 mRNA transcripts in each sample.

■ Development and testing

Development of a new vaccine proceeds along fairly standard lines. Candidate preparations are first tested in suitable small animals if available (generally mice), often followed by a trial in a non-human primate model, looking for a significant degree of protection, a lack of side effects, and if possible identifying a candidate biomarker or correlate of protection that can be used to follow responses in human populations since it is usually not ethical to deliberately infect them. Rarely this is actually done, with infection of volunteers with fully drug-susceptible isolates of *P. falciparum*, *V. cholerae*, or *Shigella spp.* allowing a rapid insight into whether a candidate vaccine might be protective in humans. Finally, the vaccine is tested in a series of clinical trials of increasing size and stringency, firstly in the country of origin (such as USA or Europe), and then where the disease is endemic, as shown in Table 28.4. Whether a vaccine will be considered successful will ultimately depend on the balance between reduction in mortality and/or morbidity on the one hand,

Table 28.4 Stages in the testing of a candidate vaccine

Animal	Aim	Comments
Mouse	Experimental model	Defined genetics and immune response; mutant strains available, but diseases may not always resemble the human equivalent
Rabbit, guinea-pig, hamster, etc.	Intermediate model	May be better mimic of human pathology (e.g. guinea-pig TB), but immunity less well characterized than for mouse
Non-human primates	Human surrogate	Closest to human for immunity, toxicity, but expensive and difficult to handle; also not genetically defined
Human		
Phase I	Safety, side effects, dose range	Small numbers of patients (e.g. 10)
Phase II	Safety, efficacy	Intermediate numbers (10–100), randomized, placebo-controlled double-blind trial where possible
Phase III	Large scale, comparison with standard therapy	Multi-centre (100–1000 patients)
IF SUCCESSFUL THEN LICENSED FOR WIDESPREAD USE		
Phase IV	Long-term efficacy, cost, safety in specific patient groups	Analysis of multiple trials following general public release

and cost, safety, and the global importance of the disease on the other. A cheap but only partially protective vaccine against malaria or HIV would probably be pursued, while an expensive and wholly protective one against Lassa fever might not. It is estimated that the cost of developing, testing, and delivering a new vaccine today is in the region of US$500 million, requiring some 10 years of development.

■ Passive ('immediate') immunization

As most people who have lived in the tropics know, the acute treatment for a snake bite is to inject antivenom, which is simply *antibody* made in advance against the relevant toxin in a horse or goat. The same principle is used for some acute infections, particularly those due to exotoxin-secreting bacteria. There are also a few other indications, the most interesting being in the case of rabies, where a combination of passive antibody and active immunization is used; the antibody to mop up virus before it gets into the nerves, the vaccine to induce a host anti-body response during the slow passage to the brain, which can take about 6 weeks. The 'last-minute' tourist injection of anti-hepatitis A antibody and the

Table 28.5 Some clinical applications of passive antibody

Disease	Species	Use
RSV	Human/mouse (mAb)	Prophylaxis; high risk infants
Cytomegalovirus	Human	Prophylaxis; e.g. kidney transplant recipients
Diphtheria	Horse	Treatment
Hepatitis A/B	Human (pooled)	Prophylaxis, post-exposure prophylaxis
Primary IgG immune deficiency	Human (pooled)	Prophylaxis/treatment
Rabies	Human	Post exposure prophylaxis
Tetanus	Human	Prophylaxis in tetanus prone wounds, treatment
Varicella	Human	Post exposure prophylaxis in high risk individuals

monthly injections of pooled normal human immunoglobulin for agammaglob-ulinaemia (see Chapter 25) also come into this category (see Table 28.5 for a more complete list of uses). Passive immunization is usually carried out using *polyclonal* antisera from either immunized animals or convalescent humans, which have the advantage of multiple specificity and isotype but the disadvantage of low activity and short supply. *Monoclonal antibodies* (also called mAbs) can be made available in unlimited amounts but their specificity for a single antigenic determinant means that in practice mixtures of several monoclonal antibodies would be needed. At present the only monoclonal antibody in clinical use for an infection is against respiratory syncytial virus. A monoclonal antibody derived from the cells of patients recovered from H5N1 influenza ('bird flu') has given promise in animals.

The frightening recent threat of bio-terrorism may prove to be the most valuable application of passive immunotherapy, and it has been suggested that pools of monoclonal antibodies against the toxins of anthrax, botulism, etc., and viruses such as smallpox and Ebola, should be stockpiled to treat susceptible individuals once a biological weapon has been identified.

■ Non-specific immunostimulation

Here the idea is to boost the general activity of the immune system, or some part of it, without reference to any particular antigen. Some ways of doing this make excellent immunological sense; the administration of cytokines, for example.

Several of these are beginning to be used clinically; IFNα is the leader because of its proven value in certain chronic viral infections (and also some tumours). IL-2 and IFNγ have also been the subject of clinical trials, mostly for chronic intracellular infections such as leprosy and leishmaniasis, but with little success so far. An alternative to cytokines is the use of TLR agonists such as CpG DNA (TLR9) and Imiquimod (TRL7). Fragments derived from antimicrobial peptides, usually expressed in epithelial cells and phagocytes (such as defensin, indolicidin, and magainin), are also in advanced clinical trials to prevent or treat bacterial infections, through a combination of their direct antimicrobial as well as immunostimulatory properties. At the opposite extreme are some remedies that seem to belong more to 'fringe' medicine, although of course this does not mean they do not work; examples are ginseng and the Chinese herbal mixtures that cause remissions in otherwise untreatable eczema. Western scientists are finally showing interest in the immunological basis of these effects. In all cases, it is important to make sure that general immune-stimulation does not induce excessive inflammation and pathology, particularly when used for treatment rather than prevention.

■ Therapeutic vaccines

So far, we have concentrated on discussion of prophylactic vaccines, given to healthy people before they are exposed to a pathogen. But another approach, that of therapeutic vaccination, aims to stimulate the immune system of an already infected individual, in order to speed their recovery or eliminate an otherwise chronic infection. There is a huge demand for such an approach—over 20 million people already infected with HIV, over 350 million with hepatitis viruses, and one-quarter and one-third of the global population are believed to harbour worms or *M. tuberculosis* respectively. Unfortunately there are no truly therapeutic licenced vaccines, apart of course from the 'passive' examples of rabies and snake-bite given above. Vaccines which work well when given prior to infection, such as the HPV vaccine, invariably fail to work in chronically infected individuals, possibly because the host immune response is impaired, and/or the organism is expressing different antigens in the chronic phase of disease. Experimental approaches to tackle these problems include temporarily blocking suppressive host molecules such as IL-10 at the time of vaccination and incorporating latency/chronic stage antigens into the new vaccine. However caution is needed as there is a potential risk of causing an overwhelming immune response leading to immune pathology.

■ Future prospects

After many years of relying on the same small set of vaccines, we are now at an exciting time in vaccine development and implementation. To consider just the five main killers we discuss in detail in this book: 1) the latest generation of polysaccharide-protein conjugate vaccines effective against up to 13 different strains of *S. pneumoniae* in developed countries are now being supplied to the tropics where they are expected to save the lives of some 7 million children by 2030; 2) two new vaccines against rotaviruses, the cause of one-third of all deaths due to diarrhoea, have been proved to reduce hospitalization by 40–94% in middle income countries and are now being tested in low-income areas; 3) there are now 12 new vaccine candidates against tuberculosis in various stages of clinical trials, the first since the introduction of BCG in the 1920s; 4) RTS,S, the leading candidate against cerebral malaria offers some 50% protection and is in the closing stages of a large Phase III trial in 15 000 children in seven different African countries; 5) unfortunately, compared to these advances, the HIV vaccine field still lags behind; a small measure of protection was seen in the latest trial of a combined viral vector plus protein in adjuvant vaccine but there is still a long way to go before any real success can be claimed (Table 27.2).

SUMMARY

- Vaccination aims to induce specific protection against a disease without inducing the disease itself. It depends on the memory function of the lymphocytes of the adaptive immune system.

- Vaccines may consist of living attenuated pathogens, killed pathogens, or chemically defined portions of pathogens, usually proteins or polysaccharides. In general, living vaccines are more effective but less safe. Vaccine production and safety testing are very time consuming and expensive.

- About 10 vaccines are in common and widespread use, whereas others are reserved for special groups and others are still experimental. There remain many major diseases for which no vaccine is available.

- Sub-unit vaccines usually require an adjuvant to boost their effectiveness.

- In cases where infection has already occurred or immunity is deficient, passive immunization, for example with antibody, can be effective.

Chapter 29

Control of infectious disease: chemotherapy

The idea of using chemicals safely to attack microbes goes back to the discovery by Paul Ehrlich (c.1900) that, because of differences in the metabolism of pathogens (mainly protozoa) and humans, certain compounds could damage one but not the other. Ehrlich baptized this 'selective toxicity'. Chemical substances are used at four levels to kill pathogens:

1. *disinfectants*, which kill microbes but may also damage human tissues, for example hypochlorite (bleach);
2. *antiseptics*, which kill microbes but are safe in contact with human tissues, for example iodine in alcohol;
3. *chemotherapy*, a general term for the treatment of infection with any kind of chemical or antibiotic given systemically;
4. *antibiotics*, substances produced by a microorganism that damage another microorganism, for example penicillin; however, the term is generally applied to synthetic substances too, for example sulphonamides.

Chemotherapy has been extremely successful against many bacteria, because their procaryotic structure offers several targets absent from eucaryotic cells (see Fig. 3.1). Antiviral chemotherapy is on the whole less effective (see below). Fortunately the opposite is true for vaccines, which are in general more effective against viruses than bacteria (see Chapter 28). It is much more difficult to devise drugs that attack eucaryotic organisms such as fungi, protozoa, and worms without damaging host cells, and unfortunately there are no human vaccines for eucaryotes either.

■ Antibacterial agents

Antibacterial agents fall into five main categories, depending on their site of action (Table 29.1). The pioneer modern antibacterials were (1) the synthetic azo-dye sulphanilamide (1935), and (2) the true antibiotics penicillin, made by the fungus *Penicillium*, discovered by Fleming in 1929 and first used in 1940, and streptomycin (1944), made by the filamentous bacterium *Streptomyces* and used mainly for TB. Earlier metal-based drugs, such as the arsenical salvarsan used for syphilis (1910), were extremely toxic, but drugs containing arsenic or antimony are still used against some protozoa (see below). Antibiotic research and production proceeds at an ever-increasing pace; about 5000 antibiotics are known, and it is said that about 300 are discovered each year, although only about 100 are in common use. It was while screening the fungus *Tolypocladium inflatum* for antibiotic activ-

Table 29.1 Some widely used antibacterial drugs, showing their site of action

Site of action	Examples	Principal uses
Cell-wall peptidoglycan synthesis	β-Lactams: penicillins, cephalosporins	Gram-positive and -negative bacteria
	Glycopeptides: vancomycin, teicoplanin	Gram-positive bacteria
Inner cell membranes	Polymyxins	Gram-negative bacteria
Protein synthesis	Aminoglycosides: streptomycin, gentamycin	TB, Gram-negative bacteria
	Tetracycline	Broad spectrum
	Macrolides: erythromycin	Gram-positive bacteria
	Clindamycin	Gram-positive bacteria
	Fusidic acid	Gram-positive bacteria
	Chloramphenicol	Broad spectrum
Nucleic acid synthesis	Sulphonamides, trimethoprim	Gram-negative bacteria
mRNA	Rifampicin	TB
DNA	Metronidazole	Anaerobic bacteria
DNA gyrase	Quinolones: ciprofloxacin	Gram-negative and atypical bacteria
Unknown (mycolic acid synthesis?)	Isoniazid	TB
	Ethambutol	TB
	Dapsone	Leprosy

The term 'broad spectrum' usually implies activity against Gram-positive and Gram-negative bacteria, and often *Chlamydia*, *Rickettsia*, etc. as well.

ity that the dramatically immunosuppressive drug cyclosporin was discovered in 1976. It is hoped that better knowledge of the genomes of bacteria (and other pathogens) will lead to the discovery of new drug targets. Meanwhile some novel possibilities are being explored; these include the use of small peptides, iron chelators, and bacteriophages. The latter, which are viruses that infect and sometimes kill bacteria (see also Fig 3.3), were in fact first used as long ago as 1918, and have remained popular in Eastern Europe ever since; they are now attracting attention in Western countries too. It is noteworthy that while bacteria and fungi have been fairly thoroughly exploited as sources of antibiotics, other sources such as insects, fish, and plants have only recently begun to be investigated scientifically—with the signal exception of the plant products quinine and artemisone, currently the leading antimalarial drugs (see below).

■ Antibiotic resistance

Considering the ability of microorganisms to elude the immune system by mutation (see Chapter 22) one might expect that they could also develop resistance to chemotherapy. Nevertheless, most people were surprised at how fast this can occur after a new drug is introduced. Gonococci became resistant to sulphonamides within 10 years, and the same happened even faster with staphylococci and penicillin. The explanation is that mutations in the genes for resistance occur spontaneously, and are selected for if they confer an advantage: in other words the bacteria *adapted* to antibiotics in just the same way as the B and T lymphocytes adapt to foreign antigens. Indeed it was while contemplating the development of antibiotic resistance that Jerne, Lederberg, and Burnet worked their way towards the clonal selection theory (see Fig.16.5).

The mechanism is not always the same, however; antibiotic resistance can develop at several levels, ranging from single point mutations to the transfer of whole sets of genes on plasmids or transposons (Table 29.2). As an example, resistance to anti-tuberculous drugs is mainly due to mutation, so it can occur in an individual at any time; the use of three or four different drugs together is an attempt to avoid the risk of multiple resistance emerging. On the other hand resistance of *Staph. aureus* to penicillin involves plasmid transfer, and can only be acquired from another individual, which is why it is so common in hospitals. The molecular basis for this resistance, a fascinating battle between microbe and drug for possession of essential components of cell wall synthesis, is illustrated in Fig. 29.1. Recently resistance has been shown to be able to spread between unrelated bacteria, for example vancomycin resistance from enterococci to staphylococci. Resistance to antibiotics is chiefly driven by their use, or overuse, so it gets worse, and never better, with time. It is estimated that in Europe alone it is responsible for some 25 000 deaths, and a cost of 1.5 billion euros, per year. It is probably safest to assume that most bacteria will develop resistance to most antibiotics in due course.

Table 29.2 Resistance to antibiotics can be achieved in several ways

Genetic basis	Mode of action	Resistance against
Chromosomal (mutation)	Alteration of target of antibiotic, e.g. ribosome	Streptomycin
	Surface permeability	Penicillin
	RNA polymerase	Rifampicin
	Membranes	Polymyxin
Plasmid (R factor)	Induction of enzymes that inactivate antibiotic	Tetracycline*, chloramphenicol*, streptomycin*, sulphonamides*, trimethoprim
	β-Lactamases	Penicillin
	Glycopeptide-binding block	Vancomycin
	Alteration of RNA target	Erythromycin[†], clindamycin[†], lincomycin[†]
	Alteration of target enzyme	Sulphonamides, trimethoprim
Transposons ('jumping genes')	As above, may act in chromosome or plasmid	Tetracycline
Integrons ('resistance cassettes')		

The location of several resistance genes on plasmids or transposons allows the very rapid spread of resistance throughout populations of bacteria.

*,[†]Resistance to these groups of antibiotics is often carried on the same plasmid. Note that antibiotic resistance genes are widely used by molecular biologists to enable a desired population of mutant bacteria to be selected in the laboratory.

Testing for resistance/susceptibility

The standard susceptibility test consists of growing the bacteria on agar with small paper discs containing various antibiotics, or various concentrations of one antibiotic. Inhibition of bacterial growth indicates susceptibility and is easily seen as a clear area in the bacterial 'lawn' around the disc. For measuring the concentration of an antibiotic in patients' serum, immunoassay is the preferred method.

Biofilms and resistance

A biofilm is a bacterial community growing on a surface and enclosed in a polysaccharide matrix and this, rather than floating free in a laboratory test tube, is how pathogenic bacteria grow in 'real life'. Mucous membranes, teeth, and surgically implanted materials are major sites, and it has been found that bacteria in a biofilm can be up to 1000 times more resistant to antibiotics than those growing free. This is partly due to the matrix itself, but also to the fact that in large colonies bacteria do not replicate so fast (and so are less affected by chemotherapy), and to

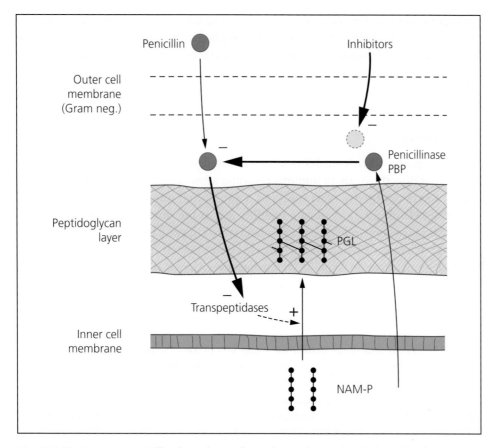

Fig. 29.1 Resistance to penicillin depends mainly on the production by the bacteria of enzymes that destroy the penicillin ring. Transpeptidases which join these together, are destroyed by penicillin. Peptidoglycan (PGL) constitutes the major cell-wall-strengthening material. Many bacterial penicillinase enzymes exist, some being more active against penicillins and others more active against cephalosporins; as a group they are referred to as β-lactamases, and there are also other penicillin-binding proteins (PBPs). One possible counter-attack is to use competitive inhibitors of the bacterial enzymes, such as clavulanic acid. NAM-P, *N*-acetyl muramic acid–peptide units.

other less well-understood changes. There is some evidence that innate immune mechanisms (e.g. iron depletion by lactoferrin from polymorphs) can inhibit biofilm formation.

Bacterial interference: the normal flora

Another aspect of 'real-life' bacterial infection is the existence of enormous numbers of non-pathogenic bacteria, also growing as biofilms, notably in the gut, which may contain up to 10^{14} organisms of 500 different species, mostly harmless *commensals* competing with pathogens for space and nutrients. Some may be actively beneficial, for example the lactobacilli which are thought to keep down pathogens, notably *Candida*, in the gut, vagina, mouth, etc. Over-zealous antibiotic treatment, by killing these, may allow pathogens to take over. Attempts have been made to deliberately colonize mucous surfaces with *Lactobacillus* and other 'good' or *probiotic* bacteria.

■ Toxicity

The other problem with antibiotics, as with all drugs, is toxicity. This can be due to the drug directly, or to an immune response against it. In fact, drugs are a major cause of hypersensitivity reactions, and a substantial number of these are due to antibiotics (Table 29.3). A third possibility is that the simultaneous destruction of many pathogens may release enough material to trigger pattern-recognition receptors (see Chapter 12), cytokine release, and intense inflammatory reactions. Examples can occur in syphilis, relapsing fever, Lyme disease, TB, and African

Table 29.3 Antimicrobial drugs account for a large proportion of drug toxicity, which may be direct or secondary to an immune response, usually to the drug bound to some body component, i.e. acting as a *hapten*

Mechanism	Examples	Clinical effects
Direct		
Renal damage	Aminoglycosides	Renal failure
	Amphotericin (antifungal)	Renal failure
Auditory nerve damage	Aminoglycosides	Dizziness, deafness
Bone marrow depression	Chloramphenicol	Infections, bleeding
	Zidovudine (antiviral)	Infections, bleeding
Changed gut flora	Tetracycline	Diarrhoea
Deposition in teeth	Tetracycline	Staining (children)
Hypersensitivity		
Type I (allergic)	Penicillin*,	Rashes
	Sulphonamides	Anaphylaxis*
Type II (cytotoxic)	Penicillin, sulphonamides	Haemolytic anaemia (autoimmune)
Type III (immune complexes)	Penicillin	Erythema
	Sulphonamides	Nephritis
Type IV (cell-mediated)	Penicillin, sulphonamides, streptomycin	Contact dermatitis

*Hypersensitivity to penicillin is the commonest cause of anaphylaxis, except perhaps among bee-keepers!

trypanosomiasis. A somewhat similar case is the sudden restoration of vigorous immune responses following treatment of HIV.

Antiviral drugs

With viruses, the problem is that many of the steps in viral replication are provided by the host cell itself, and cannot be blocked without killing the cell. One solution is that adopted by the immune system: kill both virus and cell, which is what NK cells and cytotoxic cells do (see Chapters 12 and 20). However, Nature has shown with the *interferons* that specific antiviral activity is a possibility. A few drugs are now available that exploit small differences between host and viral metabolism, usually at the enzyme level (Table 29.4). In view of the dangers of bio-terrorism and of pandemics (e.g. HIV, avian flu; see Chapter 37), there is an increased demand for the stockpiling of drugs such as HAART, Tamiflu, etc. In general, however, vaccines have proved more useful against viruses than drugs have; moreover, some viruses are able to develop resistance. The most interesting recent development, made possible by precise knowledge of viral and host genomes, is the use of small selected nucleotide fragments to bind to and inhibit

Table 29.4 Antiviral compounds are not as dramatically effective as most antibacterials, but steady progress is being made

Compound	Site of action	Effective against
Naturally occurring		
Interferon (mainly α)	Viral RNA translation	Hepatitis B and C (in carriers)
	Viral protein synthesis (plus effects on T and NK cells)	Herpesviruses, common cold*
Antibody (e.g. monoclonal)	Viral surface	RSV
Synthetic		
Amantadine	Entry into cell	Influenza A
Acyclovir	DNA polymerase	Herpesviruses, e.g. HSV, VZV
Ganciclovir	DNA polymerase	Herpesviruses, especially CMV
Zidovudine (AZT)	Reverse transcriptase	Retroviruses (e.g. HIV)
Oseltamivir (Tamiflu)	Neuraminidase	Influenza A and B
Protease inhibitors	Viral proteases	HIV
Ribavarin	Nucleic acid	RSV, Lassa, Hepatitis C
Anti-sense (experimental)	RNA	CMV

*The proved effectiveness of interferon in preventing colds has not led to clinical use because of high cost and unpleasant side-effects.

specific viral mRNA (the 'anti-sense' approach) or to interfere with gene expression ('gene silencing').

Drugs against fungi, protozoa, and worms

Most of the effective drugs against these eucaryotic infections display considerable toxicity (side effects) to their (eucaryotic) animal host, and they have to be used with caution. Tables 29.5–29.7 list the generally available ones. The story of malaria illustrates some of the problems. The effect of *quinine*, a plant derivative, has been known for over three centuries, and it is still a drug of choice for acute life-threatening malaria, despite its side effects (which include hypoglycaemia, hypotension, cardiac arrhythmias, and disturbances of hearing and vision). *Choloroquine*, a more practical drug for preventive use requiring less frequent dosage, was introduced in the 1940s, but between 1960 and 1990 chloroquine resistance emerged and spread round the world, and although new antimalarials are regularly produced, the parasites usually appear to be able to keep one step ahead. Recently, however, derivatives of a traditional Chinese herb, *artemisia*, have become standard. It is curious that few plant products other than the two major antimalarials are medically established for the treatment of infection. Another success story is the discovery of two important new antihelminthics

Table 29.5 Some drugs in use against fungi

Drug	Active against	Side effects
Cell-wall inhibitors		
Caspofungin	*Candida, Aspergillus*	Rare
Ergosterol inhibitors (damage cell membrane)		
Terbinafine	Dermatophytes	Nausea, rash
Fluconazole	Yeasts	Nausea, liver damage
Itraconazole	Yeasts, *Aspergillus*	Hepatitis
Voriconazole	Yeasts, moulds, *Aspergillus*	Visual
Ketoconazole*	Dermatophytes, *Candida*	Nausea, hepatitis
Amphotericin B*	Most moulds and yeasts	Renal toxicity
Nystatin	*Candida* (superficial)	Skin staining
Inhibitors of mitosis		
Griseofulvin	Dermatophytes	Nausea, visual
Inhibitors of protein synthesis		
Flucytosine	*Candida, Cryptococcus*	Neutropenia, jaundice

*Those asterisked are the most effective against severe systemic infection.

Table 29.6 Some drugs used against protozoal infections

Disease	Drug/regime	Comments
Malaria		
Liver stage	Primaquine/oral	
Blood stage	Chloroquine/oral	Resistance common
	Artemisinin derivatives	Resistance rare
Acute, cerebral	Quinine IM/IV	Severe toxicity
Leishmaniasis	Antimonials, pentamidine, amphotericin B	Severe toxicity
Sleeping sickness	Suramin, pentamidine	Severe toxicity
	Melarsoprol	Severe toxicity (CNS)
Chagas' disease	Nifurtimox, benznidazole	Severe toxicity
Toxoplasmosis	Pentamidine, pyrimethamine	Severe toxicity
Amoebiasis		
Intestinal	Diloxanide	Good safety
Systemic, abscess	Metronidazole	Good safety
Giardiasis	Metronidazole, tinidazole	
Cryptosporidiosis	Spiramycin, pyrimethamine, nitazoxanide	
Trichomoniasis	Metronidazole, tinidazole	

IM, administered intramuscularly; IV, administered intravenously.

(antiworm drugs), *praziquantel* and *ivermectin*, which exploit differences in neuromuscular action between worm and host. Since these drugs are relatively cheap, there are global programmes which aim to provide long-term treatment of at least 75% of all school-aged children at risk of schistosomiasis and soil transmitted helminth infection (i.e. roundworm, hookworm, and whipworms) once or twice a year. This will have a major impact on the malnutrition, anaemia, retarded growth and development, and poor performance and attendance at school, that occurs in chronic worm infections. A similar programme, using combinations of diethylcarbamazine, albendazole, and ivermectin is also targeted at eliminating lymphatic filariasis.

■ Chemotherapy and the immune system

The role of immunity in drug toxicity has already been mentioned. Many antimicrobial agents kill their target directly, but others appear to need some degree of

Table 29.7 Some drugs used against helminth infections

Disease	Drug
Flukes	
Schistosomiasis	Praziquantel, oxamniquine
Fascioliasis	Triclabendazole
Roundworms	
Filariasis	Ivermectin*, diethylcarbamazine*, albendazole*
Intestinal	Mebendazole, albendazole, levamisole
Trichinosis	Mebendazole, thiabendazole
Tapeworms	
Taenia	Praziquantel, niclosamide
Hydatid	Albendazole

*Often used in combination.

help from the immune system. As a result immunocompromised patients may need lifelong treatment for infections that would require only a short course of treatment in normal individuals. For example, pentostam (antimony sodium gluconate) is not effective against leishmaniasis in the absence of a T-cell response. The powerful immunosuppressive effect of the otherwise promising antibiotic cyclosporin has already been mentioned. Some drugs accumulate in macrophages, making them more effective against intracellular pathogens. The same effect may be achieved by encapsulating them in lipid vesicles, an example being liposomal amphotericin B. Finally, some antibiotics are themselves immunostimulatory.

SUMMARY

- Drug treatment (chemotherapy) is used against all classes of pathogen, but is most successful against bacteria.

- Antibacterial agents may be natural products of bacteria or fungi (e.g penicillin), or synthetic molecules (e.g. sulphonamides).

- Bacteria commonly develop resistance against antibacterials, by mutation or plasmid exchange. Resistance is encouraged by inadequate treatment, and can often be overcome by using drugs in combination.

- There are a few effective antiviral drugs, including (natural) interferon.

- Antimicrobial drugs, particularly those effective against fungi, protozoa, and worms, are commonly quite toxic to the patient.

Chapter 30

Control of infectious disease: public health measures

According to Dr Samuel Johnson, 'Decent provision for the poor, is the true test of civilization'. One might update this to say that a concern for the health of others could be considered as one of the hallmarks of a civilized society. Nowhere is this truer than in the field of infectious disease.

■ Science, politics, and ethics

For centuries before the invention of vaccines or antibiotics, societies have explored ways of limiting infectious disease. In the previous two chapters we described how TB can now, in some parts of the world (but sadly not in the tropics), be largely controlled both by vaccination and by chemotherapy, yet a careful study of the disease in England and Wales shows the surprising fact that the incidence, particularly in younger people, had already fallen by about a third between 1850 and 1900, before either vaccine or drug treatment had started. This improvement was due to the general improvement in health that accompanied better nutrition and food handling, better housing and housing regulations, stronger legislation, and a more enlightened attitude to social problems, which continued throughout the 20th century, helped in the case of *M. bovis* by Pasteur's milk-heating technique (Fig. 30.1). The elimination of cholera in Europe and the USA, and its reduction elsewhere, owed far more to proper separation of sewage and drinking water than to the not-very-effective vaccine.

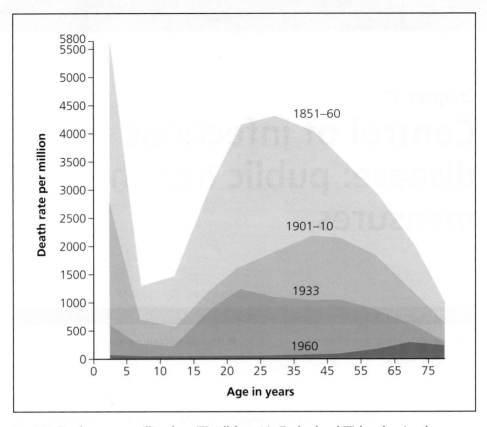

Fig. 30.1 Death rates per million from TB (all forms) in England and Wales, showing the changing pattern of infection. Note that chemotherapy was not introduced until 1944, whereas the BCG vaccine, though produced in the 1920s, was not used widely until the 1950s, yet the disease had already declined by about 80%, particularly in the younger age group.

Some other success stories that have nothing to do with vaccines or drugs are listed in Table 30.1. For example, the global campaign to eradicate Guinea worm is on the verge of success: by providing access to clean water, the incidence of this debilitating condition (caused by the *Dracunculus* parasite) has been reduced by 99% with 192 countries now certified free of disease and only some 1000 cases still reported in 2011, mostly in South Sudan. It can be seen that most of these would have made little sense in the days before the *germ theory* of Koch and Pasteur (*c.*1880) highlighted the crucial role of infectious microbes in transmitting disease.

From then on, it was clear that control of infectious disease was a matter of both scientific understanding and political will. Some of the necessary measures imply prolonged or continuous efforts and a certain restriction of normal human activity, with a tendency to relax these as they are seen to take effect and disease begins to retreat. Often a degree of self-sacrifice is required; for instance not everybody with a cold or influenza is prepared to stay at home or wear a mask, although this would clearly benefit others. The famous Typhoid Mary, a New York cook who

Table 30.1 Some examples of attempted disease control through public health measures

Disease/organism	How controlled
Leprosy (Middle Ages)	Quarantine of cases (in lazarettos)
Leprosy (Middle Ages)	Isolation of cases (in leprosaria)
Cholera (London, 1855)	Identification of contaminated water source
Typhoid	Water purification, quarantine of cases
Legionella	Maintenance of air-conditioning cooling systems
Hospital staphylococci	Screening of possible carriers (nurses, etc.)
HIV, hepatitis B, malaria	Screening of blood donors
TB (bovine)	Heating of milk (pasteurization)
Brucellosis	Heating of milk (pasteurization)
Sexually transmitted diseases	Advice, condoms
Malaria (Rome, 1935)	Draining of marshes where mosquito vector breeds
Malaria (tropical)	Killing of mosquitoes by DDT, etc.
Malaria (tropical)	Insecticide-impregnated mosquito nets
Malaria (non-tropical)	Fumigation of aircraft
Plague, typhus	Control of rat reservoir/insect vector
Rabies	Killing of rabid dogs
Hydatid disease	Reduced contact with dog reservoir
Schistosomiasis (China)	Draining of ditches where snail vector breeds
Schistosomiasis (Africa, S. America)	Education about danger of barefoot paddling
Onchocerciasis	Spraying insecticide on rivers to kill fly vector
Guinea worm	Access to clean water

was a typhoid carrier, repeatedly refused to abandon cooking, even in the face of a prison sentence. Nurses with virulent staphylococci in their noses are taken off duty and treated. Especially vigorous control measures are needed in hospitals since (1) conditions are unusually crowded, with hundreds of person–person contacts per day, (2) patients frequently bring infection in with them, (3) antibiotic-resistant and opportunist infections are more common in hospitals than in the community as a whole, and (4) many patients will be relatively immunodeficient because of their disease or surgery. Also to be considered, of course, is the psycho-logical effect of catching a serious disease while in a place supposedly dedicated to improving health.

By contrast vaccines and antibiotics, apart from occasional side effects, nor-mally benefit the individual without any inconvenience, although here, too, there are ethical issues; for example whether patients with drug-resistant infections should be isolated and/or obliged to take appropriate antibiotics, a problem high-lighted by the appearance of multiple or extensive drug-resistant TB. There is also the question whether vaccination should be compulsory, which has come to the fore most recently in connection with the measles vaccine. Even in the most politi-cally and scientifically sophisticated societies there is not always agreement on such issues.

Note that even when a vaccine or a drug has been developed and introduced, public health organizations are still an important element in disease control. The numbers treated, the numbers who seroconvert, and the numbers who develop disease will all have to be accurately monitored and the results studied by epide-miologists experienced in handling such data. Moreover, if the treatment fails and is abandoned, it is vital for the alternative means of disease control to continue being enforced. The somewhat relaxed International Health Regulations intro-duced in 1951 and revised in 1969 were tightened up again in 2005 (IHR2005), with a view to a prompt response to a threatening outbreak anywhere in the world. Under this new scheme global resources were mobilized to deal with a yel-low fever outbreak (Paraguay 2008) and the H1N1 flu pandemic originating in Mexico (2009).

■ Vector control

The importance of insects in the transmission of infectious diseases, including some of the most serious, is emphasized in Chapters 7 (*ectoparasites*) and 11 (*entry and exit*). In fact about half of the public health measures listed in Table 30.1 are directed at insect or larger animal vectors.

Some idea of the challenges involved can be judged by considering *malaria* (see Chapter 27). Here, despite half a century of research, vaccination has yet to make an impact and chemotherapy, though effective, is continually being thwarted by the development of parasite drug resistance. The spotlight has therefore turned once again on mosquito control—which would have the added advantage of reducing some important virus diseases such as dengue, yellow fever, Chikungunya, West Nile virus. Originally it was hoped that insecticides such as DDT, sprayed on larval breeding sites, would virtually eliminate mosquitoes, and this has indeed been achieved in specific limited areas since as long ago as 1900. However mos-quitoes can develop resistance, and in any case damage to wildlife and possible human toxicity has led to DDT being banned in most countries since the 1970's. So a number of newer strategies are being considered that seemed quite far-fetched when they were first proposed. For example mosquitoes have been (1) irradiated so that the males are sterile, (2) genetically engineered to block parasite development in their gut, (3) engineered to block sperm production, (4) transfected with the endosymbiotic bacterium *Wohlbachia* which halves their lifespan; this approach has been shown to be effective in dengue. The key question whether such genetic abnormalities would spread through the mosquito population sufficiently to have a real effect 'in the wild' has been the subject of sophisticated mathematical modelling.

Another example that highlights the public health approach is the helminth disease *schistosomiasis* (see Chapter 6). Here the vector is a freshwater snail and in addition to an effective drug—praziquantel—control methods are aimed at preventing skin contact with water containing the infective cercariae. These include (1) various molluscicides, (2) plants and fish with supposed anti-snail activity, (3) avoidance of large dam construction with the consequent standing lake formation and, most important of all, (4) education and prominent public advertising about the risk of catching what should theoretically be a preventable disease.

■ Animals without pathogens?

Continuous advances in vaccine and antibiotic technology, combined with ever more draconian public health control of food, water, vectors, etc., might tempt the unwary to dream of a world without pathogens. This seems an extremely unlikely prospect. In the first place, *bacteria* appear in general to be beneficial to higher animals; no less a scientist than Pasteur stated that 'microbes are essential for normal life'. He was certainly right in the sense that animals deprived of their normal flora—particularly that of the intestine—or born and raised in the total absence of any form of microbe, show reductions in weight, metabolic rate, cardiac output, immune development, etc. Such 'germ-free' or *gnotobiotic* animals can be kept alive and reasonably healthy, provided they do not become exposed to pathogens, which in practice means very careful and expensive housing and feeding. Indeed, such animals, mainly mice, have been of great value in understanding infection, nutrition, cancer, ageing, and many other areas where host and pathogen normally both make a contribution. However, it is impossible to imagine a way in which the germ-free state could come about or persist naturally, given the limitless reservoir of freeliving bacteria, any of which could theoretically become adapted to a parasitic existence and some of which, being newcomers to the human ecosystem, would probably cause pathology.

In fact, it is much easier to imagine a world of microbes without higher animals, which after all existed for billions of years and could again, if the worst predictions of nuclear Armageddon were ever to come about, because there are bacteria that can survive at extraordinary ranges of temperature (from −12 to 120 °C), oxygen concentration (including none), radiation (1–2 megarads, the fatal dose for humans being well under 1 kilorad), water and salt concentration, etc. The evolution of higher animals would then, presumably, have to start all over again, a depressing but intriguing thought.

SUMMARY

- Public health measures are in many cases at least as important as drugs or vaccines in controlling disease and its spread, and in some cases they are the only prospect of control.

- However, they depend to an even greater degree on political stability and social compliance.

- With vector-borne diseases, control or elimination of the vector may sometimes be the most practical approach. The prospect of eliminating a pathogen altogether, as occurred with smallpox, is restricted to a small number of viruses.

Chapter 31

Viral and prion disease and immunity

The general features of viruses and prions are discussed in Chapters 2 and 8, and Chapters 10–26 describe the immune mechanisms that combat them. These are summarized in Fig 31.1. During their intracellular phase, viruses are generally dealt with most efficiently by interferon, NK cells, and cytotoxic T cells, whereas, when spreading from cell to cell, they become susceptible to antibody. Most viruses have well-developed *escape mechanisms*, they frequently cause *immunopathology*, and some are *opportunists*. Fortunately, there are some excellent antiviral *vaccines*. In this chapter we will survey the individual features of the principal virus infections, considered from a clinical, pathological, and immunological viewpoint.

■ The common childhood viruses

Measles, rubella, and chickenpox are similar in being spread by the respiratory route and infecting a high proportion of contacts, measles especially, with prominent skin

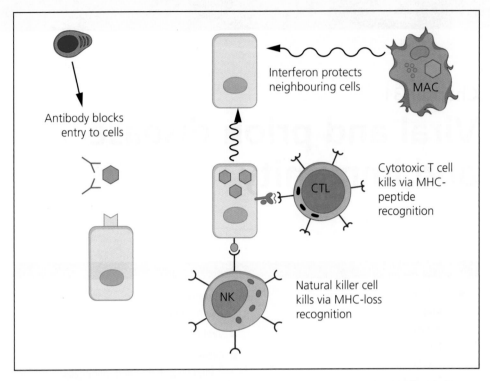

Fig. 31.1 Antiviral immunity; an overview. Antibody, interferon, CTLs, and NK cells are the main antiviral defences.

lesions. Since there is only one antigenic type of each, the immunity following recovery is virtually lifelong. Attenuated vaccines against measles, mumps, and rubella (the MMR vaccine) are highly effective, although the 1998 'scare' about a link with autism, which was never confirmed, led to a decreased uptake, and some resurgence of measles has already occurred, which is unfortunate because it is among the diseases being considered as a possible candidate for complete eradication.

Measles

In healthy children, measles is self-limiting, with ear and conjunctival infection the major complication. However in the poorly nourished, for example in the tropics, it can lead in addition to pneumonia, which is frequently fatal. The virus can infect T cells and dendritic cells, and causes a transient immunosuppression, with increased susceptibility to, for example, TB.

Rubella

Rubella, otherwise a fairly mild disease, is particularly important because of its effect on the growing fetus during the first 3 months of pregnancy: blindness, deafness, heart defects, and mental retardation occur in up to a quarter of cases (other viruses that can cause congenital malformation are CMV and chickenpox).

Mumps

Mumps virus is unique in localizing to the parotid and other glands, and to the testis. It is thus a major cause of parotitis, and occasionally of autoimmune orchitis.

Chickenpox

The herpesvirus HHV3 (VZV) gives lifelong immunity to the primary disease chickenpox (varicella) but can persist in nerve cells and reappear many years later in the form of localized shingles (zoster), with painful vesicular skin lesions on the trunk from which susceptible children can catch chickenpox. There is an effective vaccine but its use is not routine in all countries. It is too soon to know whether it prevents the later development of zoster, but an anti-zoster vaccine for the elderly has been shown to give about 50% reduction in incidence and/or severity. Note that despite its name, chickenpox is quite unrelated to the pox viruses such as *smallpox*, now eradicated.

Skin rashes

Whereas the vesicular rash of chickenpox is due to the destruction of cells by the virus, the rashes of measles and rubella appear to be immunopathological and probably T-cell-mediated. This is illustrated by the fact that children with T-cell deficiency do not develop a measles rash but suffer a fatal systemic infection instead. Other viruses involving the skin include HSV (see below), Coxsackie A, and (before its elimination) smallpox.

■ The common cold

Colds can be caused by a variety of viruses, notably rhinovirus, coronavirus, Coxsackie virus, adenovirus, parainfluenza, respiratory syncytial virus, and echovirus. Since there are from two to 100 antigenic types of each, one can suffer hundreds of colds without meeting the same type twice, so that in effect there is no useful immunity following recovery and very little prospect of a vaccine. Fortunately most colds are short-lived, mainly due to the local activity of interferon and NK cells, and simple anticongestants will relieve most of the symptoms. It has been shown that intranasal IFNα will prevent most colds, if administered before the virus!

Most of these viruses, and several herpesviruses (see below) can also cause pharyngitis (sore throat), although about 30% of sore throats are bacterial.

■ Influenza

Of the three types of influenza (A, B, and C), influenza A is the most serious, because of the *antigenic variation* (see Chapter 22) that affects its haemagglutinin

(H) and neuraminidase (N) surface antigens, preventing the build-up of B- and T-cell memory. Minor variants produced by accumulated mutations (*antigenic drift*) are responsible for the fact that each year's outbreak is antigenically different, and for the major epidemics that occur every decade or so. The much larger *antigenic shifts* that occur when the human virus exchanges RNA with one from a bird (the recombination usually occurring in pigs, which are susceptible to both bird and human flu) give rise to global pandemics. Even more dangerous are the natural bird flu viruses (e.g. H5N1) that have infected humans and could, if human–human transmission became more efficient, give rise to massive pandemics like the one that followed the First World War, killing more people than the war itself. An inactivated *vaccine* is nowadays given to those in the high-risk category (the elderly, nurses, doctors, and cardiac, diabetic, and immunodeficient patients, etc.), but it has to be made afresh every year because of antigenic drift. A stable attenuated vaccine, given by the nasal route, is also available which may provide broader coverage of different strains. A 'universal' vaccine against all strains might one day be possible, given greater knowledge of the viral genome and the detailed molecular structures formed between the viral antigens and host antibodies (so called 'structural vaccinology'). The drugs amantadine and oseltamivir (Tamiflu) are effective if given early in infection.

Other respiratory viruses

Most of the viruses affecting the nose and throat can spread to the bronchi and lungs. *Respiratory syncytial virus* (RSV) is a very common cause of bronchiolitis and pneumonia in young children. A killed vaccine was tried, but upon infection caused enhanced disease with pulmonary eosinophilia (the first measles vaccine also increased pathology due to production of non-neutralizing antibodies resulting in immune-complex (Type III) hypersensitivity). However an RSV monoclonal antibody has given good results, the only one currently licensed for use against any infection.

■ Glandular fever

This unpleasant disease bristles with interesting immunology. It is caused by the herpesvirus HHV4, usually called EBV after its discoverers (Epstein and Barr, in 1964), and is also known as *infectious mononucleosis* because of the 'atypical monocytes' seen in the blood. These are in fact cytotoxic T lymphocytes directed against the EBV-infected cells, which are mainly B lymphocytes and the pharyngeal mucosa, a clear-cut example of useful CD8 T-cell immunity (see Chapter 20). Because it is easily spread by saliva and affects mainly teenagers, it is sometimes called 'kissing disease'. Recovery is the rule, but can take several weeks; very rarely the disease can be acutely fatal or become chronic. In tropical countries EBV infection is more likely to occur unnoticed in childhood, and glandular fever is rare. Instead, in conjunction with repeated malaria infection, EBV can predispose to

Burkitt's lymphoma, a B-cell tumour mainly of the jaw. In the Far East EBV is involved in nasopharyngeal carcinoma, and in AIDS patients it can give rise to B-cell tumours in the brain. Finally, EBV has also been thought by some to be responsible for a proportion of cases of the mysterious *chronic fatigue syndrome*. Progress in developing a vaccine against EBV in the half century since its discovery has been disappointingly slow, partly due to the lack of an animal model. Attention is mainly focussed on the gp350 antigen, which binds to the B cell target but several other surface antigens are under study.

Other herpesviruses

The herpes simplex viruses HSV1 and HSV2 cause cold sores and genital herpes, and like VZV they can persist in nerve cells and reappear as painful demarcated skin lesions. There is no vaccine but prolonged treatment with *acyclovir* is very effective. Cytomegalovirus (CMV or HHV5), mainly important as an opportunist, causes severe pneumonitis in AIDS patients and in those immunosuppressed for bone-marrow transplantation. HHV8 is the cause of Kaposi's sarcoma in AIDS patients.

■ Poliomyelitis

This once feared paralytic enterovirus disease is another candidate for eventual eradication, thanks to two highly effective vaccines: inactivated (IPV, Salk 1954) and attenuated (OPV, Sabin 1957), each of which has its advantages and disadvantages, IPV being safer but less effective at immunising the gut, where the virus enters, OPV being potentially capable of reversion to the virulent wild-type virus, but also of inducing 'herd' immunity in the non-vaccinated population. Both vaccines work by preventing viral replication in host cells, e.g. the brain. Preferences have varied with time, e.g. in the UK, IPV from 1956, OPV from 1962, IPV from 2004. The most recent IPV formula, targeted at only virus types 1 and 3 (type 2 is considered to have been eradicated) is giving very encouraging results in isolated parts of Africa where the vaccine was temporarily resisted on wrongly perceived issues of safety (see Box 31.1 for further details).

Other enteroviruses

Echovirus and Coxsackie virus have been mentioned as causes of colds; they can also, like polio, cause meningitis. *Hepatitis A* is discussed below. Note that the name *enterovirus* describes the site of spread (oral–faecal) and replication, rather than the site of infection. In fact most viral diarrhoea is caused by the unrelated *rotaviruses*, an important source of 'nursery' epidemics in the developed world and of childhood death in the tropics. Rotavirus is one of the rare pathogens for which a live heterologous (bovine) vaccine may prove effective.

Box 31.1 Polio: a suitable case for eradication?

The target

Following the eradication of smallpox in 1980, the World Health Organization in 1988 announced a polio vaccination campaign to eradicate the disease by 2000. Neither this target nor the modified one of 2005 could be met, but enormous progress has been made. Over 70% of children now live in polio-free countries, and annual cases (2011) are in the region of 650, a 99% reduction since 1998. Of the three serotypes, type 2 has been eradicated since 1999. The majority of cases are in Pakistan (40%) or West and Central Africa.

The vaccines

Unusually, two different vaccines are in use, each with its advantages and disadvantages. (1) Most countries have in the past relied on the live oral (Sabin; OPV) vaccine, but this is susceptible to reversion of the mutations introduced during attenuation and the resulting emergence of circulating vaccine-derived poliovirus (cVDPV), especially in areas where vaccine coverage is inadequate. Outbreaks with human–human transmission, sometimes leading to paralysis, have occurred in several countries—at an estimated rate of 1 case per 2.5 million doses. There is also the risk that symptomless vaccinees may continue shedding infective virus. (2) Some countries, particularly in Scandinavia, have always preferred the inactivated (Salk; IPV) vaccine, and others, including the UK since 2004, have switched over from OPV to IPV which, though more expensive and requiring four further booster injections, is safer.

Objections

Polio vaccines have been subjected to more negative propaganda than any other vaccine. The total refusal of all vaccines on principle by fundamentalist religious groups (e.g. the Amish) will perhaps never be overcome. More serious, because it is more widespread, is the belief that polio vaccine was deliberately contaminated by HIV. Originating among Nigerian Muslims, this 'genocide conspiracy' theory led to a major outbreak of type 1 polio in 2004, which then spread to the Middle East and as far as Indonesia. Some 1500 paralytic cases resulted, suggesting at least 100 times as many infections. A somewhat similar campaign in Uganda blamed OPV for all cases of polio there. Clearly such developments threaten the whole eradication programme, but steps have generally been taken to overcome these objections.

A change of direction?

In recent years the emphasis has shifted slightly from total eradication (which would be a major triumph but also quite hard to prove) to simply including IPV among the other vaccines routinely given to children—diphtheria, tetanus, pertussis, *Haemophilus*, measles, mumps, rubella, and hepatitis B. Even without eradication, a reduction of all these diseases would save an estimated 3 million children per year. The drawbacks would remain: *production* of enough IPV to go round (barely 50% at present) and *expense*; a course of IPV costs at least 20 times a single dose of OPV. Where these drawbacks cannot be overcome, and in endemic areas, use of OPV with an uptake rate of 100% remains the only alternative.

■ Viral hepatitis

There are at least five hepatitis viruses, giving a similar clinical pattern—fever, nausea, jaundice—but with different outcomes. *Hepatitis A*, spread mainly by the oral–faecal route, is normally a self-limiting infection. There is a good inactivated vaccine, recommended for travellers to the tropics; passively injected pooled immunoglobulin also gives effective short-term protection. *Hepatitis B* is more serious. Normally transmitted from mother to child, or via contaminated blood or needles, it is eliminated mainly by cytotoxic T cells that kill the infected liver cells (which the virus itself does not), but can persist in about 10% of patients, who become *carriers*, able to infect others. Further complications are chronic active hepatitis, cirrhosis, and liver carcinoma. Fortunately there is a highly effective vaccine, the first to be produced by recombinant DNA technology. IFNα has some effect in preventing carrier status, and there are several useful drugs. *Hepatitis C*, previously known as 'non-A non-B', is similar but is even more likely to lead to chronic active hepatitis and cirrhosis. No commercial vaccine is available, but current research is encouraging. Hepatitis D resembles and can enhance Hepatitis B, while Hepatitis E is more like Hepatitis A, but with particular severity during pregnancy.

■ Rabies

This virus is celebrated for Pasteur's extraordinarily lucky vaccine experiment (see Tutorial 4). Rabies is unusual in that the virus travels slowly along nerves, taking weeks to get from the site of infection (usually a dog bite) to the brain, where it infects and damages neurons (encephalitis). This allows time for both passive antiserum and active vaccination to give protection.

Viral encephalitis and meningitis

Other viral causes of encephalitis include herpesviruses, mumps, polio, HIV, and togaviruses such as Japanese encephalitis and West Nile virus (see below). Most of these viruses can also cause meningitis, but the disease is usually milder than the bacterial variety (see Chapter 32).

■ Other viral zoonoses

In addition to rabies, some of the most acutely fatal viral diseases are derived from animal hosts, in which they are usually much milder infections. *Lassa* fever (from African bush rats), *Hanta* virus (from American and Scandinavian rodents), and *Marburg* and *Ebola* fever (from as yet unidentified African animals) are characterized by severe haemorrhages into the skin and internal organs.

■ Yellow fever and dengue

These viral haemorrhagic viruses are spread by mosquitoes, like the encephalitis viruses mentioned above. Bleeding defects are a major feature and in dengue a particularly severe haemorrhagic shock syndrome can occur, in which non-neutralizing antibodies enhance the entry of the virus into monocytes, triggering the release of inflammatory cytokines. For this reason progress towards a vaccine has been cautious. The very effective attenuated yellow fever vaccine (17D) is remarkable in having remained stable since 1937, despite changes in the virus. There is no effective dengue vaccine yet but recent trials are encouraging.

Papilloma viruses

Ten of the more than 70 types of human papilloma viruses (HPVs) are associated with various kinds of warts (types 1 and 4), and others with cancer of the cervix and, more rarely, penis, anus, and larynx. The recently introduced (2006) vaccines for young girls are mainly effective against types 16 and 18. HPV vaccination is also recommended for young males.

Other 'cancer viruses'

The link between EBV and Burkitt's lymphoma and nasopharyngeal carcinoma is mentioned above. Hepatitis B and C are responsible for many liver carcinomas. The human T-cell lymphocytic viruses HTLV-1 and HTLV-2 cause rare cases of T-cell leukaemia (see below). Kaposi's sarcoma appears to be caused by HHV8. Vaccines against hepatitis B and human papilloma virus at present constitute the only vaccines available against cancer.

Retroviruses

HIV and the vaccine and drug prospects for its control are discussed in Chapter 26. There is currently great interest in the possibility of using the small interfering RNA (siRNA) sequences, which help to regulate gene expression, to inhibit specific HIV genes. Although promising, the effect seems at the moment to be transient and the virus appears to be able to escape it. A recent vaccine against SIV, based on vaccinia virus carrying HIV genes, has had some success in macaque monkeys.

The only other retroviruses of significance to humans are HTLV-1 and HTLV-2. HTLV-1 causes T-cell leukaemia and lymphoma, but only in about 1% of infected people. It appears to promote the growth of T cells by stimulating IL-15.

Prion diseases

The first prion disease (or transmissible spongiform encephalopathy; TSE) to be clearly shown to be infectious was *kuru*, a neurological condition seen only among the Fore people of New Guinea and transmitted by ritual eating of the brains of

Table 31.1 Human prion diseases and their transmission

Disease	Mode of transmission
Iatrogenic (iCJD)	Contamination of growth hormone, dura mater grafts, corneal grafts, surgical instruments
Familial (fCJD)	Germ-line mutation in PrP gene (more than 20 known)
Sporadic (sCJD)	Somatic mutation in PrP gene; transmission?
New-variant (vCJD)	Contaminated beef from BSE-infected cattle
Kuru	Cannibalism

ancestors. Very much as with bovine spongiform encephalopathy (BSE; so-called 'mad cow disease') in cattle, the disease gradually died out as this practice was abandoned. The main symptom was a Parkinsonian tremor, indicating involvement of the cerebellum. Shortly after, *Creutzfeldt–Jakob disease* (CJD) was also shown to be transmissible (see Chapter 8 for the history). In this condition, after an incubation period of many years, dementia and ataxia are the commonest presenting symptoms, usually fatal within a year. The main pathological finding is spongiform vacuolation in the cerebral cortex. Four varieties are currently recognized (see Table 31.1). Although it is possible to raise antibodies experimentally against prion proteins, there is no good evidence for the development of protective immunity in the natural disease, so that active immunization (i.e. a vaccine) seems at present a rather remote possibility. It has been proposed that T cell tolerance to prion antigens is the main stumbling-block.

SUMMARY

- Immunity to intracellular viruses is normally mediated by interferon, NK cells, and CTLs, whereas in the extracellular phase they are susceptible to antibody.

- Many virus infections (e.g. measles) stimulate good memory responses, leading to a slighter or absent secondary infection. However, antigenic variation and other escape mechanisms ensure that others (e.g. colds, influenza) can cause repeated infections.

- Several good vaccines exist against viruses, whereas chemotherapy, though sometimes effective, is much less so than against bacteria.

- In prion infections, immunity has not yet been shown to play a useful or a harmful role.

Chapter 32

Bacterial disease and immunity

First, re-read Chapter 3 to remind yourself of the key properties of bacteria and the all-important distinction between extracellular and intracellular habitat. In general, extracellular bacteria are dealt with by the combination antibody+complement+phagocytic cells, and intracellular ones (usually resident in macrophages) depend largely on T cells+cytokines such as IFNγ for their control (Fig. 32.1). In this chapter we review the immunological and therapeutic features of the most important pathogenic bacteria.

■ Staphylococcal infection

The Gram-positive extracellular staphylococci, transmitted by contact and air-borne droplets, are the cause of most pyogenic (pus-forming) infections of the skin

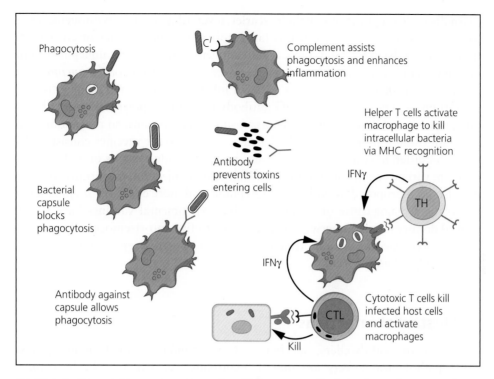

Fig. 32.1 Antibacterial immunity: an overview. Phagocytes, antibody, and complement are the main defences against extracellular bacteria, whereas macrophages activated by T-helper cells/IFNγ, and CTLs, are dominant in immunity to intracellular bacteria.

and soft tissues, sometimes spreading to lungs and bone. Healthy nasal carriers of *Staph. aureus* are a major source of infection, especially in hospitals. Many strains produce numerous exotoxins, with both local effects (tissue destruction, coagulation of serum, abscess formation) and more distant ones (food poisoning, toxic shock). Other virulence factors include the anti-phagocytic capsule and the IgG-neutralizing Protein A. Deficiencies of neutrophil function (see Chapter 15) predispose to severe chronic staphylococcal infections. Penicillin was originally effective but most staphylococci, particularly in hospitals, are now resistant, these being usually referred to as methicillin-resistant *Staph. aureus* (MRSA); some are now resistant to the newer antibiotic vancomycin too. Several vaccine trials are in progress, involving such antigens as capsular polysaccharides and various toxins, including the superantigen of toxic shock, TSS1 (see Chapter 18), but so far success has been limited.

■ Streptococcal infection

Group A streptococci are a common cause of sore throats and, less often, of spreading skin infections (including the 'flesh-eating superbug' beloved of popular journalism). Complications include scarlet fever (due to an erythrogenic exo-toxin), rheumatic fever, myocarditis (an autoimmune consequence of cross-reac-tion between bacterial and myocardial antigens), and glomerulonephritis (an immune-complex-mediated hypersensitivity reaction). *Streptococcus pneumoniae* (formerly *Pneumococcus*), a major cause of lobar pneumonia and meningitis, has an anti-phagocytic capsule, but IgG antibody to capsular polysaccharides allows phagocytosis and destruction of the organisms by neutrophils, so pneumonia is a common complication of antibody deficiency. The current vaccines consist of 23 of the 84 different strain-specific capsular polysaccharide variants or 7, 10, or 13 different variants conjugated to protein. Rather than injection, the intranasal route has also been proposed as both more acceptable and more effective. *Streptococcus mutans* is a major cause of dental caries but experimental vaccines have so far proved disappointing. Otherwise there are no effective anti-streptococcal vaccines. *Streptococcus faecalis*, an important cause of post-operative septicaemia, has been reclassified as *Enterococcus*.

■ Clostridial infections

Clostridia are soil-dwellers, surviving adverse conditions by forming spores. Their pathological effects are due to exotoxins (see Chapter 9). In *tetanus* (*Clostridium tetani*), the effect is on nerve–muscle transmission, blocking the inhibition of contraction; the result is spasm of voluntary muscles, fatal if untreated. In acute cases antitoxin is effective and there is a good toxoid vaccine, introduced during the early months of the Second World War and nowadays given together with diphtheria toxoid and pertussis and *Haemophilus* vaccines. The toxin of *Clostridium botulinum* (botulism) has the opposite effect of 'floppy paralysis'. Antitoxin can be life-saving but the disease is so rare that no vaccine is available. *Clostridium perfringens* causes gas gangrene, with tissue destruction in deep wounds, where conditions are anaerobic. Oxygenation of the wound and antibiotics are the standard treatment. *Clostridium difficile* has come to the fore as a cause of hospital diarrhoea following destruction of the normal gut flora by antibiotics.

■ Anthrax

Mainly a disease of farm animals and farmers (see Box 32.1), anthrax has achieved notoriety as a possible weapon of biological warfare. A major feature is that spores can persist for decades in the environment. It begins as an ulcerating skin lesion which may proceed to septicaemia and death from the effects of the exotoxin. There is an effective attenuated vaccine (as Pasteur demonstrated in 1883) but there is considerable controversy as to both the safety and the need for the current human vaccine, a cell-free culture filtrate, other than in the military and high-risk individuals. High-dose penicillin is an effective treatment.

Box 32.1 Robert Koch, the father of bacteriology

A surgeon and a patriot

In 1870, at the age of 27, Koch was operating at the front of the Franco-Prussian war and listening to the theories of Semmelweiss and Billroth about wound infection. His belief that germs caused disease and his hatred of the French (and Louis Pasteur in particular) never left him.

Black sheep disease

Back in civilian life he opened a practice in Wollstein (now in Poland) and in the intervals between patients devoted himself to the study of anthrax, a major blight of the local sheep farms. Meticulous work with mice, plus the best available microscope, convinced him that it was caused by a specific identifiable bacillus. Here he evolved his famous Four Postulates, the basis of microbial aetiology ever since.

A spiral of fame

A well-prepared demonstration at the celebrated University of Breslau in 1876 impressed the local staff so much that his fame spread rapidly around the German medical world. Next he applied himself to tuberculosis, and thanks to the young genius of microscopic staining, Paul Ehrlich, he was able to prove that tuberculosis too had its own specific bacillus. This time (1882) his fame was instant and international. His triumph over the French microbiologists was completed the following year by the successful identification of the cholera *Vibrio*, first in Egypt and then in India (the British effort was restricted to trying to show that the disease had not spread via the Suez canal, which would have necessitated expensive quarantine procedures there). Only Rudolf Virchow, the great pathologist, refused to accept Koch's theory of 'one germ one disease'.

Romance and first mistake

In 1888, at the age of 45, Koch finally separated from his wife, with whom he had become increasingly unhappy, and took as mistress a 17-year-old actress and model, whom he married 5 years later. To answer the criticism that he had lost interest in science, he produced what was intended as the crowning glory of his work: the treatment of tuberculosis with the protein 'vaccine' extract tuberculin. This not only didn't work but made many victims worse (probably by inducing a pathological immune reaction—the so-called 'Koch phenomenon'). It was left to the French to sort out the mess: Mantoux showed that a tiny dose of tuberculin was useful in diagnosing previous tuberculosis, while Calmette and Guerin produced the only effective vaccine, the attenuated BCG organism.

Tropical finale

With his pretty and adventurous young wife, Koch embarked on a series of visits to Africa, where he studied rinderpest ('cattle plague'), malaria, and sleeping sickness, not to discover the organism—that was being done by others, following his lead—but to lay down the correct public health strategies for containment and control. Honours were heaped on him and, the final act of forgiveness, the Nobel Prize in 1905.

Other bacterial skin infections

Leprosy

Mycobacterium leprae resembles *Mycobacterium tuberculosis* in many ways but is restricted to skin and superficial tissues, causing terrible deformities to the face and extremities. It is the classic example of the balance or 'spectrum' between T_H1

(cell-mediated) and T_H2 (antibody-mediated) immunity. A predominantly T_H1 response results in killing of the bacteria with scarring and destruction of peripheral nerves (tuberculoid leprosy); a predominantly T_H2 pattern leads to uncontrolled growth of bacteria in superficial tissues (lepromatous leprosy); several intermediate stages are recognized and patients may move from one to another as a result of treatment (see Figure 22.4). The immune mechanisms by which about a third of infected individuals control the disease without symptoms are not understood. The BCG vaccine gives some protection, from 80% (Uganda) to only 20% (Burma), with a worldwide average of about 50% protection, but the main hope for elimination is by combination chemotherapy (dapsone, rifampicin, plus one other drug).

Acne

Propionobacterium acnes, a normal skin commensal, plays a large part in the adolescent skin infection acne, in which excessive sex hormones cause sebaceous glands to become blocked.

■ Diphtheria

Destruction of pharyngeal epithelium by the exotoxin of *Corynebacterium diphtheriae* gives rise to a 'false membrane' which can cause respiratory obstruction. Sometimes there is also damage to the heart and nervous system. The disease is now rare thanks to the universal use of the toxoid vaccine (see above).

Other corynebacterial infections

Of the many other corynebacteria, *Corynebacterium jeikeium* is emerging as an important opportunist.

■ Tuberculosis

TB is the most important mycobacterial infection and one of the world's major health problems (see Box 32.1 and Chapter 27). Spread by droplet (mainly from coughs), *Mycobacterium tuberculosis* is the classic example of a bacterium capable of surviving for long periods in macrophages, which enables it to cause chronic and often lifelong infections. Being aerobic, it prefers the well-oxygenated parts of the lung, but can spread to almost any other organ if cell-mediated immunity becomes inadequate, and can also survive at low oxygen concentrations in granulomas. This capacity for survival makes it a major problem in undernourished or immunodeficient patients. In nineteenth-century Britain tuberculosis was responsible for about 20% of deaths, and the AIDS epidemic has caused a resurgence of the disease in the tropics.

The pathology, based on tissue necrosis and granuloma formation, is also due to cell-mediated mechanisms (Type IV; see Chapter 23). Broadly speaking, T_H1 cells, secreting IFNγ, and CTLs, are beneficial, and T_H2 cells (and antibody) useless or harmful once already infected (although there is a new interest to see if generating antibodies directly in the lung by a mucosal vaccine could actually prevent infection). T_H17 cells have been implicated on both protection and in pathology depending on the model. However, all the elements in the balance between health and disease are not fully understood. A positive Mantoux (delayed hypersensitivity) skin test denotes previous exposure but does not guarantee immunity. The attenuated vaccine (BCG), derived from *Mycobacterium bovis*, is widely used but varies markedly in its effectiveness in different parts of the world; e.g. UK 75%, South India 0%. In the tropics it is effective in children but strikingly less so in adults. Several replacement vaccines are at the trial stage, including those based on DNA, recombinant TB antigens, genetically engineered vaccinia virus, improved versions of BCG, and even a live attenuated *M. tuberculosis* strain (Table 27.3). Chemotherapy requires combinations of up to four drugs, maintained usually for six months. *M. bovis* was a cause of human TB before pasteurization of milk; *Mycobacterium avium intracellulare* emerged as an important pathogen in AIDS patients before the establishment of HAART.

■ Whooping cough

Bordetella pertussis causes the childhood disease pertussis, or whooping cough. The bacterium is rich in virulence factors, including an endotoxin, an exotoxin, a toxin that damages phagocytes, and another that inhibits the beating of cilia in the bronchi and trachea, thus arresting the 'muco-ciliary escalator'. There is an effective whole-cell vaccine, given with tetanus and diphtheria toxoids, but it has been suspected of dangerous side effects, notably convulsions and brain damage, probably due to the endotoxin. As a result, during the 1970s many parents refused the vaccine and in the winter of 1978–1979 the death rate from whooping cough rose dramatically. Several new approaches have been tried, the present preference being for an acellular vaccine containing inactivated toxin and other bacterial components.

Other respiratory infections

Streptococcus pneumoniae is mentioned above as a common cause of pneumonia.

Haemophilus

Haemophilus influenzae infection is most common in children from about 6 months to 3 years old, since during this age period maternally transmitted antibody has waned and they do not yet produce their own IgG antibody against the capsular polysaccharide. Infections of the lungs, bronchi, sinuses, middle ear, and epiglottis are usually secondary to virus infection. Another species of *Haemophilus*, *Haemophilus ducreyi*, causes genital 'soft chancre'. *H. influenzae* is normally present in the throat, but of the six types, the capsulated Type b ('Hib') may spread to the lungs and/or the meninges (see below). The name is due to the fact that it was once thought to be the cause of influenza. A good capsule-protein conjugated vaccine is available, but only against Type b.

Legionella

Only discovered in 1976, the intracellular bacillus *Legionella pneumophila* grows in water from industrial cooling towers, hot water, and air conditioning systems, from which it is spread by aerosol. Legionnaire's disease presents as an 'atypical' pneumonia; the name *atypical* derives from its failure to respond to penicillin as 'classic' pneumococcal pneumonia does and the name of the disease refers to a convention of the American Legion where the first outbreak occurred. A rare complication is encephalitis. There is no vaccine but erythromycin is effective.

Pseudomonas

Pseudomonas aeruginosa has become important as an opportunist infection of the lungs in patients with cystic fibrosis, and in burns.

Burkholderia

Burkholderia (formerly *Pseudomonas*) *mallei* and *pseudomallei*, have been proposed as potential agents of biological warfare, and the latter causes septicaemia in south-east Asia. *B. cepacia* causes serious infection in children with cystic fibrosis.

■ Meningococcal meningitis

Neisseria meningitidis (the meningococcus) is a Gram-negative capsulated diplococcus carried in the nasopharynx of some 20% of healthy people, which for ill-understood reasons can occasionally spread to the meninges (meningitis) or the blood (septicaemia). Based on the polysaccharide capsular antigens, three serotypes are recognized (A, B, C), of which B is the commonest cause of disease. Unfortunately the type B polysaccharide is the least immunogenic, since it is mainly sialic acid and may cross-react with host tissues. There are already good polysaccharide conjugate vaccines against A and C however a new protein-based vaccine against B is close to being licensed. Unlike most other bacteria, *Neisseria* are largely eliminated by antibody plus the lytic complement pathway, so people deficient in C5–C9 are more susceptible. Meningococcal septicaemia is a dangerous complication, associated with a skin rash, vascular collapse, and acute renal and adrenal failure; excessive production of cytokines, especially TNF, is thought to be responsible (see Case Study 14.1 Meningococcal meningitis and septicaemia).

Other causes of meningitis

Pneumococcal infection

Meningitis is a rare complication of pneumococcal infection, but carries a high mortality.

Haemophilus infection

Haemophilus meningitis is commonest in children from about 6 months to 3 years old, since during this age period maternally transmitted antibody has waned and they do not yet produce their own IgG antibody against the capsular polysaccharide.

Listeriosis

Listeria monocytogenes, usually acquired from animals via uncooked food, is an opportunist, an important cause of meningitis in immunodeficient patients and, since it is transmitted across the placenta, the newborn. The organism is mainly intracellular, spreading from macrophage to macrophage by a form of budding that allows it to remain totally concealed. T_H1 cells, cytotoxic T cells, and NK cells are all thought to play a part in immunity, both via activation of macrophages (by IFNγ) and by direct cytotoxicity. No vaccine is available.

■ Gonorrhoea

Neisseria gonorrhoeae (the gonococcus) resembles *N. meningitidis* in susceptibility to complement lysis and the use of pili, in this case to attach to the genitourinary mucosa. An anti-phagocytic capsule, two pore-forming proteins, and an IgA-destroying enzyme complete a formidable list of virulence factors. Infection is usually limited to the genitourinary tract, leading in women to pelvic inflammatory disease and lifelong infertility, with rare systemic complications (arthritis, endocarditis). Congenital infection can cause blindness and death of young infants. There is no vaccine but in the past a variety of antibiotics were effective. However, antibiotic resistance has been an ever-increasing problem, with a recent report of completely drug resistant bacteria causing major concern. Although the infection is normally self-limiting, there is little evidence of lasting immunity.

Other venereal diseases

For chlamydial diseases, see page 324.

■ Syphilis

Caused by the spirally coiled spirochaete *Treponema pallidum*, syphilis was the major venereal disease before the advent of penicillin. It was much feared because of its slow and inexorable course, often taking 20–30 years to kill an adult patient from damage to the brain, heart valves, bones, or other organs. The organism induces numerous antibodies, including one that cross-reacts with the normal mammalian phospholipid cardiolipin (the Wasserman reaction), but although about a third of patients recover spontaneously, it is not known what immune response if any is responsible, nor how the bacteria survive in the patients who progress. Early treatments with metals (arsenic, bismuth, mercury) led to the cynical summary of syphilitic infection as 'one night with Venus, a lifetime with Mercury'. Less well known is the major impact of congenital syphilis in tropical countries, causing over 750 000 stillbirths and deaths in early childhood per year. This could be prevented by implementation of simple, rapid tests and treatment of all pregnant women in these countries, perhaps alongside existing HIV testing schemes, and would make a substantial impact on the Millennium Development Goals of reducing childhood mortality in poor countries. It is also important to note that sexually transmitted bacterial infections such as gonorrhea and syphilis increase the transmission of HIV, making STD management an important aspect of HIV control.

Other spirochaete infections

Leptospirosis

Leptospirosis, or Weil's disease, caused by the spiral bacterium *Leptospira interrogans*, is a multi-system zoonosis caught from rats and domestic animals via contaminated food or water. In a small number of cases there may be haemorrhages in the brain, eye, liver, and kidney, leading to liver and/or kidney failure. Penicillin and tetracycline are effective.

Borrelia infection

Borrelia recurrentis, the cause of relapsing fever, a spiral bacterium spread by body lice, was one of the first bacteria in which antigenic variation was shown, allowing it to escape the antibody response, much as influenza and African trypanosomes do (see Chapter 22). *Borrelia burgdorferi* is spread by ticks and causes Lyme disease, a migrating skin rash followed weeks or years later by brain, heart, and joint lesions, possibly autoimmune in origin. Treatment is as for Weil's disease.

■ Typhoid

Salmonella typhi, the cause of typhoid fever, survives within macrophages and is disseminated to lymph nodes and, via the bloodstream, to other organs. Without treatment about 15% of patients die, and following recovery up to 3% continue to excrete the organisms; these *carriers* are responsible for fresh outbreaks. The original killed typhoid vaccine was unpleasant (due to the endotoxin content) and only partly effective; more recent candidates are (1) an attenuated organism with deletion of genes needed for long-term survival (GalE, AroA), and (2) a purified capsular polysaccharide, the Vi (virulence) antigen. Both give about 50–80% protection, but the disease is rarely fatal thanks nowadays to antibiotics (e.g. cephalosporins) and oral rehydration (see Chapter 27).

Other gastrointestinal infections

The enterobacteria group includes a number of organisms spread by the oral–faecal route, capable of causing diarrhoea and/or urinary infection with occasional systemic spread. Some, such as *Proteus* and *Klebsiella*, are part of the normal gut flora, while *Salmonella* and *Shigella* are not. Some strains of *Escherichia coli* occur normally, while others are enterotoxic (ETEC), enteropathogenic (EPEC), invasive (EIEC), or haemorrhagic (EHEC, which includes the most severe serotype O157). Vaccines against *Shigella* and *E. coli* are still at the experimental stage.

   Bacteroides fragilis, a normal gut commensal, is a common cause of peritonitis following trauma to the gut or surgery. Treatment is with gentamicin.

Cholera

Vibrio cholerae (see Box 32.1) gives rise to the characteristic rapid watery diarrhoea ('rice water stool') of cholera by secreting a toxin that raises cAMP levels in intestinal epithelial cells, causing them to lose water and electrolytes - up to a litre per hour. Thus the patient, if untreated, dies of dehydration. The most effective vaccine is an oral combination of whole killed bacteria and a recombinant B toxin, but it is only recommended for those at high risk.

Campylobacter infection

Campylobacter jejuni and *Helicobacter pylori* (formerly known as *Campylobacter pylori*) are common causes of diarrhoea and gastritis, respectively. *H. pylori* survives in the highly acid environment of the stomach by producing urease which breaks down urea to ammonia. The resulting inflammation is thought to underlie not only gastric and duodenal ulcers but also gastric carcinoma. Immunity may contribute to the ulcers through the local production of cytokines and the attraction and activation of neutrophils. In mice, immunity appears to depend on CD4 T cells, possibly via an effect on the character and secretion of mucus.

■ Plague

Yersinia pestis, a mild infection in rats transmitted by fleas, periodically causes human epidemics, in which either the bubonic (lymph node) or the pneumonic form may predominate. Both carry a high mortality, but survivors are immune to reinfection and there is a fairly effective killed vaccine which protects better against bubonic than pneumonic disease. Newer vaccines based on capsular antigens are under trial. Tetracycline gives good prophylactic protection.

■ Tularemia

A multi-system infection caused by *Francisella tularensis*, this has been proposed as an agent of biological warfare. It is normally acquired from wild animals, either directly or by tick bite.

■ Brucellosis

Normally an infection of animals (*Brucella abortus*, cattle; *Brucella melitensis*, sheep and goats; *Brucella suis*, pigs), *Brucella* infect humans by contact or food contamination (e.g. milk). An undulant pattern of fever results, the organism residing and spreading in macrophages. Diagnosis is by blood culture, and treatment is by antibiotics. Although there is an attenuated vaccine for animals, it has not been used in humans. Since very few organisms are needed for infection, laboratory-acquired infection is a possibility.

■ Actinomycosis

Actinomyces israeli is often found in dental plaque and tooth caries. It resembles a fungus in its filamentous morphology but is related to the corynebacteria in the structure of its cell wall and its response to penicillin.

■ Chlamydial infection

These small obligate intracellular parasites have a curious lifestyle involving an initial infective elementary body, and a reticulate body which replicates to release more elementary bodies. *Chlamydia trachomatis*, primarily a genital infection, can spread to the eye to cause conjunctivitis and trachoma, the commonest cause of blindness; there are perhaps 5 000 000 cases worldwide. *Chlamydia psittaci* (acquired from birds) and *Chlamydia pneumoniae* are among the causes of atypical pneumonia.

■ Rickettsial infection

Rickettsiae are also obligate intracellular parasites because of a requirement for certain host cell factors (NAD, ATP, coenzyme A). They are acquired from animals or indirectly via insect bites. Brain, liver, and skin (vasculitis) are the organs chiefly affected. Different species cause slightly different diseases in different parts of the world (*Rickettsia rickettsii*, Rocky Mountain spotted fever; *Rickettsia conorii*, Mediterranean spotted fever; *Rickettsia typhi*, *Rickettsia prowazekii*, typhus; *Rickettsia tsutsugamushi*, scrub typhus; *Coxiella burnetii*, Q fever). Rickettsial infections induce good immunity, mediated largely by IFNγ, TNF, H_2O_2, and NO (see Chapter 12). A killed vaccine was used in the Second World War, but vaccination is currently only recommended in the case of a bioterror attack.

■ Mycoplasma infection

Mycoplasma are atypical in not possessing a normal bacterial cell wall. *Mycoplasma pneumoniae* is an important cause of bronchitis and pneumonia. *Mycoplasma hominis* may cause genital infections although this is disputed. Mycoplasma pneumonia is followed by a transient period of immunity to reinfection.

SUMMARY

- Extracellular bacteria are normally dealt with by antibody, complement, and phagocytic cells, generally acting together. Bacteria that survive in macrophages (e.g. *M. tuberculosis*) can be eliminated if the macrophages are activated by IFNγ from T cells.

- Bacteria of both kinds display escape mechanisms so that bacterial infections can become chronic.

- The main therapeutic strategy against bacteria is chemotherapy, although resistance is increasingly common. There are some good bacterial vaccines, mainly based on subcellular components such as toxins or protein-polysaccharide conjugates.

- Anthrax, plague, and some other bacteria have been proposed as biological agents of warfare.

Chapter 33

Fungal disease and immunity

Look back to Chapter 4 to be reminded that fungal diseases fall into three main patterns: *primary* infections in healthy individuals, *viz*: (1) filamentous moulds infecting the superficial and subcutaneous tissues, (2) a dimorphic group causing systemic, mainly lung, infections; and (3) *secondary* infections caused by a number of important opportunists which have come to the fore with the increase in immunocompromised patients, in which they can cause disseminated and even fatal disease (Table 33.1). It is the latter group for which there is the greatest need for vaccines, a real challenge in view of their deficient immune system. The mechanisms of host defence are generally similar to those that act against bacteria, namely the intact skin and membranes; antibody, complement, neutrophils, and macrophages for extracellular organisms; and T_H1 cells and cytokines for those that survive in macrophages. It is significant that many of the pathogen-associated molecular patterns (see Chapter 12) recognized by phagocytic and antigen-presenting cells are found on fungi. Escape mechanisms/virulence factors include immunosuppression (e.g. of T cells by dermatophytes), the production of capsules (by *Cryptococcus*), and inhibition of intracellular killing (e.g. by *Histoplasma*). In general, T_H1-type immunity correlates with effective immunity and T_H2-type with susceptibility; antibodies have been shown to be protective only in some cases, e.g. *Cryptococcus*.

■ Primary superficial and subcutaneous infections

Tinea (ringworm) is more common in children than adults, partly because of the antifungal effect of post-pubertal sebaceous secretions. The occurrence of disseminated infection with *Trichophyton* spp. in immunocompromised patients suggests a role for immunity in normal individuals, but the precise mechanisms are unknown.

Table 33.1 Some conditions predisposing to fungal infection

Condition	Common infections
T-cell defects	
AIDS	*Aspergillus, Candida, Cryptococcus*
Immunosuppressive drugs	*Pneumocystis, Penicillium*
Neutrophil defects	*Aspergillus, Candida, Zygomyces*
Diabetes	*Candida, Zygomyces*
Tumours	*Candida, Aspergillus*
Cystic fibrosis	*Aspergillus*
Antibacterial drug therapy	*Candida*
Surgery, catheters	*Candida*

Similarly, the mycetoma of *Madurella* and other species of mould (Madura foot) and the nodular lesions of *Sporothrix* (sporotrichosis), despite their granulomatous pathology, are more common in patients with impaired cell-mediated immunity. *Candida albicans* is a rather special case, being a normal commensal of skin and mucous membranes, which can exacerbate to cause the itching and discharging lesions of *thrush*, frequently under the influence of antibiotic treatment, which suppresses the normal bacterial flora. However, systemic dissemination can occur in the immunocompromised (see below), intravenous drug users, and patients with central lines.

■ Systemic infections

The dimorphic fungi *Histoplasma*, *Blastomyces*, and *Coccidioides*, mainly restricted to the American continent, exist in a filamentous form in soil, from which the spores, inhaled into the lung, develop into the yeast phase, giving rise to a pneumonia-like illness from which recovery is usual. A similar disease occurs following inhalation of the yeast *Cryptococcus*. Further dissemination, especially in the immunocompromised, may be fatal (see below). Thus, once again, there is good evidence for protective immunity. The increased susceptibility of AIDS patients, plus experiments in animal models, suggest a major role for CD4 T cells, mainly through their effect in activating the intracellular killing mechanisms in macrophages and neutrophils. *Histoplasma* is particularly prone to remain dormant for years after apparent recovery, and to flare up if immunodeficiency occurs.

■ Opportunistic fungi

Here the evidence for protective immunity is most convincing, since the fungi do not cause disease except in the immunocompromised (see Table 33.1).

Candidiasis

This is the predominant opportunistic fungal infection, particularly in hospitalized patients. It is common in T-cell deficiencies, particularly AIDS, but also in patients on steroids or antibiotics, drug abusers, those with diabetes or leukaemia, and post-operatively. The lesions may affect the skin and mucous membranes (chronic mucocutaneous candidiasis; CMC) or the gastrointestinal tract or, in severe cases, dissemination can occur to any organ, including the eye and heart. Because exposure to *Candida* is so common, a delayed skin test using candidin is often used to monitor T-cell immunity in general.

Cryptococcus

Unlike most fungi, *Cryptococcus neoformans* is susceptible to antibody and complement, since IgG against the polysaccharide capsule can overcome its antiphagocytic effect. However, T_H1 cells and cytokines are also involved in its control, and spread outside the lung, particularly to the meninges and brain, is common in AIDS patients.

Pneumocystis carinii

This organism, once considered a protozoan, has the dubious distinction of having led to the discovery of AIDS (see Chapter 26). In small numbers it is probably a normal resident of the lung in most individuals, but multiplies to cause severe pneumonia in T-cell-deficient patients. There is debate as to whether this constitutes a reactivation of pre-existent organisms or a true reinfection.

Aspergillus

This filamentous mould can cause symptoms in four situations: (1) normal people may become allergic to the spores, mainly of *Aspergillus fumigatus*, and develop asthma; (2) in patients with pre-existing lung infection (e.g. cavitating TB) the hyphae may grow into a large *fungus ball*, worsening the respiratory problems; (3) in immunocompromised, particularly neutropenic, individuals primary infection is often in the lungs and dissemination can occur to brain, heart, gut, and bone, with frequently fatal results; and (4) the exotoxin (aflatoxin) of *Aspergillus flavus*, a contaminant of stored grain or nuts, is a risk factor for liver cancer.

Zygomycosis

A variety of filamentous fungi that are prone to infect and proliferate in injured, burned, malnourished, diabetic, and other debilitated patients, though less often in those with AIDS. Reduced neutrophil and macrophage function appears to be the common predisposing factor.

■ Treatment and vaccines

Antifungal chemotherapy is aimed predominantly at cell-wall synthesis, but there are a few drugs that act against protein and nucleic acid synthesis; for further details see Table 29.5. There are no vaccines in use at present, but in experimental vaccine models both antibody-mediated immunity (e.g. for *Cryptococcus*, *Candida*, and *Aspergillus*) and cell-mediated immunity (e.g. for *Histoplasma*, *Blastomyces*, and *Coccidioides*) have been successfully induced. Vaccines against *Candida*, blastomycosis, and *Pneumocystis* are the most advanced at present, and seem likely before long to come to clinical trial. Another possibility is the use of monoclonal antibodies for passive immunization. Recently a 'generic' antifungal vaccine has been proposed, based on antigens common to several species, such as β-glucan or the heat-shock or 'stress' protein HSP60. It is not impossible to imagine a future vaccine effective against *all* fungi.

SUMMARY

- Immune responses to fungi are broadly similar to those against bacteria, though frequently less effective.

- Antifungal drugs are effective but toxic.

- Antifungal vaccines are still at the experimental stage.

Chapter 34

Protozoal disease and immunity

The common features of the protozoal pathogens described in Chapter 5 are that (1) the diseases they cause are extremely chronic, with spontaneous recovery a very rare event and only partial immunity at best, and (2) no effective vaccines are currently available. The problem lies in their highly developed *immune evasion* mechanisms, which make use of virtually all the devices discussed in Chapters 13 and 22.

■ Malaria

In populations regularly exposed to malaria, most deaths and severe complications (e.g. anaemia, cerebral malaria) and the highest parasitaemias are seen in children, suggesting that older patients have acquired some degree of immunity to both the parasite and the disease. This immunity is maintained by continued exposure to infection and can be lost after only a few months of non-exposure. Experiments in mice suggest that T cells, antibody, and cytokines all play a role (Fig. 34.1). The continued survival of parasites in patients with high levels of antibody and activated T cells is due to a number of factors, as listed below.

1. Following a mosquito bite, the survival of only a few sporozoites is enough to initiate a liver-stage infection.

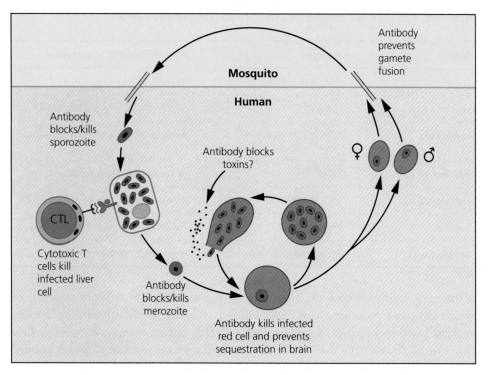

Fig. 34.1 The malaria life cycle offers numerous points of attack for the immune system, all of which are potential targets for a vaccine.

2. The free-living blood stages (sporozoite, merozoite) are very brief: seconds or minutes.

3. The intracellular liver stage is susceptible to killing by CD8 T cells, but only a few released merozoites are needed to initiate the next (blood) stage of infection.

4. Both the free merozoite and the infected red blood cells carry dominant antigens which are highly polymorphic and may undergo variation. Polymorphism is enhanced by the presence of a sexual stage in the cycle.

5. In the case of *Plasmodium vivax*, the liver stage may survive in the dormant form of hypnozoites, to relapse years later.

6. Malaria infection is immunosuppressive (see Chapter 27).

Natural resistance to malaria is discussed in Chapter 27.

Prospects for a vaccine

A vaccine that prevented malaria, or prevented the million or more deaths per year from malaria, or even reduced transmission, would be of enormous benefit. There is no shortage of potential parasite antigens, as Table 34.1 shows, but most trials to-date have been disappointing, showing barely statistical levels of protection insufficient to justify large-scale manufacture. Current hopes are pinned on combinations

Table 34.1 Potential target antigens for malarial immunity and vaccination

Source	Antigen	Role of immunity if successful
Sporozoite	CSP, (RTS,S),TRAP	Antibody blocks entry into liver cell
Liver cell	LSA-1, 3	CD8 T cells kill infected liver cell
Merozoite	MSP-1, 2, 4, EBA-175, AMA-1, GLURP, RESA	Antibody blocks entry into red cell
Infected red cell	PfEMP-1	Antibody blocks sequestration
Gametocyte	Pfs 230, 48/45	Prevents sexual stage and transmission
Gamete	Pfg 25/27	Prevents sexual stage and transmission
Malaria toxins (?)	Phospholipid (?; GPI)	Protects against toxic symptoms

of three or more antigens or, alternatively, the use of novel delivery systems, of which the most promising is RTS,S, which consists of a recombinant sporozoite antigen fused to hepatitis B surface antigen (HBs antigen) and combined with a detoxified LPS analogue (MPL) plus QS21, a plant-based saponin adjuvant derived from *Quillaja saponaria*. This combination has given up to 50% protection in young children in several regions of Africa. Ironically, the best protection ever achieved was 40 years ago, using radiation-attenuated sporozoites, an approach which has recently come under fresh consideration, but which poses huge problems of mass availability since sporozoites can only be grown within living mosquitoes.

Immunopathology

Apart from the anaemia, which is partly due to direct destruction of red cells, the symptoms and complications of malaria are related to immune activity, particularly (1) immune-complex formation, leading to glomerulonephritis, and (2) excessive release of inflammatory cytokines such as TNFα, IL-1, IL-6, and IFNγ, which underlie the fever, the hypoglycaemia, and probably the cerebral changes. Unfortunately, several anti-TNF antibody trials in humans have only reduced fever and not mortality. The reason for the chronic nephrotic syndrome caused by *Plasmodium malariae* is not understood. The link between malaria, EBV, and Burkitt's lymphoma is thought to be at least partly due to suppression of the CTL response to EBV-infected B lymphocytes. Early in the twentieth century, controlled *P. vivax* infection ('fever therapy') was used to treat late-stage syphilis, on the basis that treponemes survive poorly at high temperatures.

Treatment

Both the liver and the blood stage are susceptible to drugs, but resistance has developed to most of these (see Chapter 29).

■ Leishmaniasis

The critical element in leishmaniasis is survival of the amastigote stage of the parasite within macrophages, which can be overcome by vigorous activation of the macrophages by cytokines, particularly IFNγ and TNF; hence the importance of T cells of the T_H1 subset. By contrast, T_H2 cells, by releasing IL-4, tend to promote non-protective antibody formation. In line with this, recovery and resistance correlate with strong delayed hypersensitivity responses. Encouragingly, only about 5% of exposed individuals develop disease. In immunodeficient patients (e.g. AIDS) both cutaneous and visceral disease are much more severe. The search for a vaccine has been encouraged by the fact that mild cutaneous cases of *Leishmania tropica* ('oriental sore') are immune to reinfection after recovery; deliberate exposure has traditionally been practised in the Middle East, a process known as 'leishmanization', analogous to the use of variolation against smallpox. There have been numerous trials of more sophisticated vaccines, but none has yet been adopted as standard. In their absence, treatment relies on antimonial drugs and the more expensive amphotericin B, or miltefosine and paromomycin.

■ African trypanosomiasis

The two species of *Trypanosoma brucei* are unique among protozoa in living and multiplying free in the blood, where they are exposed to virtually every element of the immune system, including antibody, complement, PMNs, and lymphocytes. Their survival is due to a remarkable form of antigenic variation in which the parasite repeatedly changes its entire surface coat of 'variant-specific glycoprotein' (VSG) by a gene-switching mechanism; the genome contains about 1000 different genes for this purpose. As a result, following an antibody response, many parasites are eliminated but a new variant population emerges. The host is thus obliged to mount a series of primary responses at approximately weekly intervals (see Fig. 22.3). Massive polyclonal IgM production adds further to the inefficiency of immunity, the parasite stimulates inflammatory changes in the CNS, and the patient eventually succumbs to the coma of *sleeping sickness*. The prospects for a vaccine seem rather remote, and treatment was for long mainly based on arsenical drugs, hardly different from those introduced by Ehrlich over 100 years ago.

Ironically the major effort is being applied to the disease in cattle, an important contributor to malnourishment in Africa. The existence of resistant strains of cattle gives a hint that some degree of immunity is possible.

■ South American trypanosomiasis (Chagas' disease)

In its early stage in macrophages, *Trypanosoma cruzi* behaves like *Leishmania*, inhibiting both intracellular killing mechanisms and their stimulation by IFNγ. The succeeding blood stage is resistant to lysis by complement, and the final stages in heart and nervous tissue are thought by some to be partly autoimmune; the chronic destructive effects (cardiomegaly, megaoesphagus, megacolon), which may progress for decades, are due to *cross-reaction* between parasite and host antigens. Clearly a vaccine which enhanced this would be disastrous, and although arsenicals and other drugs are of some benefit, ultimate control of the disease lies in the hands of those responsible for the slum housing in which the reduviid bug vector flourishes.

■ Toxoplasmosis

Toxoplasma is of special interest as an intracellular parasite, able to develop in many types of cell and many species of animal. It is also an important *opportunist*, taking advantage of weakened immunity to reactivate and proliferate, particularly in the brain (encephalitis) and eye (chorioretinitis). Toxoplasma is also one of the few pathogens able to cross the placenta, infect the fetus, and cause malformations or neonatal infection; others being rubella virus, CMV, HIV, hepatitis B, syphilis, leprosy, and *Listeria* (see Table 11.5). Various drugs are used for treatment and prophylaxis, notably pyrimethamine–sulphonamide combinations such as co-trimoxazole. Care in handling pet cats, the definitive hosts and frequent carriers, is important for susceptible individuals.

■ Amoebiasis

Infection with *Entamoeba histolytica* can range from symptomless carriage in the large intestine, mild attacks of diarrhoea, and dysentery with intestinal ulceration and bleeding, to peritonitis and abscesses in liver, lung, etc., with only slight evidence of useful immunity. *Acanthamoeba* spp. are an increasingly important cause of eye infections. Treatment with antibiotics and normal hygienic measures are the mainstay of control.

Other protozoal diarrhoeal diseases

Giardiasis

Giardia lamblia causes a self-limiting attack of diarrhoea, except in some immunodeficient patients when it may be prolonged and debilitating.

Cryptosporidiosis

Infection with *Cryptosporidium parvum*, which normally induces a brief episode of profuse diarrhoea, has emerged as an important cause of disease in AIDS patients, with additional dissemination to liver and lungs. Anti-HIV drugs give the best hope of recovery.

Cyclosporosis, Isosporosis

As with the above infections, these can be a major problem in immunodeficient patients.

SUMMARY

- Protozoal infections are usually chronic and spontaneous recovery is rare.
- With the exception of malaria, the prospects for effective vaccines are still remote. However, a vaccine giving some protection against malaria does look possible.
- Treatment relies on anti-protozoal drugs, many of them fairly toxic.

Chapter 35

Helminth disease and immunity

As emphasized in Chapter 6, these large multicellular parasites represent a formidable challenge to the immune system, and any effective immunity is usually directed against the more delicate larval stages. Though differing in detail, worm infections have several features in common: (1) well-developed *evasion* mechanisms leading to chronicity; (2) a bias towards the T_H2 type of adaptive response, featuring the cytokines IL-3, IL-4, IL-5, IL-9, and IL-13, elevated numbers of mast cells and eosinophils, and high levels of IgE; (3) a tendency to induce strong *immunopathology*; and (4) varying degrees of *immunosuppression*.

■ Schistosomiasis

Estimates of the adult worm burden, derived from counting eggs in the faeces, show that in endemic areas the burden peaks in the mid-teens and then declines. This used to be attributed to differences in contact with the lake water in which the snail vector releases the infective cercaria (see Fig. 6.1 for the life cycle), plus a possible effect of pubertal sex hormones, but careful epidemiological studies suggest that there is also an element of true immunological resistance. This appears to act against the larval stage (schistosomulum), involving (1) killing in the skin by combinations such as specific IgE–eosinophils–major basic protein, specific IgG–macrophages–NO, and (2) interference with migration of the larvae through the lungs by inflammatory reactions. Younger stages are more susceptible than older ones, so that established worms survive in the presence of immunity against subsequent infections, a situation known as *concomitant immunity*. This survival by organisms lying within blood vessels is aided by the acquisition of host molecules, including blood group and MHC antigens, fibronectin, cholesterol, and non-specific immunoglobulins; thus the worm becomes 'camouflaged' by what to the host is 'self' material. Production of factors that interfere with the complement pathway is another protective mechanism for the worms.

Immunopathology

Schistosomiasis would not be such a serious disease but for the fact that some eggs, instead of penetrating host tissues to reach the exterior, become trapped in organs such as the gut wall, liver (*Schistosoma mansoni, Schistosoma japonicum*), and bladder (*Schistosoma haematobium*). Here they provoke granuloma formation, again predominantly involving T_H2 cells, and cytokines (IL-4, IL-5, IL-13), and eosinophils. In the bladder this can lead to haematuria, urinary obstruction, calcification and, particularly in North Africa, bladder cancer. In the liver the granulomata may coalesce around the portal tracts to produce the classic 'pipe-stem fibrosis', leading to portal hypertension, dilated oesophageal varices, and haematemesis. There is some evidence that T_H1 cytokines (e.g. IFNγ) can slow the process of granuloma formation, but with this comes the danger of liver damage by molecules released by the eggs, since one of the effects of the granuloma is to wall off these toxic factors (Fig. 35.1).

Control and vaccine prospects

The evidence for at least partial immunity during natural infections is encouraging, and in animal models infection with X-irradiated cercariae, which mature to the lung stage and then die, induces up to 90% protection against subsequent challenge. Human studies have concentrated on purified or recombinant vaccine candidate antigens, notably the enzyme glutathione S-transferase (GST) and the muscle protein paramyosin. Immunity to GST appears to be largely directed against fecundity, as measured by egg output and viability. An alternative idea, still experimental, is to try and reduce immunopathology by boosting T_H1 responses; an 'anti-disease' vaccine which might reduce the amount of fibrosis around trapped eggs. Fortunately there are safe, effective, and inexpensive drugs, notably praziquantel, which kill adult worms. Public health measures to prevent contact between humans and cercariae would constitute the ideal control strategy.

Other fluke infections

Clonorchis and *Paragonimus*, infecting the liver and lung respectively, and the animal liver fluke *Fasciola*, are treatable by praziquantel and are not candidates for vaccine development.

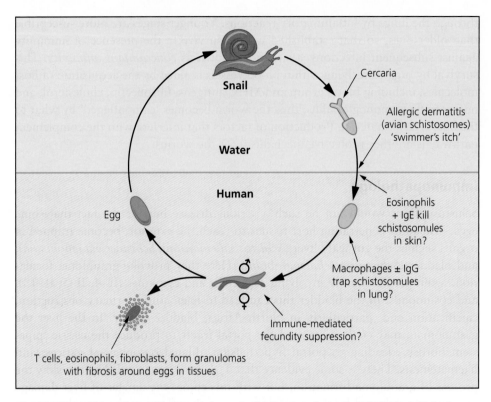

Fig. 35.1 Immunity against schistosomiasis can be both protective and pathological. Only the cercarial stage (irradiated) has so far been really effective as a vaccine (in animals).

■ Filariasis

More is known about pathological than protective immunity against filarial nematodes, but encouragingly only a small proportion of exposed individuals actually develop symptoms, suggesting that immunopathological responses are under the influence of genetic and/or environmental factors.

Lymphatic filariasis

Simple blockage of lymphatics by adult *Wuchereria* worms is not enough to explain the swelling and hardening of tissues seen in elephantiasis, and there is probably an element of chronic inflammation due to superimposed bacterial and fungal infection. The presence in the soil of quartz, which is toxic to macrophages, is thought to be another factor. However, elephantiasis is rare, and many exposed individuals clear their worms, retaining high levels of specific IgE and T_H2 cytokine responses. Others have circulating microfilariae and only minor lymphatic pathology, with suppressed T_H1 responses (e.g. IFNγ), not only to worm antigens but unrelated antigens such as BCG; this is associated with high levels of

IL-10. Interestingly, most filarial worms carry the endosymbiotic rickettsia *Wolbachia*, which produces an LPS that may contribute to inflammation. A few patients with extremely high levels of IgE and eosinophils develop a severe allergic response to microfilariae in the lung known as tropical pulmonary eosinophilia. As with schistosomiasis, both an irradiated larval and a GST vaccine have given substantial reductions in worm burden.

Onchocerciasis

The most serious complication of onchocerciasis, caused by *Onchocerca volvulus*, is *river blindness*, so named because the fly vector breeds in running water and the microfilariae migrate to the skin and eye, where they provoke damage which may be partly immunological; types I, III, and IV hypersensitivity have all been postulated. In endemic areas 2–5% of children and 4–14% of adults are blind, an incidence three times higher than for trachoma. Treatment with diethylcarbamazine, which kills microfilariae, used to be followed by an acute reaction in the skin (Mazzotti reaction) apparently due to allergy to released worm antigens. Vaccine development is still experimental, but an attenuated larval vaccine has given good results in cattle.

Current therapy for filariasis favours the drug ivermectin and programmes have been proposed for its free distribution.

Intestinal nematode infections

Evidence for a role of immunity in human nematode infections comes from the effect of *immunodeficiency* on strongyloidiasis, which became apparent with the introduction of steroid treatment in the 1960s, resulting in massive body-wide fatal larval burdens. Whether this is due to reduced larval killing (e.g. by IgE) or increased worm fecundity is not clear. A similar effect is not seen with *Ascaris*, *Trichuris*, etc., but about 10% of normal individuals have unusually high worm counts, possibly for genetic or immunological reasons. In animal models, a number of factors contribute to the killing and expulsion of worms, including the activity of T_H2 cells in increasing IgE, mucin production, smooth muscle contraction, and lipid peroxidation of the worm membrane. There is some evidence that IgE can reduce the egg output of female *Ancylostoma* (hookworms). Passage of *Ascaris* through the lungs can trigger pulmonary eosinophilia with asthma (Loeffler's syndrome). Drug treatment of *Ascaris* has been shown to improve the response to a cholera vaccine and to BCG, suggesting that here, too, the suppression of T_H1 responsiveness, for example by IL-10, is of general significance. Vaccine studies have so far been mainly carried out in sheep, using a variety of enzyme antigens, but a hookworm vaccine, composed of radiation-attenuated larvae, was for some years available for dogs. Its abandonment appears to have mainly been due to resistance on the part of vets to adopt it rather than to ineffectiveness. More recently a haemoglobinase antigen has shown promise as a vaccine in animals.

■ Hydatid disease

The hydatid cysts of *Echinococcus granulosus* (see Chapter 6) may rupture, particularly during surgical removal, releasing worm antigens into the circulation. Because of the already-present high levels of specific IgE on mast cells, massive life-threatening anaphylaxis may follow (see Fig. 23.2). It has been shown that injection of serum from a patient into his own cyst can result in killing of the worms in it; thus the cyst constitutes a protected site for the worms in an otherwise hostile environment. An experimental vaccine based on the early larval stage in dogs and sheep, and in mice, a recombinant oncosphere antigen, EG95, have given good protection, suggesting that a human vaccine may be possible.

Other tapeworm infections

Taenia saginata (in cattle) is normally harmless, but *Taenia solium* (in pigs) eggs can hatch into cysts in the muscles, eye, or brain.

■ Worms, IgE, and allergy

The increase in IgE levels and eosinophil counts in worm infections has been mentioned, and is attributed to a preponderance of T_H2 over T_H1 cell activity and the corresponding cytokines IL-4, IL-5, and IL-13. This probably allows more effective killing of the worms than PMNs, macrophages, or CTLs would be capable of, but brings with it the penalty of immunopathological (type I) reactions. Anaphylaxis in hydatid disease and asthma in *Ascaris* infection are just two examples.

Ironically, it has frequently been observed that allergies are less common in the tropics, but the earlier hypothesis that the high levels of circulating IgE blocked Fcε receptors on mast cells has not been universally upheld; alternative proposals are (1) raised levels of IL-10 by T_{reg} and B cells, and (2) direct effects of worm products on eosinophils. It has even been argued that the apparent increase in inflammatory bowel disease in developed countries is due to a lessened burden of intestinal worms. Thus innocuous worms, or worm antigens, might eventually be useful in the treatment of allergies.

SUMMARY

- Worm infections are associated with high levels of IgE and eosinophils. However, the development of effective immunity is rare.
- The best vaccines to date have consisted of larval stages attenuated by irradiation.
- Worm infections tend to inhibit allergic responses, which if fully understood might lead to effective treatment of allergies.

Chapter 36

Ectoparasites and immunity

Chapter 7 describes how arthropods can be irritating skin parasites, but also, much more importantly, vectors for many major pathogens (look back to Table 7.1). Since transmission usually occurs very rapidly, host immunity is not likely to be able to block it effectively, but will normally operate, successfully or otherwise, against the pathogen itself. However evidence is accumulating that vector-derived substances, largely in saliva, can influence the subsequent host response to the pathogen once transmitted—an interesting example of synergy between three different species which may contribute to the stability of their relationship.

■ Leishmaniasis and the sandfly

Sandflies puncture the skin to feed on blood, so their primary need is to circumvent the clotting mechanism. For this purpose, their saliva contains anticoagulants and vasodilators. It also contains molecules that induce inflammatory and antibody responses, particularly involving PMN, antigen-presenting cells and cytokines. Effects on immunity to the pathogen have been noted in both directions in different animal models—(1) enhancement of disease via inhibition of PMN, expansion of the macrophage population and the immunosuppressive cytokine IL-10, and (2) reduced disease by increasing antibody, IFNγ, and cell-mediated immunity. The CD4 T cell balance between T_H1 (protection) and T_H2 cells (susceptibility) may be critical. It has been suggested that, properly understood, saliva-derived molecules might be incorporated into a vaccine.

■ Ticks and immunomodulation

Ticks, the vectors for several viral, bacterial, and Rickettsial diseases (see Table 7.1), produce similar molecules to sandflies in their saliva, with similarly confusing effects. Tick saliva has been shown to facilitate the development of Lyme disease in mice, apparently through an inhibitory effect on antigen-presenting dendritic cells. However a specific tick protein, which associates with the pathogen within the tick, has been shown to be an effective vaccine in mice.

■ Mosquitoes and malaria

Individuals vary greatly in the number and severity of mosquito bites in the same environment, suggesting some form of natural immunity. Very intense reactions are often termed 'allergic' and anaphylaxis can occur. It has been claimed that repeated bites by non-infected mosquitoes induce a level of protection, but this is controversial. Note: repeated bites by *infected* mosquitoes X-irradiated to prevent the full parasite life cycle occurring in the human host remain the single most effective vaccine against malaria (see Chapter 34). The insect vector also plays a part in transmission-blocking vaccines, which aim to induce host antibodies against the sexual stages that interrupt the cycle in the mosquito.

■ Tsetse flies and trypanosomiasis

Again, inflammatory and immunomodulatory molecules are found in the saliva, which tend to promote T_H2-type host responses (IgE, disease progression). In animal experiments, drug-cure at the 10–15-day skin chancre stage led to resistance to reinfection.

■ Simulium (blackfly) and onchocerciasis

Repeated *Simulium* bites can give rise to severe allergic reactions ('blackfly fever') but little is known about effects on the infection in humans.

■ Chagas' disease and the reduviid ('kissing') bug

Since the manifestations of human infection with *T. cruzi* may take years to develop, it is hard to estimate the effect of vector bites and saliva on the disease.

■ Mites, allergy, and resistance

Mites in house dust, beds etc are notorious causes of hay fever, asthma, and dermatitis. Evidence for immunity in *scabies* comes mostly from animal experiments, where T_H1 responses (DTH, IFNγ) are associated with resistance to reinfection, and T_H2 (IgE) with lack of resistance. Whether significant immunity occurs in the human disease is still controversial.

Chapter 37

Emerging and future infectious diseases

The delicate balance between infectious organisms and human populations, as we have described it in this book, has been gradually established over hundreds of thousands of years. However, it is still possible for the infectious-disease profile of a population to undergo sudden alterations for a number of reasons:

1. the causative organism may be identified for a previously unrecognized disease;
2. a pathogen previously restricted to animals (zoonosis) may cross into humans;
3. new opportunistic infections may appear in immunocompromised patients;
4. a known organism may increase its virulence by mutation or gene transfer;
5. a new organism may be created accidentally or deliberately;
6. an organism may change its resistance to chemotherapy;
7. a successful vaccine campaign may be abandoned;
8. public health measures may break down;
9. travel and immigration may bring host and pathogen together for the first time;
10. climatic changes, including global warming, may expose populations to new pathogens.

In this chapter we will consider the major changes that have occurred within living memory, always bearing in mind that all infections make more impact on their first appearance in a population. For example, the arrival of plague from the East in 1347 or of syphilis from South America in 1493 must have been even more unexpected and terrifying to Europeans than the arrival of HIV to us. However, plague, syphilis, and HIV are rather exceptional and probably most of today's human diseases go back to prehistoric times; polio, schistosomiasis, and TB can be clearly recognized in ancient Egyptian documents. Domestication of animals and the setting up of closely packed urban communities around 10 000 years ago were probably the major factors in establishing the present pattern of human infections.

■ Newly identified pathogens

Several microorganisms have only been identified as the cause of disease in recent years; Tables 37.1 and 37.2 list the most important of these.

■ Newly acquired zoonoses

Unusual contacts with animals—for example African monkeys shipped to laboratories in Europe—have caused sporadic cases of severe viral disease, often haemorrhagic and fatal (Table 37.2). The proposed use of animal organs for transplantation, and in particular those of pigs, which have been genetically modified to be more suitable donors, is an obvious potential source of new virus infections, although no evidence for this has yet emerged.

Table 37.1 Some recently identified human pathogens

Organism	Disease
Chikungunya virus (1952, reemerged 2005)	Arthritis
Borrelia burgdorferi (1975)	Lyme disease
Legionella pneumophila (1976)	Legionnaire's disease
Helicobacter pylori (1983)	Gastric ulcer and cancer
Hepatitis C (1989), D, E	Hepatitis
HHV6 (1988), HHV7	Roseola infantum
HHV8 (1995)	Kaposi's sarcoma
SARS coronavirus (2003)	SARS

SARS, severe acute respiratory syndrome.

Table 37.2 Some recently identified zoonotic infections

Organism	Source	Disease
West Nile virus (1937)	Birds	Encephalitis
Chikungunya (2005)	Monkeys	Arthritis
Marburg virus (1967)	African green monkeys	Haemorrhagic fever
Lassa fever virus (1969)	Rodents	Haemorrhagic fever, shock
Monkeypox (1970)	Monkeys, squirrels	Like smallpox
Ebola virus (1976)	Bats?, monkeys	Haemorrhagic fever
Hanta virus (1978)	Rodents	Pulmonary syndrome
HIV-1, HIV-2 (1981)	Chimpanzees, monkeys	AIDS
Hendra virus (1994)	Horses	Respiratory
Variant CJD (1995)	Cattle	Spongiform encephalitis
Nipah virus (1998)	Pigs	Encephalitis
Coronavirus (2003)	Bats?	SARS

■ Opportunistic infections

During the last 50 years the number of immunocompromised individuals in the population has increased tremendously, for three reasons: (1) improved diagnosis, treatment, and survival of primary immunodeficiencies; (2) the widespread use of immunosuppressive drugs for transplantation, cancer therapy, and inflammatory disease; and (3) the AIDS pandemic. In such patients, in addition to unusually severe infections with normal pathogens, a variety of organisms previously considered harmless can become pathogenic (Table 37.3).

■ Changes in virulence

Here the classic example is influenza, where each pandemic is due to what is essentially a new recombinant virus (antigenic shift; see Chapter 22); some, such as the 'Spanish' H1N1 strain of 1918, the 'Asian' H2N2 of 1957, and the 'Hong Kong' H3N2 of 1968, have been particularly virulent. The latter two strains were recombinants between avian and human viruses, but the 1918 strain, which killed 5% of the world population, is believed to have been an unaltered porcine virus and should therefore be considered as a zoonosis. The many small outbreaks of avian flu in humans during the past decade are currently a cause of anxiety (see Box 37.1).

Table 37.3 Some important opportunistic infections (see also Table 26.7)

Organism	Disease in immunocompromised host
CMV (HHV5)	Pneumonitis, fetal abnormalities
HSV	Generalized herpes
VZV	Generalized VZV, shingles
EBV	Burkitt's lymphoma
Mycobacterium avium intracellulare	Disseminated infection
Pseudomonas aeruginosa	Skin infection, pneumonia, septicaemia
Proteus	Pneumonia
Candida albicans	Chronic mucocutaneous candidiasis
Cryptococcus neoformans	Pneumonia, meningitis
Pneumocystis carinii	Pneumonia
Penicillium marneffei	Skin lesions, systemic infection
Cryptosporidium	Diarrhoea
Giardia lamblia	Diarrhoea
Toxoplasma gondii	Brain, eye defects, also in fetus
Strongyloides	Diarrhoea, malabsorption, dissemination

Severe acute respiratory syndrome (SARS)

In 2003 a new coronavirus, originating in China, caused an outbreak of *severe acute respiratory syndrome* (SARS) with around 900 deaths, mainly in China. This is worrying because coronaviruses, a common cause of colds, are not normally fatal. One possibility is that, as with flu, an animal or bird virus was involved. If so, this is a further warning that close human–animal contact is a potent source of danger. However in this case, thanks to prompt action by WHO, the epidemic was rapidly halted, though the virus has not been eliminated.

■ Artificial creation of new pathogens

Every attenuated vaccine is in effect a new organism, deliberately created to be immunogenic but not virulent. However, when inadvertently given to immunocompromised individuals, it can give rise to a new disease (e.g. disseminated BCG-osis in T-cell-deficient babies). With the development of recombinant DNA technology

Box 37.1 Avian flu: the next pandemic?

Reminder: virology (see also Chapter 22)

Influenza is caused by an RNA virus with a genome in eight separate segments. Of the three *types*, only A is able to infect both birds and humans, B and C being confined to humans. The viral surface is coated with haemagglutinin (H) and neuraminidase (N) protein molecules, which can be one of several *subtypes*: 1–16 for H and 1–9 for N. Within each subtype (e.g. H3N2, H5N1, etc.) there are *strains* showing small antigenic differences, which may be of low or high pathogenicity.

Reminder: immunity (see also Chapter 31)

Because of frequent mutation, H and N antigens constantly undergo small changes (antigenic drift), rendering immunity much less effective. In addition, human and animal viruses can exchange RNA segments in a common host (e.g. pigs), producing a quite new combination (antigenic shift). For this reason, vaccines can only be prepared after the next expected subtype has been identified, usually only months before its arrival in the community.

Avian influenza

Wild birds are the natural host of influenza A, typically showing no symptoms, but many other hosts can also be infected, including pigs, horses, poultry, and humans, in which the infection can be severe or fatal. Recent avian flu outbreaks that spread to humans include H7N2, H7N3, H5N2, H3N2, H2N2, H1N1, and H1N2. In addition, H1N1, H1N2, and H3N2 have caused outbreaks in pigs, and H3N8 and H7N7 in horses. H3N2 has also spread from humans to pigs, and H3N8 from horses to dogs. H5 and H7 subtypes are the most pathogenic, and have been responsible for high mortality in poultry (up to 100%).

Avian and swine influenza in humans

There was considerable concern when an H5N1 outbreak in 1997 was shown to be able to infect humans and subsequently to spread from human to human, although only following very close contact. A second outbreak in 2003 has persisted up to the present, with some 600 human cases and 350 deaths, predominantly in Indonesia and China, but also as far away as Egypt. This is an unusually high mortality for influenza (about 60%); the 1918 pandemic killed 'only' about 2.5% of infected cases. How much the virus would need to change in order for human–human spread to be as efficient as with the endemic human viruses, such as H1N1, H1N2, and H3N2, is not known, but it is clearly a possibility. This raises the spectre of a global pandemic, since previous immunity to H5N1 is virtually non-existent, human–human spread is possible, and pathogenicity is high. An H1N1 'swine flu' pandemic derived from pigs occurred in 2009, with 1.6 million cases and over 19 000 deaths (a 1.2% death rate), but was declared in 2010 to be 'over'—that is, H1N1 infections, which are probably descended from the original 1918 pandemic strain, were back to their normal occasional epidemic level.

Planning for an avian flu pandemic

Seldom has a disease engendered such uncertainty. If human–human transmissability does not increase, the risk is minor. But if it does, estimates of 500 000 deaths in the UK alone are quite plausible. As with most infections, both *prevention* and *treatment* must be considered. Preventive measures include discouraging bird–human contact, banning imports, and culling infected or 'at-risk' birds. Preventive vaccination of birds is a disputed topic, the disadvantage being that a less than perfect vaccine might suppress symptoms and mortality, but allow continuing infectivity; thus it would become impossible to control spread. Vaccines for human use though available, have to be precisely tailored to a still unknown strain, and the enormous number of doses that would be

Box 37.1 (*Continued*)

required would be difficult and expensive to produce. A novel approach, the generation of monoclonal antibodies from the cells of recovered patients, looks promising in experimental animals. Antiviral drugs such as amantadine and oseltamivir (Tamiflu) would probably be effective if enough doses were available; however, production is currently held back by patent restrictions.

it has unfortunately become possible to create new organisms of increased virulence for use in biological warfare, for instance by incorporating genes for immune or antibiotic resistance. Increased virulence can also be introduced accidentally; for example a vaccinia virus incorporating the gene for IL-4, which was expected to improve its antigenicity, was actually *more* lethal in mice; in effect it was a new 'killer virus'. Recent experiments which identified how the transmission of H5N1 influenza could be increased in ferrets (the closest animal model to humans) raised the question of whether such research should be published in detail in case the information could be used for bioterrorism. A related issue is whether stocks of 'eliminated' pathogens such as smallpox should be preserved for research purposes, and if so, what the level of secrecy should be. Meanwhile, a number of naturally occurring pathogens are already considered as potential biological weapons of mass destruction and subject to stringent control (Table 37.4).

■ Drug resistance

The widespread use of antibiotics has had an enormous effect on the world of pathogens, promoting the emergence of resistant strains that may eventually

Table 37.4 Some candidate agents for biological warfare

Pathogen/disease	Type of agent	Comments
Anthrax	Bacterium	Easily spread, high mortality
Plague	Bacterium	Easily spread, high mortality
Tularemia	Bacterium	Easily spread, low mortality
Botulism	Bacterial toxin	High mortality
Smallpox	Virus	Easily spread but vaccine available
Haemorrhagic fevers	Virus	Easily spread, no available treatment
Burkholderia mallei, Burkholderia pseudomallei	Bacteria	Aerosol spread, often fatal
Ricin	Plant toxin	More suitable for use on individuals

replace the original population. Multiple-drug-resistant staphylococci and tubercle bacilli are leading examples (see Chapter 29). If the drug-resistant strain also happens to have a growth advantage in normal hosts, it would spread through untreated populations very rapidly; this may have been the case with chloroquine-resistant malaria. The emergence of *Clostridium difficile* in 2005 as a major cause of diarrhoeal disease was due to the sudden development of resistance to previously effective antibiotics which had disturbed the normal balance of bacteria in the gut.

■ Vaccine uptake

The reduction in disease following a successful vaccine campaign can easily be reversed if for some reason vaccine uptake is reduced. This is usually either because the disease is no longer seen as a threat (e.g. diphtheria in developed countries) or because the vaccine is considered, rightly or wrongly, to be dangerous. Examples of this are the pertussis 'scare' of 1978 (see Chapter 28) and the 1998 claim of a link between the MMR vaccine, bowel disease, and autism, which, though not upheld by further studies, prejudiced some parents for up to 6 years against the measles component of the vaccine, and led to an increase in cases of the disease. Some other examples of what has been aptly termed the 'vaccine confidence gap' are given in Table 37.5. Careful research in the affected areas has shown that it is not enough to have an effective vaccine, but that local customs, beliefs, fears, rumours, and media coverage need to be borne constantly in mind. Even so, every medical intervention does, of course, carry a risk, however small, and very large trials are needed before the fears of the public can be categorically dismissed.

■ Public health

Public health measures require considerable political will for their maintenance. Food and water hygiene and vector control can easily break down in the face of other priorities such as war or revolution. Even in peacetime, education of the public about the cause and transmission of disease is not always the priority it should be, and here newspapers do not help by publishing inaccurate stories and spreading unjustified 'scares'. On the other hand, delay by health authorities or governments in admitting that outbreaks have occurred, usually because of embarrassment, can seriously endanger attempts at proper control. Recent examples are BSE in the UK, SARS in China, and AIDS in South Africa.

■ Travel and immigration

Most infectious diseases have a sufficiently long incubation for a tourist or immigrant to start his or her journey healthy and become ill after arrival. There have

Table 37.5 Some reasons for the lack or decline of vaccine uptake

Reasons cited	Examples
Fear of complications:	
Autism	MMR, thiomersal (mercury additive)
Sterilization	Polio, tetanus
Encephalitis	Pertussis
Multiple sclerosis	Hepatitis B
'Unexplained death'	HPV
Disease uncommon, cost not justified	Haemophilus
Belief vaccine no longer needed	Diphtheria
Belief vaccine not effective	Flu
General objection to compulsory medical treatment	
General suspicion of government-sponsored schemes	
General suspicion of pharmaceutical industry	
Religious beliefs and traditions	

been cases where tourists have spent a single night in a tropical hotel and died of malaria, sometimes undiagnosed and not even suspected, on their return home. In the absence of breeding mosquitoes, this would not pose a danger to the public, but many pathogens can maintain themselves in a new habitat, for example the West Nile encephalitis virus in humans and animals, recently imported for the first time (1999) into the USA and now successfully established there.

■ Climate change

One of the perils of global warming will probably be the appearance of 'tropical' diseases in temperate countries whose inhabitants, genetically and immunologically unprepared for the new pathogens, would be expected to suffer worse disease than those in the tropical areas that have had thousands of years to adapt. For example, the spread of mosquito breeding north and south of the traditional tropical zone has already led to cases of malaria and dengue being seen in parts of the USA and Australia where the diseases were previously unknown and health services unprepared. Yellow fever, West Nile virus, and several forms of viral encephalitis are also expected to increase. It is possible that immigrant populations from the traditionally endemic areas would then find themselves at an advantage.

Without wishing to appear unduly fatalistic, we hope we have made clear in this chapter that the host–pathogen balance is never stationary. The tireless efforts of generations of microbiologists, epidemiologists, immunologists, and health workers of all kinds have achieved reductions in infectious disease undreamed of in earlier times, but there is plenty of opportunity for the trend to be reversed if vigilance is not maintained.

SUMMARY

- The pattern of infectious disease does not stand still. New pathogens are discovered, known pathogens may change their virulence or cross from animals to humans, or be deliberately used as weapons of war.
- Travel and immigration may introduce pathogens to populations not prepared for them, while climate change can allow pathogens to spread to previously unaffected areas.
- The successful control of infectious disease requires political stability, social compliance, constant vigilance, and considerable expense.

Tutorial 4

This section of the book has a more clinical feel which may disconcert those with no medical knowledge. By attempting the following essays, you may find you know more than you thought about the clinical implications of infection. In any case there is no harm in knowing about medical and health matters, provided you remember to let your doctor feel he/she knows more than you do. Some guides to a possible answer for each question are given on page 374.

1. 'Money should go into public health measures rather than drugs or vaccines.' Should it?

2. *... the death of the child appearing to be inevitable ... on July 6 ... little Meister was inoculated ... with a half-full syringe of spinal cord from a rabbit dead of rabies ... preserved in a dry air flask ... Joseph Meister escaped the rabies ... (Pasteur 1885)* Explain this happy outcome.

3. 'The golden age of antibiotics is past.' Is it?

4. 'Eucaryotic infections are the worst.' Are they?

5. 'AIDS is the most serious infectious disease we have ever encountered.' Do you agree?

6. What further improvements in the immune system might evolve, given time?

Further reading and information

Textbooks

Cook, G.C., Zumla, A. (eds) *Manson's Tropical Diseases.* W. B. Saunders, 21st edn., 2002.

Gill, G.V., Beeching, N. *Tropical Medicine (lecture notes).* Wiley Blackwell, 6th edn., 2009.

Giesecke, J. *Modern Infectious Disease Epidemiology.* Edward Arnold, 2nd edn., 2002.

Mandell, G. L., Bennett, J. E., Dolin, R. *Mandell, Douglas and Bennett's Principles and Practice of Infectious Diseases.* Churchill Livingstone, 7th edn., 2009.

Mayers, D. L. *Antimicrobial drug resistance: Clinical and epidemiological aspects, Volume 2.* Human Press, 2009.

Plotkin, S. A., Orenstein, W. A., Offit, P. A. (eds.) *Vaccines.* Saunders, 5th edn., 2008.

Scholar, E. M., Pratt, W. B. *The Antimicrobial drugs.* Oxford University Press, 2nd edn., 2000.

Websites

www.bmn.com/infectious-diseases (BioMedNet gateway to reviews and articles in infectious diseases.)

www.who.int/health_topics/hiv_infections/en/ (WHO HIV Infections web site.)

www.unaids.org/ (The Joint United Nations Programme on HIV/AIDS.)

www.who.int/topics/tuberculosis/en/ (WHO Tuberculosis web site.)

www.cdc.gov/ncezid (CDC Emerging Infectious Diseases web site.)

www.cdc.gov/nip/publications/pink (Epidemiology and prevention of vaccine-preventable diseases.)

http://www.cdc.gov/vaccines/ (has general information on vaccine schedules.)

http://www.who.int/topics/vaccines/en/ (a good source on vaccine preventable diseases.)

http://www.gavialliance.org/ (The Global Alliance for Vaccines and Immunization (GAVI) website.)

www.dh.gov.uk/en/Publichealth/Immunisation/Greenbook (the government document which describes the immunization procedures in the UK.)

www.tbvi.eu (European consortium for TB vaccine development.)

www.gatesfoundation.org (provides an overview of Gates funded vaccine and other public health programmes.)

www.vaccine.confidence.org (a site which monitors public confidence and scientific issues in immunization programmes.)

www.un.org/millenniumgoals/pdf/MDG (Report 2010. The Millennium Development Goals report 2010. United Nations [online (2010)].)

Recent reviews and articles

Andrade, B. B., de Oliveira, C. I., Brodskyn, C. I., Barral, A., Barral-Netto, M. 'Role of sand fly saliva in human and experimental leishmaniasis: current insights'. *Scandinavian Journal of Immunology*. 2007, 66: 122–7.

Beeching, N. J., Dance, D. A., Miller, A. R., Spencer, R. C. 'Biological warfare and bioterrorism'. *BMJ*, 2002, Feb. 9; 324 (7333): 336–9.

Bush, K., Courvalin, P., Dantas, G., Davis, J., Eisenstein, B., Huovinen, P., Jacoby, G. A., Kishony, R., Kreiswirth, B. N., Kutter, E., Lerner, A. A., Levy, S., Lewis, K., Lomovskaya, O., Miller, J. H., Mobashery, S., Piddock, L. J. V., Projan, S., Thomas, C. M., Tomasz, A., Tulkens, P. M., Walsh, T. R., Watson, J. D., Witkowski, J. W., Wright, G., Yeh, P., Zgurskaya, H. I. 'Tackling antibiotic resistance'. *Nature Reviews Microbiology*, 2011, 9, 894–6.

Casares, S., Brumeanu, T. D., Richie, T. L. Brumeanu, T. D., Richie, T. L. 'The RTS,S malaria vaccine'. *Vaccine*. 2010, Jul 12; 28 (31): 4880–94.

Cole, S. T., Riccardi G. 'New tuberculosis drugs on the horizon'. *Curr Opin Microbiol*. 2011, Oct.; 14 (5): 570–6.

Diemert, D. J., Pinto, A. G., Freire, J., Jariwala, A., Santiago, H., Hamilton, R. G., Periago, M. V., Loukas, A., Tribolet, L., Mulvenna, J., Correa-Oliveira, R., Hotez, P. J., Bethony, J. M. 'Generalized urticaria induced by the Na-ASP-2 hookworm vaccine: Implications for the development of vaccines against helminths'. *J Allergy Clin Immunol*. 2012, May 25.

Fighting child mortality (Editorial) *Nature Reviews Microbiology* 9:146 (2011).

Hancock, R. E. W., Nijnik, A., Philpott, D. J. 'Modulating immunity as a therapy for bacterial infections'. *Nature Reviews Microbiology*. 2012, 10: 243–54.

Holmgren, J., Svennerholm, A. M. 'Vaccines against mucosal infections'. *Curr Opin Immunol*. 2012, May 11.

Hotez, P. 'Enlarging the "Audacious Goal": elimination of the world's high prevalence neglected tropical diseases'. *Vaccine*. 2011, Dec. 30; 29 Suppl. 4: D104–10.

Iannitti, R. G., Carvalho, A., Romani, L. 'From memory to antifungal vaccine design'. *Trends Immunol*. 2012, May 28.

Justin, D. R., Caimano, M. J., Stevenson, B., Hu, L. T. 'Of ticks, mice and men: understanding the dual-host lifestyle of Lyme disease spirochaetes'. *Nature Reviews Microbiology*, 2012, 10, 87–99.

Kaufmann, S. H., Hussey, G., Lambert, P. H. 'New vaccines for tuberculosis'. *Lancet*. 2010, Jun. 12; 375 (9731): 2110–9.

Kman, N. E., Bachmann, D. J. 'Biosurveillance: a review and update'. *Adv Prev Med*. 2012; 2012: 301–408.

Larson, H. J., Cooper, L. Z., Eskola, J., Katz, S. L., Ratzan, S. 'Addressing the vaccine confidence gap'. *Lancet*. 2011, Aug 6; 378 (9790): 526–35.

Levine, O. S., Bloom, D. E., Cherian, T., de Quadros, C., Sow, S., Wecker, J., Duclos, P., Greenwood, B. 'The future of immunisation policy, implementation, and financing'. *Lancet*. 2011, Jul. 30; 378 (9789): 439–48.

Lienhardt, C., Glaziou, P., Uplekar, M., Lönnroth, K., Getahun, H., Raviglione, M. 'Global tuberculosis control: lessons learnt and future prospects'. *Nature Reviews Microbiology*, 2012, Jun., 10: 407–16.

Livermore, D. M. 'Fourteen years in resistance'. *Int J Antimicrob Agents*. 2012, Apr.; 39 (4): 283–94.

Livermore, D. M. 'British Society for Antimicrobial Chemotherapy Working Party on The Urgent Need: Regenerating Antibacterial Drug Discovery and Development. Discovery research: the scientific challenge of finding new antibiotics'. *J Antimicrob Chemother*. 2011 Sep.; 66 (9): 1941–4.

Marlow, R. D., Finn, A. 'The promise of immunisation against rotavirus'. *Arch Dis Child*. 2012, May 18.

McElrath, M. J., Haynes, B. F. 'Induction of immunity to human immunodeficiency virus type-1 by vaccination'. *Immunity*. 2010, Oct. 29; 33 (4): 542–54.

McMichael, A. J., Lindgren, E. 'Climate change: present and future risks to health, and necessary responses'. *J Intern Med*. 2011 Nov; 270 (5): 401–13.

McMichael, A. J., Haynes, B. F. 'Lessons learned from HIV-1 vaccine trials: new priorities and directions'. *Nat Immunol*. 2012, Apr. 18; 13 (5): 423–7.

Medina, R. A., García-Sastre, A. 'Influenza A viruses: new research developments'. *Nature Reviews Microbiology*, 2011, 9: 590–603.

Moffitt, K. L., Malley, R. 'Next generation pneumococcal vaccines'. *Curr Opin Immunol*. 2011, Jun.; 23(3): 407–13.

Oliviera, C. J. F., Sa-Nunes, A., Francischetti, I. M., Carregaro, V., Anatriello, E., Silva, J. S., Santos, I. K., Ribeiro, J. M., Ferreira, B. R. 'Deconstructing tick saliva'. *J. Biol. Chem*. 2011, 286: 10960–9.

Plotkin, S. A. 'Vaccines: past, present and future'. *Nat Med*. 2005, Apr.;11 (4 Suppl): S5–11.

Plotkin, S. A. 'Correlates of vaccine induced immunity'. *Clin Inf Diseases*, 2008; 47: 401.

Plotkin, S. A., Plotkin, S. L. 'The development of vaccines: how the past led to the future'. *Nature Reviews Microbiology*, 2011, 9: 889–93.

Poland, G. A., Jacobson, R. M., Tilburt, J., Nichol, K. The social, political, ethical, and economic aspects of biodefense vaccines. *Vaccine*. 2009, Nov. 5; 27 Suppl. 4: D23–7.

Prichard, R. K., Basáñez, M. G., Boatin, B. A., McCarthy, J. S., García, H. H., Yang, G. J., Sripa, B., Lustigman, S. 'A research agenda for helminth diseases of humans: intervention for control and elimination'. *PLoS Negl Trop Dis*. 2012, Apr; 6 (4): e1549.

Prudencio, C. R., Marra, A. O. M., Cardoso, R., Goulart, L. R. 'Recombinant peptides as new immunogens for the control of the bovine tick'. *Veterinary parasitology*. 2010. 172: 122–31.

Rinaudo, C. D., Telford, J. L., Rappuoli, R., Seib, K. L. 'Vaccinology in the genome era' *J Clin Investigation*, 2009, 119: 2515.

Siddiqui, A. A., Siddiqui, B. A., Ganley-Leal, L. 'Schistosomiasis vaccines'. *Hum Vaccin*. 2011 Nov.; 7(11): 1192–7.

White, O. J., McKenna, K. L., Bosco, A., van den Biggelaar, H. J. A., Richmond, P., Holt, P. G. 'Agenomics-based approach to assessment of vaccine safety and immunogenicity in children'. *Vaccine*. 2012, Feb. 27; 30 (10): 1865–74.

Whittle, J. R., Zhang, R., Khurana, S., King, L. R., Manischewitz, J., Golding, H., Dormitzer, P. R., Haynes, B. F., Walter, E. B., Moody, M. A., Kepler, T. B., Liao, H. X., Harrison, S. C. Broadly neutralizing human antibody that recognizes the receptor-binding pocket of influenza virus hemagglutinin. Proc Natl Acad Sci USA. 2011, Aug. 23;108 (34): 14216–21.

Willadsen, P. 'Vaccination against ectoparasites'. *Parasitology*. 2006, 133: S9–S25.

Williamson, E. D., Titball, R. W. 'Vaccines against dangerous pathogens'. *Br. Med. Bull.*, 2002, 62: 163–73.

Williamson, E. D., Duchars, M. G., Kohberger, R. 'Predictive models and correlates of protection for testing biodefence vaccines'. *Expert Rev Vaccines*. 2010, May; 9 (5): 527–37.

Willing, B. P., Shannon, L., Russell, S. L., Finlay, B. B. Shifting the balance: antibiotic effects on host–microbiota mutualism. *Nature Reviews Microbiology*, 2011, Apr., 9, 233–43.

GLOSSARY OF TERMS AND ABBREVIATIONS

acute phase (response, protein) Early response to infection, involving macrophages, cytokines, and liver

ADA adenosine deaminase

adaptive (of immunity) Lymphocyte-based, showing high specificity and memory

ADCC antibody-dependent cellular cytotoxicity

adjuvant A substance (e.g. alum, saponin) that increases the response to a vaccine given with it

aerobic Growing in the presence of oxygen

aerosol Airborne water droplet which may contain viruses, bacteria, etc.

AFB acid-fast bacilli

affinity (of antibody) A measure of binding strength to antigen

agammaglobulinaemia Absence of gammaglobulins (antibody) from serum

AIDS acquired immune deficiency syndrome

allergy Pathological antibody response resulting in acute inflammation

amino acids The building blocks of proteins

anaerobic Growing in the absence of oxygen

anaphylaxis Extreme form of allergy, often resulting in shock

anergy Lack of an expected response

antibiotic Naturally occurring antimicrobial agent

antibody Lymphocyte-derived protein molecule contributing to immunity

antigen Portion of foreign object (e.g. pathogen) recognized by a lymphocyte

antitoxin Antibody preparation for neutralizing toxin

APC antigen-presenting cell

ARC AIDS-related complex

attenuated (of vaccine) Living but with absent or reduced pathogenicity

atypical (of bacteria) Lacking some feature of normal bacteria

autoimmunity Immune response (cellular or humoral) against 'self' components

autosomal (of mutation) On a chromosome other than X or Y

AZT azidothymidine (also known as zidovudine)

Bacillus Rod-shaped bacterium

bacteriophage Virus specialized for infecting bacteria

B cell Bone-marrow-derived lymphocyte

BCG bacille Calmette–Guérin (the attenuated TB vaccine)

biofilm Layer of bacteria growing as a unit

BSE bovine spongiform encephalopathy

C (gene, region) Constant

capsid Outer protein layer of a virus

capsule Anti-phagocytic outer coat, for example of bacterium, usually polysaccharide

carrier Symptomless individual infectious to others; (in a vaccine) protein component to which, for example, sugars are attached

CD cluster of differentiation (numbering system for cell-surface molecules)

CDR complementarity-determining region (e.g. of antibody)

cell The basic structural element of animals and plants

cellular (of immune response) Mediated by T lymphocytes but not antibody

CGD chronic granulomatous disease

chemokine A cytokine that promotes cell movement

chemotherapy (of infection) Treatment by natural or synthetic antimicrobial compounds

chitin Stiffening polysaccharide component of fungal wall

chloroplast Organelle in plant cell containing respiratory enzymes

chromosome Structure along which a cell's genes are organized

cirrhosis Destruction of liver tissue by fibrosis

CJD Creutzfeld–Jakob disease

class (of antibody) Subdivision with particular biological function (*see also* Ig)

clonal selection Mechanism by which lymphocytes responding to a particular antigen are expanded into a larger number (originally a theory)

CMV cytomegalovirus

CNS central nervous system

coccus A spherical bacterium

combining site (of antibody) Region that binds to antigen and defines specificity

commensal Harmlessly parasitic

complement Series of serum proteins involved in immune defence

complex (immune-) *See* immune complex

co-stimulation The requirement for two or more stimuli

CR complement receptor

CRP C-reactive protein (an acute phase protein)

CSF colony-stimulating factor

CTL cytotoxic T lymphocyte

cyst (e.g. of protozoa, worm) Hollow structure facilitating survival

cytokine Molecule mediating cellular interactions in the immune system

cytopathic Causing damage to cells

cytoplasm Contents of cell, other than the nucleus

cytotoxic Able to kill cells; also a subdivision of T lymphocytes, usually carrying CD8 molecules

DAF decay-accelerating factor

DC dendritic cell

decoy Protective microbial analogue of immune molecule

DNA deoxyribonucleic acid (genetic material, composed of nucleotides)

dominant (of mutation) Producing effect in a single dose

DPT The triple diphtheria–pertussis–tetanus vaccine

DTH delayed-type hypersensitivity

dysentery Diarrhoea containing blood

EBV Epstein–Barr virus

ectoparasite An arthropod parasite inhabiting the skin

endemic (of infection) Constantly present in a population

endocytosis The taking in of an object by a cell

endoplasmic reticulum A membrane system in eucaryotic cells

endosome Internal cell structure involved in endocytosis

endotoxin Toxin released by a dead organism, usually a bacterium

enzyme A protein that catalyses a particular chemical reaction

eosinophil A white blood cell containing granules toxic to, for example, worms

epidemic (of infection) Occurring at an unusually high frequency

eucaryote Single or multicellular nucleated organism, such as a protozoan or mammal

exotoxin Toxin secreted by a living organism, usually a bacterium

Fab Antigen-binding fragment (immunoglobulin)

Fc Crystallizable fragment (immunoglobulin)

FcR Fc (of antibody) receptor

FDC follicular dendritic cell

fibrosis Replacement of normal tissue structure by fibres of, for example, collagen

filaria A thread-like roundworm

fimbria (plural: fimbriae) Bacterial attachment organ similar to a pilus

flagellum (plural: flagella) Thread-like organ of, for example, bacterial movement

GALT gut-associated lymphoid tissue

GCSF granulocyte colony-stimulating factor

gene Unit of heredity, composed of DNA

genome The total of all genes in the cell or animal

germ-line (gene, mutation) In sperm or ova and therefore inherited

germ theory Theory proposed by Koch that microbes caused specific diseases

glucan Polysaccharide of glucose, for example cellulose and starch

granuloma Chronic inflammatory focus mainly composed of macrophages

H- N- Haemaglutinin and neuraminidase antigens of flu virus

HAART highly active anti-retroviral therapy

helminth A name covering the parasitic classes of worms

helper cell Subdivision of T lymphocytes that activate B lymphocytes, macrophages, etc. by secreting cytokines; usually carry CD4 molecules

herd immunity Freedom from infection of the unprotected minority in a mainly immune population

HHV human herpesvirus (eight types)

HIB *Haemophilus influenzae* type B

HIF hypoxia inducible factor

HIV human immunodeficiency virus (two types, HIV-1 and HIV-2)

HLA human leucocyte antigen (*see also* MHC)

hormone Molecule regulating cell functions, for example insulin and thyroxine

HPV human papilloma virus

HSV herpes simplex virus (two types, HSV1 and HSV2)

HTLV human T-cell lymphotropic virus

humoral (of immune response) Mediated by antibody

hybrid vigour Improved qualities produced by crossing two different strains

ICAM intercellular adhesion molecule

IFN interferon

Ig immunoglobulin (e.g. IgM, IgG, etc.)

IL interleukin (e.g. IL-1, IL-2, etc.)

immune (to a pathogen) Resistant to infection; (to an antigen) Able to mount an enhanced response

immune complex Combination of antigen and antibody

immunity The state of being immune

immunize To induce immunity, for example by vaccination

immunoglobulin (Ig) Synonymous with antibody (*see* Ig)

immunopathology Tissue damage caused by the immune system

inflammation Local tissue response to injury or infection, with increased blood flow and pain

innate (of immunity) Initial non-adaptive, non-lymphocyte-based

integrins A group of cell-adhesion molecules

interferon (IFN) Family of antiviral cytokines (three types, α, β, γ)

interleukin (IL) Numbered member of the cytokine family

in vitro In laboratory culture (literally, 'in glass')

in vivo In the living animal

ISCOM immunostimulatory complex

isotype (of antibody) Class or subclass

J (gene, chain) Joining

KIR killer cell immunoglobulin-like receptor

latent (e.g. of virus) Persistent but symptomless

lectin Plant or animal molecule that binds to particular sugars

leucocyte White blood cell

LFA lymphocyte function antigen

lichen a symbiotic fusion of fungi and algae

ligand Molecule with specific binding properties

lipid Fat-based water-insoluble molecule

LPS lipopolysaccharide (the major bacterial endotoxin)

LT leukotriene (one of a group of inflammatory molecules)

lymphatic Vessel transmitting fluid and cells from tissues to and between lymph nodes lymphocyte White cell of the blood, the cell of adaptive immunity

lysis Damage-induced leakage of cell contents

lysosome Intracellular vesicle containing killing and digestive material

lysozyme An enzyme in blood, tears, and saliva that kills some bacteria

macrophage Large phagocytic cell, mainly found in tissues

MALT mucosa-associated lymphoid tissue

mannan Polysaccharide of mannose

mast cell Tissue cell containing inflammatory mediators

MBL mannose-binding lectin

MBP major basic protein

memory (in immunology) Ability to respond more vigorously to a second identical stimulus

meninges Lining layer between skull and brain

messenger RNA (mRNA) RNA carrying information to make protein

metabolic Related to biochemical processes in the cell

MHC major histocompatibility complex (a set of highly diverse genes; MHC molecules are responsible for transport of intracellular peptides for recognition by T lymphocytes, and thus also for graft rejection)

miasma Hypothetical medium transmitting infection (before germ theory)

mitochondrion Intracellular organelle containing respiratory enzymes

MMR The triple measles, mumps, and rubella vaccine

molecule Chemical unit of (in biology) protein, carbohydrate, fat, or nucleic acid

monoclonal (of antibody) Produced by a single clone of identical B lymphocytes

MRSA methicillin- (or multiple-drug-) resistant *Staphylococcus aureus*

mutation Change in DNA affecting one or a few bases, which can be inherited if it arises in the germ-line

mycosis Fungal infection

myeloid A lineage of marrow-derived cells; includes PMNs and monocytes

natural selection Evolution based on mutation and survival of the fittest variants

NBT nitroblue tetrazolium (assay)

network (in immunology) A set of interacting cells or molecules (e.g. cytokines)

neutropenia Low level or absence of neutrophils in the blood

neutrophil *see* PMN

NK cell natural killer cell

NLR NOD-like receptor

NOD nucleotide oligomerization domain-containing protein

normal flora The microbial content of the normal body (intestine, skin, etc.)

nosocomial Disease acquired in hospital

nucleic acids *see* DNA *and* RNA

nucleolus Structure within the cell nucleus, rich in RNA

nucleotide A single unit of a nucleic acid (purine or pyrimidine)

nucleus Membrane-bound region of eucaryotic cell containing chromosomes

oncogene Gene predisposing to tumour development

opportunist Organism pathogenic only in immunodeficient host

opsonin Molecule capable of enhancing phagocytosis, for example antibody or complement

PAMP pathogen-associated molecular pattern

pandemic A worldwide epidemic

parasite A living organism depending on another for some or all of its requirements

passage (pronounced as in French) A cycle of growth *in vitro* or *in vivo* during, for example, the attenuation of a vaccine

passive (of immunity) Transferred from another source, for example by serum

pathogen A parasite causing disease

peptide Molecule composed of two or more amino acids

PG prostaglandin

phagocytosis Ingestion of particles by, for example, a protozoan or phagocytic cell

pilus (plural: pili) Thread-like bacterial attachment organ

plasma Blood minus the cells

plasmid Non-chromosomal DNA, for example in bacterium

PMN polymorphonuclear neutrophil (the major phagocytic cell of blood)

polyclonal Affecting many different clones (e.g. of lymphocytes)

polymerase Enzyme involved in synthesis of RNA and DNA

polymorph *see* PMN

polymorphism Coexistence in a population of two or more versions of the same gene

polysaccharide Complex sugar molecule

presentation (e.g. of antigen) Delivery to an effector cell

primary (of immune response) Following first contact with antigen; (of immunodeficiency) genetically determined

prion Infectious particle containing protein only (*see also* BSE, CJD)

procaryote Single-celled organism without nucleus, for example a bacterium

prostaglandin (PG) One of a family of small lipid molecules involved in inflammation

protein Molecule composed of amino acids and coded in DNA

proteome The sum of all proteins expressed by an organism

PrP prion protein

PRR pattern-recognition receptor

purine One type of nucleotide (pyrimidine is the other type)

pyrimidine One type of nucleotide (purine is the other type)

pyrogen Molecule stimulating fever

receptor Molecule on a cell surface to which a virus, cytokine, etc. binds

recessive (of mutation) Producing an effect only in double dose

recirculation (of lymphocytes) Passage from blood to tissues and back

recognition (by immune cell or molecule) Specific binding

recombinant (of DNA) Combined from two or more sources

reservoir (of infection) Alternative (e.g. animal) source of infection

retrovirus RNA virus able to insert DNA into host cell genome

reverse transcriptase An enzyme used by retroviruses to transcribe their RNA into DNA

ribosome Site of protein synthesis from messenger RNA template

RIG retinoic acid-inducible gene

RNA ribonucleic acid (intermediary between DNA and protein synthesis, composed of nucleotides)

ROI reactive oxygen intermediates

RSV respiratory syncytial virus

SAP serum amyloid A protein

SARS severe acute respiratory syndrome

SCID severe combined immune deficiency

secondary (of immune response) Following second or later contact with antigen; (of immunodeficiency) environmentally caused

selectin One of a group of cell-adhesion molecules

self (of antigen) Derived from host

sepsis Septicaemia with multi-organ involvement

septicaemia Invasion of the bloodstream, usually by bacteria

serum Blood minus cells and clotting factors

sex-linked (of disease) Occurring in one sex only; *see also* X-linked shock Vascular collapse, with low blood pressure and often organ failure

SIV simian immunodeficiency virus

somatic (of mutation) In a cell other than germ-line; not inherited

SP surfactant protein (SP-A, SP-D)

specific (in immunology) Denoting restriction to one or a few antigens

spleen Large abdominal organ with haematological and immune functions

spore Resistant resting form of bacteria or fungi

Staph. Common abbreviation for staphylococcus

stem cell Cell able to give rise to many or all other cell types

strain Genetically identical subdivision of a species (e.g. mouse, *Staphylococcus*)

Strep. Common abbreviation for streptococcus

superantigen Antigen that stimulates multiple clones of lymphocytes

symbiosis Association between living organisms that is beneficial to both

taxonomy Science by which living organisms are classified

TB tuberculosis

T cell Thymus-derived lymphocyte

TCR T-cell receptor

TGF transforming growth factor (a mainly inhibitory cytokine)

T_H T helper cell (T_H1, T_H2, T_H17)

thymus Lymphoid organ in the neck, the source of T lymphocytes

TLR Toll-like receptor

TNF tumour necrosis factor (an inflammatory cytokine)

tolerance (in immunology) Unresponsiveness to a normally antigenic stimulus

toxin Microbial product, usually protein, able to damage host cells

toxoid Inactivated toxin able to induce immunity as a vaccine

transcriptome Sum of all RNAs transcribed

transduction Gene transfer in bacteria by a bacteriophage virus

transposon Chromosome or plasmid gene(s) transferable between bacteria

TSST toxic shock syndrome toxin

V (gene, region) Variable

vaccine A preparation able to induce immunity, usually a killed or attenuated microorganism or portion thereof

vacuole Membrane-bound, fluid-containing intracellular structure

vCJD new-variant Creutzfeld–Jakob disease

vector (of pathogens) Transmitting insect or animal; (of genes) transmitting element, for example plasmid, bacteriophage

vesicle Membrane-bound, fluid-containing intracellular structure

Vibrio A group of curved bacteria, of which *Vibrio cholerae* causes human disease (cholera)

virulence Ability of a pathogen to survive in and/or damage host

VZV varicella zoster virus (the virus of chickenpox and shingles)

wild-type Normal or predominant (e.g. not mutant) type of organism

X-linked (of disease) Due to mutation on the X chromosome

zoonosis An animal disease that can affect humans

APPENDIX 1
The major causes of human infection

Upper respiratory tract

Rhinovirus
Coronavirus
Adenovirus
Echovirus
Coxsackie virus
Epstein–Barr virus (EBV)
Influenza virus
Streptococcus pyogenes
Haemophilus influenzae
Diphtheria

Lower respiratory tract

Influenza, parainfluenza
Respiratory syncytial virus (RSV)
Measles virus
Adenovirus, rhinovirus
Streptococcus pneumoniae
Bordetella pertussis
Haemophilus
Staphylococcus aureus
Mycobacterium tuberculosis
Legionella
Pseudomonas

Ear infection

Mumps virus
Respiratory syncytial virus (RSV)
Streptococcus pneumoniae

Eye infection

Adenovirus
Measles virus
Streptococcus pneumoniae

Trachoma
Toxoplasma
Onchocerca

Meningitis and encephalitis

Herpesvirus
Varicella zoster virus (VZV)
Measles virus
Human immunodeficiency virus (HIV)
Polio virus
Rabies virus
Mycobacterium tuberculosis
Neisseria meningitidis
Haemophilus
Malaria
Trypanosomiasis
Toxoplasma

Gastroenteritis

Rotavirus
Salmonella spp.
Shigella
Escherichia coli
Vibrio cholerae
Campylobacter
Helicobacter
Entamoeba
Giardia
Cryptosporidium
Strongyloides

Food poisoning

Staphylococcus aureus
Bacillus cereus
Clostridium botulinum

Urinary infection

Escherichia coli
Proteus
Staphylococci

Sexually transmitted

Herpesvirus (HHV1, HHV2)
Human immunodeficiency virus (HIV)
Hepatitis B
Papilloma virus
Neisseria gonorrhoeae
Syphilis
Chlamydia
Candida
Trichomonas

Skin

Measles virus
Rubella virus
Herpes simplex virus
Chickenpox/zoster virus
Papilloma virus
Staphylococcus
Streptococcus
Clostridium perfringens
Propionibacterium acnes
Mycobacterium leprae
Candida albicans
Dermatophyte spp
Leishmaniasis
Onchocerciasis
Lice
Scabies

Bones and joints

Hepatitis B virus
Chikungunya virus
Staphylococcus

Streptococcus
Mycobacterium tuberculosis
Neisseria gonorrhoea

Liver

Hepatitis viruses
Yellow fever virus
Leptospirosis
Amoebiasis (abscess)
Schistosoma

Heart and other muscles

Coxsackie virus
Corynebacterium diphtheriae
Trypanosoma cruzi
Taenia solium
Echinococcus granulosus
Trichinella spiralis

Sepsis and shock

Dengue
Neisseria meningitidis
Escherichia coli
Staphylococcus
Streptococcus

Pyrexia (fever) of unknown origin

Human immunodeficiency virus
EB virus
Hepatitis viruses
Rickettsia typhi (typhus)
Mycobacterium tuberculosis
Salmonella typhi (typhoid)
Brucella
Borrelia spp. (Lyme disease; relapsing fever)
Malaria
Amoebiasis

APPENDIX 2
Cytokines featured in this book (See also Tables 12.4, 19.1, and 20.1.)

Cytokine	Main cell source	Main functions
IL-1	Mac	Acute phase response, fever
IL-2	T	B-cell activation, T- and NK-cell proliferation
IL-3	T	Haemopoiesis
IL-4	T_H2, NKT	T_H2 differentiation, B-cell activation, Ig switch
IL-5	T_H2	B cell, eosinophil growth, IgA switch
IL-6	T, Mac	B cell, plasma cell differentiation, acute phase response
IL-7	Bone marrow	Early T- and B-cell maturation
IL-8	Leucocytes	Cell migration
IL-10	T_H2, T_{reg}	B-cell proliferation, macrophage inhibition
IL-12	Mac, DC	T_H1, NK activation
IL-13	T_H2	IgE switch, macrophage inhibition
IL-15	Mac	T- and NK-cell proliferation
IL-17	T_H17	Induction of IL-1, TNF, chemokines
IL-18	Mac, DC	T- and NK-cell activation
IL-23	Mac, DC	T_H1, memory T differentiation
IFNα	Mac	Antiviral, T_H1
IFNβ	Fibroblasts	Antiviral
IFNγ	T_H1, NK, CTL	Antiviral, B-cell IgG switch, macrophage activation
TNF	T, DC	Acute phase response, inflammation
TGF-β	T, Mac	B-cell IgA switch, inhibit T cells and macrophages

DC, dendritic cell; IFN, interferon; IL, interleukin; Mac, macrophage; NK, natural killer; T, T cell; TGF, transforming growth factor; TNF, tumour necrosis factor.

APPENDIX 3
Cluster of differentiation (CD) antigens

Over 250 CD antigens have been identified. The following are those mentioned in this book.

CD number	Other names	Cell distribution	Main functions/comments
1		T, B, DC	Presentation of glycolipid antigens
2	LFA2	T, NK	Co-stimulation
3		T	Linked to T-cell receptor
4		T helper	Binds to MHC II; also receptor for HIV
8		Cytotoxic T	Binds to MHC I
14		DC, Mono, Mac, Gran	LPS binding
16	FcγRIII	NK, Mac	Aids phagocytosis
19		B	Co-stimulation of B cells
21	CR2	B	Aids antigen uptake
23	Fcε receptor	B, Mac	Low-affinity IgE receptor
28		T, B	Co-stimulation
32	Fcγ RII	Mac, B, Eos	Aids phagocytosis
35	CR1	Mac, B	Aids phagocytosis
40		Mac, B	Interaction with T_H cells
44		Memory T	Leucocyte adhesion
45		Leucocytes	Lymphocyte activation
46		Widespread	Regulates complement; also receptor for measles virus
64	FcγRI	Mac	Aids phagocytosis
81		B	Co-stimulation
89	FcαR	Mac	Cytotoxicity

B, B cell; CR, receptor for complement; DC, dendritic cell; Eos, eosinophil; FcR, receptor for Ig Fc region; Gran, granulocyte; HIV, human immunodeficiency virus; Mac, macrophage; MHC, major histocompatibility complex; Mono, monocyte; NK, natural killer; T, T cell.

APPENDIX 4
Some methods used in studying infection and immunity

■ Microbiological methods

A highly desirable step in the investigation of any suspected infectious disease is the identification of the responsible pathogen, which is usually a pointer to the most suitable treatment. Methods in common use include (1) **microscopy**, frequently preceded by **culture** and assisted by **staining,** and (2) **genetic** analysis.

Microscopy

Bacteria and all larger organisms are well within the resolving power of the light microscope. Microscopy is usually combined with **staining** to make bacteria visible and help in diagnosis. The Gram stain, which classifies bacteria by their cell wall structure into **positive** (e.g. staphylococci) and **negative** (e.g. meningococci) is particularly useful. Immediate microscopy can be life-saving; e.g. in the examination of cerebrospinal fluid in suspected meningitis. The Ziehl-Neilsen (acid-fast) stain is valuable for identifying mycobacteria; e.g. in sputum. When specific monoclonal antibodies are available, they can be coupled to fluorescent dyes and positively stained bacteria visualized under ultraviolet light. With larger pathogens such as fungi, protozoa, and helminths, microscopy alone is often sufficient for identification.

Culture

Generally, samples for bacterial analysis contaminated with other material are first grown on suitable culture media (e.g. blood agar or liquid media) in such a way that individual clonal bacterial colonies can be isolated for study. Sputum, faeces, urine, and blood are commonly treated in this way. Incorporation of antibiotic-impregnated paper discs into culture plates allows bacterial sensitivity to antibiotics to be evaluated.

Electron microscopy

Viruses can only be clearly seen in the electron microscope, but methods are expensive and elaborate for routine use. Standard identification of viruses is by specific monoclonal antibodies coupled to an enzyme that can be visualized colorimetrically in the presence of its substrate (**ELISA**), a test that lends itself to the rapid analysis of large numbers of samples. The specific antibody is bound to plastic wells followed by the suspected antigen and finally a second antibody 'labelled' with the enzyme. Unbound second antibody is washed off and the colour change read automatically. A variation of this technique can also be used to detect antibody, e.g. in serum (see below).

Genetic methods

Very precise characterization of microorganisms is possible by analysis of their genomic DNA via the binding of complementary labelled oligonucleotide probes. It is generally necessary to expand the DNA sequences available for testing by the use of the polymerase chain reaction (**PCR**), an ingenious technique that can replicate a chosen DNA sequence by a factor of millions. Modern, high-throughput sequencing technology, including 'deep sequencing' where each sequence is read multiple times to reduce error, allows complete and rapid analysis of multiple genomes at a fraction of the cost and time of previous methods. By incorporating a reverse transcriptase step, mRNA sequences can also be measured. This can either be done for specific genes of interest using for example real-time PCR or for the entire transcriptome using microarray chips such as those from Affymetrix or Illumina. The newest technology of RNASeq, where high throughput sequencing of cDNA is used to determine RNA expression, is now increasingly used but requires expensive equipment and the ability to analyse extremely large data sets. Genetic analysis can be useful at all levels, from the rapid identification of a bacterial or viral species to the detection of very small changes, e.g. in the expression of a particular virulence factor or, in epidemiological studies, to pinpoint the source and timing of new or emerging variants.

■ Immunological methods

Both humoral (serological) and cellular arms of the immune system can be assessed by laboratory assays, often using **antibodies** for detection and **automated** machines for rapid large-scale results.

Serology

Levels of immunological serum components are frequently requested, particularly where immunodeficiency is suspected. Total immunoglobulins (Ig), separate Ig classes, complement components, acute-phase proteins (e.g. CRP) and, more rarely, individual cytokines, can all be measured using **ELISA**. To measure antibody specific for an individual pathogen the test is modified by coating the plastic wells with the antigen, followed by the serum to be tested and finally labelled anti-human Ig antibody. To detect antigen (e.g. a particular virus) the order is reversed, thus: specific antibody, suspected antigen, second specific antibody.

In suspected autoimmunity, serum can be applied to a panel of human tissue sections or a blood film, followed by labelled anti-human Ig—usually labelled with a fluorescent dye to enable precise localization of binding within the cells or tissues; e.g. in kidney: the glomerular tuft in glomerulonephritis, the basement membrane in Goodpasture's disease.

Cellular analysis

Gross abnormalities can often be seen in a simple stained blood film; e.g. abnormal red cells, absent polymorphs, an excess of lymphocytes in leukaemia. However the standard 'blood profile' is obtained by **flow cytometry**, in which blood is passed through a fine jet and across one or more laser beams; 'forward' and 'side' light scatter of each cell being plotted graphically to give a distribution diagram of cell size and granularity, from which the relative numbers of the major cell types can be calculated and plotted. A more powerful machine, the fluorescence-activated cell sorter (**FACS**) counts and separates cells on the basis of single or multiple monoclonal antibodies labelled with different coloured fluorochromes and binding to cell-surface 'markers' characteristic of T cells, B cells, etc., and their subpopulations. Similar laser-based assays such as Cytokine Bead Array (CBA) and Luminex are also used to measure multiple cytokines in one assay, using very small sample volumes.

Functional assays

These are particularly useful for assessing T cell function *in vitro*, and include responses to mitogens (e.g. PHA), to specific antigens, or in transplant patients, to cells from a proposed donor. Typical responses include proliferation (measured by 3H thymidine incorporation into DNA or more recently by dilution of the cell-bound dye CFSE as each round of cell division occurs), cytokine release (measured by ELISA or by ELISPOT, the latter providing the frequency of cells which produce a cytokine), and occasionally cytotoxicity against tumour cells. There is a simple and rapid test for the 'oxidative burst' in neutrophils, depending on their ability during phagocytosis to reduce a yellow dye, nitroblue tetrazolium (**NBT**) to granular blue formazan.

Genetic methods

Rather than detecting very small amounts of some proteins (e.g. cytokines) in the blood, it is often better to measure expression of the relevant gene (DNA) directly via the amount of corresponding mRNA (the transcriptome, see p. 57). Complete transcriptional profiling of peripheral blood cells from individuals responding to vaccines or infected with pathogens is now frequently used in a research setting and provides a detailed picture of which genes are expressed during immune responses. Another useful role for DNA analysis is in typing 'tissue' antigens, mainly HLA, before transplantation, where genetic methods have largely replaced the earlier and slower microcytoxicity and mixed-lymphocyte tests.

In vivo testing

Two categories of immune responsiveness can be evaluated in the clinic by skin testing for hypersensitivity. In allergies, the offending antigen can usually be identified by a skin prick test using a panel of standard allergens; a reddened weal appearing within minutes (**immediate** reaction) denotes the presence of specific IgE antibody on the local mast cells.

In contrast, a **delayed** reaction (2–3 days) to intradermal injection of antigen occurs when a sufficiently large population of memory T cells exists, indicating previous exposure. Delayed tests are mainly used in tuberculosis, leprosy, and some protozoal infections.

HINTS AND SUGGESTIONS FOR ANSWERS TO TUTORIAL QUESTIONS

Tutorial 1

Here are some hints and pointers to answering the tutorial questions for Part 1. Remember, there is never one single perfect answer to an essay question.

1. The minister was incorrect in that (1) malaria is caused by a protozoan, not a virus, (2) it is not spread by uncooked meat but by a mosquito, and (3) vaccines against it are still experimental. He was correct in that (1) it was once widespread in Europe and could be again if the mosquitoes could breed there, and (2) it is definitely unwise to eat uncooked meat abroad, mainly because of contamination with bacteria and worms. (As a matter of additional interest there is no malaria in Nairobi because of its height above sea level.) Descriptions of infectious organisms in the newspapers are often full of errors.

2. Do not assume the question means only *parasitic* bacteria! It would be wise to include a discussion of the vital importance of bacteria in the evolution of life on Earth, in the maintenance of ecosystems, of carbon, nitrogen, sulphur cycles, etc., and in modern molecular biology. You could mention that some antibiotics come from bacteria (although of course they might not be needed if there were no bacterial diseases). Then you could consider the role of bacteria in ruminants, in which they are responsible for digesting cellulose (a cow's rumen contains over 100 litres, with 10^{10} or more bacteria per millilitre). This would lead on to the human gut flora, generally considered to have an important, although not vital, function. Finally the comparatively few bacteria that cause human disease could be discussed; it would be reasonably safe to conclude that, as individuals, we would be better off without these, although the increased lifespan that has already resulted from reducing infectious disease is causing medical and social problems at the population level.

3. A tricky question and really a matter of definition. What is life? If the ability to infect and self-replicate is sufficient, they are certainly living. But if metabolic activity is also a requirement, they are not, since they depend on their host cell to supply this. A safe compromise would be to regard them as mobile sets of genes with their own reproductive capacity, although this gets very close to including bacterial plasmids in the definition. In fact, this is an academic rather than a seriously important question.

4. Again, the short answer is that the best parasites do not make their hosts ill, and certainly do not kill them in large numbers. This might lead on to the argument that host–parasite pairs, given time, will evolve towards the most mutually beneficial relationship, the lethal parasites being only recently, or accidentally, acquired. But is this true? Some bacterial toxins may have to destroy tissues to allow the bacteria to spread. An organism may have to cause diarrhoea to get back into the water supply. Does the occasional host death matter to such organisms? In Part Two you will see that the role of the immune system has to be taken into account too, but even at this stage you could build up an interesting debate. Keeping the examiner *interested* is half the battle: you can lose far more marks by being boring (or illegible) than by the odd error of fact.

5. This is a good example of a question to which nobody knows the complete answer, since we can never know what would have happened if higher animals had not evolved. Nevertheless, there is a lot to say. You might perhaps divide your higher animals into *humans* and the rest. Clearly humans, with our vaccines and antibiotics, have made a huge impact: the elimination of smallpox being a really major triumph. When you know more about antibiotics, however, you will see that they are a two-edged weapon, with the ability to drive microbial evolution faster (penicillin resistance, etc.). Then there is the amazing power of genetic engineering to create mutant or recombinant microbes that never existed before, whose possibilities make yesterday's science fiction today's fact. But leaving humans aside, higher animals have been useful to microbes rather than the opposite; think of the difficulty the malaria parasite would have in spreading from person to person without the help of mosquitoes (or, as some parasitologists would put it, in spreading from mosquito to mosquito without help from humans). The expansion of higher species must have opened up possibilities for the development of new viruses, since many of these are quite species-specific.

Tutorial 2

Here are some ideas for you to consider.

1. This is from Metchnikoff's classic paper in which he described phagocytes eating fungal particles in a transparent water flea. Fundamentally, he was right; the phagocyte is probably the single most valuable antimicrobial element. But it is of course not the only one! In Metchnikoff's day, scientists were sharply divided into proponents of cells as the major defence mechanism, and champions of humoral factors such as antibody. Since both are important, frequently acting together (as proposed by Sir Almroth Wright in 1903), the debate eventually died out. Amazingly enough, it was not until the 1950s and 1960s that lymphocytes were proved to be involved in immunity at all!

2. Alexine was the original name for complement, and the clumping substance was *antibody*. Put into modern language, what Bordet was saying was that injecting rabbit blood (i.e. red cells, a safer substitute for bacteria) into a guinea-pig induced the formation of antibody against the red cells, which would clump them in a test tube. But in order to destroy (i.e. lyse) the red cells, something from normal rabbit serum is needed, namely complement: actually a series of interacting proteins that can punch holes in membranes. This experiment illustrates perfectly the distinction between innate (complement) and adaptive (antibody) immunological molecules.

3. This is a useful analogy, emphasizing the fact that cytokines are small soluble molecules that convey instructions from cell to cell. Thus thyroid-stimulating hormone (TSH) 'tells' the thyroid to secrete thyroxine; the cytokine IFNγ 'tells' macrophages to secrete TNF; the 'target' cells carry receptors for TSH and IFNγ, respectively. However, TSH is made only in the pituitary, and acts only on the thyroid, whereas IFNγ is made by several cell types (T cells, NK cells), acts on many cells, and produces many different effects. Also it exerts most of its activity on cells in the immediate vicinity, whereas with TSH it is the blood level that matters, since pituitary and thyroid cells cannot make direct contact. Note that there are molecules such as erythropoietin that are often classified as both hormones and cytokines, so the definitions are not really precise, and either a 'yes' or a 'no' answer to the question could be justified, provided the facts were right and the case well argued.

4. It depends what you mean by better. For a rapid response to, for example, bacterial infection, the more cells that can be involved the better, which means that some cells must recognize more than one type of bacterium. Phagocytes and (for viruses) NK cells do this; that is, they are non-specific. But for developing memory, to deal progressively better with infections that are not got rid of rapidly and recur frequently, it is more economical for only a few cells to respond initially and then build up their numbers, leaving others to deal with infections with other microbes. Lymphocytes do this: they are specific. Each approach has its strengths and weaknesses, and higher animals seem to require both for healthy life. The analogy with a police force (street patrol versus detectives) is useful: try and imagine a force restricted to one or the other type of officer.

5. A typical overstatement but it contains a germ of truth. The earliest organisms are thought to have developed in the absence of oxygen, and even today some, notably the anaerobic bacteria, are killed by it. The evolution of electron-transport chains using oxygen permitted the emergence of aerobic respiration, but even aerobic cells are susceptible to the toxic effects of ROI: superoxide, hydrogen peroxide, hydroxyl radicals, singlet oxygen. In phagocytic cells, these are generated following phagocytosis and kill the majority of bacteria and fungi. The cell itself is protected by catalase, glutathione, etc., but escaping ROI are thought to be responsible for degenerative diseases of blood vessels, lung, brain, etc.

6. NK cells are so named because, like all other components of the innate ('natural') immune system, they act rapidly and use germ-line-encoded receptors. By contrast the cytotoxic T lymphocytes, which kill in the same way but carry specific receptors and develop memory, might be called 'adaptive killer cells'. The distinction between innate and adaptive immune mechanisms is not just for the convenience of teachers and students, but represents two fundamentally different ways of going about the job of recognizing and disposing of foreign invaders, in this case intracellular viruses.

Tutorial 3

Here are some suggestions for your answer to each question.

1. Pauling was the most famous proponent of the *instructive* or *template* theory, whereas Burnet thought out the *clonal selection* theory, to which everyone now subscribes. The problems for instructive theories were (1) different antibodies do not in fact have the same amino acid sequence, (2) they could not explain memory or tolerance, (3) once the genetic code was understood there was no mechanism for an antigen to induce a permanent change in DNA, (4) eventually it was shown that individual lymphocytes recognized different antigens. The problem for clonal selection was considered to be that it was incredibly wasteful to carry around millions of lymphocytes that might never be used. However, this was a short-sighted argument because the world of microorganisms is constantly throwing up new antigenic types and selecting the most successful; Burnet's theory simply says that the immune system does the same. As he himself said: 'It is a Darwinian approach'.

2. For clonal selection to work, each lymphocyte (B or T) must retain its specific antigen receptor through numerous divisions, otherwise some members of the clone would be no use against the original triggering antigen. Thus in each B cell, only one combination of V, D, and J genes is chosen to code for the immunoglubulin heavy chain (and only one

for the light chain). However, it cannot be known in advance which class of immuno-globulin (i.e. which type of Fc region) will be most effective; IgM, IgG, IgA, and IgE all have their advantages in particular situations. Therefore every B cell must retain the ability to switch classes—from IgM to IgG, etc.—without losing its antigen specificity.

3. Purely from the viewpoint of the immune system, this statement appears to be true. The function of MHC molecules is to display antigenic peptides on the surface of cells in such a way that T cells recognize them and take appropriate action: cytotoxicity in the case of class I MHC and help in the case of class II. In the thymus, MHC molecules play a major part in deciding which T-cell receptors are to be deleted and which 'permitted'. If T cells had not evolved, there would seem to be no point in displaying MHC in the thymus or MHC–peptide complexes on B cells, macrophages, etc. However, it has been suggested that MHC molecules have other, non-immunological roles, for example in cell association in primitive animals and even in mating preference (dogs can unerringly smell and distinguish foreign MHC molecules in urine).

4. Clearly antigenic variation contributes to the success of many pathogens in avoiding elimination by the immune system, including some that might otherwise have great difficulty surviving, such as the African trypanosome living free in the blood. It is also presumably useful to organisms that may need to infect the same host repeatedly, such as influenza in humans. But there is no reason to suppose that *all* successful pathogens need to vary their antigens, although those that do not may run the risk of being eliminated by vaccination campaigns, as smallpox was. (It might be worth pointing out that the attenuated viruses used as vaccines are selected for variation of virulence but *not* of surface antigens.) Another point of interest is that not all antigenic variation is driven by the immune system; the free-living protozoan *Paramecium* varies its surface antigens in response to temperature, salinity, etc., without ever having to worry about immunity.

5. Certainly memory is one of the unique and valuable features of the lymphocyte, but not the most characteristic. Some extremely useful lymphocyte functions, such as the IgM response to bacterial polysaccharides, do not show significant memory. Recirculation is probably equally important, since without it antigen and lymphocyte would seldom meet. But the real hallmark of the lymphocyte is *specificity*, which can in turn be traced back to rearrangement of receptor genes. Whether the immunoglobulin or T-cell receptor genes are in the coding (rearranged) or germ-line (non-rearranged), configuration is the clinching test of whether the cell in question is a B cell, a T cell, or neither.

6. There is much truth in this, although often the damage is trivial and rapidly repaired; the one-day runny nose in some colds for example. However, by definition a pathogen implies *disease*, and disease implies tissue damage. The important thing is that many of the symptoms of disease *are* side effects of the processes that lead to elimination of the pathogen (or sometimes fail to achieve this). Only in the case of microbial toxins or direct cell destruction can one say that the symptoms are nothing to do with the immune system.

7. This is the celebrated case in which Bruton (1953) first demonstrated the association between repeated bacterial infection and absence of gammaglobulins in an electrophoretic analysis of serum. The boy lacked B cells, a condition now known as Bruton's agamma-globulinaemia which, because it is caused by a gene on the X chromosome, is inherited by boys from their mothers. Chickenpox, a viral disease, was no problem because his T cells were normal. Monthly injections of pooled normal human gammaglobulin kept him healthy, and the treatment is still used today.

Tutorial 4

Here are some guides to a possible answer for each question.

1. In a Utopia where everyone has unlimited access to clean water and properly cooked food, every wound is promptly sterilized, and everyone with the slightest infection is rigorously isolated until they either recover or die, we probably could manage quite well without vaccines or antibiotics. However, it is hard to imagine such conditions ever being established, let alone maintained. There is certainly an argument for *fewer* drugs and perhaps fewer vaccines, and there is a strong argument for much more information on, and enforcement of, public health measures. A safe guide might be that the latter should replace the former *when possible*.

2. Pasteur was amazingly lucky! His dried rabbit spinal cord contained dead rabies virus, a very hazardous way of killing an organism which nobody at that time had ever seen. He was using it as a vaccine in a child already exposed by the bite of a rabid dog. In any other infection this would be too late for active immunization, but rabies has an unusually long incubation period, giving the immune system time to respond before symptoms appear. Killed virus is still used to protect against rabies, combined with passive antibody if exposure has already occurred.

3. This frequently heard statement reflects the fact that resistance eventually develops to virtually all antibiotics, especially when they are used carelessly. It is somewhat over-defeatist, in that millions of lives are still saved every year by the correct use of antibiotics, and the pharmaceutical industry is continually producing new antibiotics, based on ever-improving knowledge of microbial biology. If there ever was a golden age, it was founded more on ignorance and optimism than on fact. In any case, where eucaryotic organisms are concerned, the golden age has hardly begun.

4. It depends what you mean by *worst*. The top killers at present (HIV, TB, infantile diarrhoea) are viruses or bacteria—*not* eucaryotes—although the top eucaryote (malaria) runs them close. The thought behind this statement was probably that eucaryotic infections (fungal, protozoal, helminth) are the hardest to *treat*, either with drugs or vaccines, whereas there is a steadily increasing list of effective drugs and/or vaccines against viruses and bacteria. Another problem is that because of their means of transmission, protozoal and helminth infections tend to be commonest in tropical countries, where adequate funding for health care is not always available.

5. One is certainly tempted to agree with this statement. What is so alarming about HIV is that, as a newcomer to the human race and already the leading single infectious cause of death, what it will do next is still unknown. Really vigorous public health measures and the provision of cheap effective drugs will undoubtedly slow its progress, and reduction of secondary infections will prolong lives (in fact the really devastating threat is the combination of HIV and tuberculosis). An effective vaccine would change everything though the prospects are not too good (why is this?). In the *very* long term there will probably be selection for resistance genes. You could argue that plague in the Middle Ages and influenza in 1918 were almost as bad, and if they had been sexually transmitted they might have been. But if one wished to invent a truly ruthless and terrifying pathogen, it would be hard to improve on HIV.

6. A fascinating challenge, tempting the unwary to invent all kinds of exotic new cells and molecules. However, you will find that most 'improvements' bring with them new risks in

the shape of immunopathology, autoimmunity, etc. In the process, you will come to appreciate just how well designed the immune system is. The safest bet is probably a continuation of existing trends such as (1) more V genes in the germ line (a rare event, requiring a useful mutation during gametogenesis), (2) another immunoglobulin C gene, conferring some new biological property on the antibody molecule: different species of mammals already differ considerably in their IgG subclass genes, showing that they are fairly recent developments, (3) some more natural inhibitors of endotoxin and other life-threatening molecules, (4) further diversification of the MHC (which would benefit the species rather than the individual). In the very long term, it would be nice to imagine some way in which the brain could acquire more control over the immune system. Looking at it from the therapeutic viewpoint, we might expect to see (1) a reliable way of directing vaccines at T_H1, T_H2, T_H17, and B cells, (2) a safe way of switching on and enhancing NK-cell activity, (3) safe, efficient gene replacement for the congenital immunodeficiencies, (4) a range of monoclonal antibodies against infectious organisms, although admittedly the existing monoclonal antibodies have not been as successful as was hoped.

INDEX

Numbers in **bold face** refer to figures, boxes, or tables.

Infection and Immunity

This book is due for return on or before the last date shown below.